T0262705

Selected Researches in Anemia

Selected Researches in Anemia

Edited by **Rudy Willis**

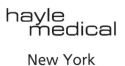

New York

Published by Hayle Medical,
30 West, 37th Street, Suite 612,
New York, NY 10018, USA
www.haylemedical.com

Selected Researches in Anemia
Edited by Rudy Willis

International Standard Book Number: 978-1-63241-349-9 (Hardback)

Printed in the United States of America.

Contents

Preface

Over the recent decade, advancements and applications have progressed exponentially. This has led to the increased interest in this field and projects are being conducted to enhance knowledge. The main objective of this book is to present some of the critical challenges and provide insights into possible solutions. This book will answer the varied questions that arise in the field and also provide an increased scope for furthering studies.

Anemia is a common blood disorder. This book presents a complete summary of many developments in the field of anemia. It discusses anemia linked to pregnancy, the fetus and the infant. Some general infections that cause anemia in rising nations, malaria and trypanosomiasis, have been discussed thoroughly. Hence, this book gives a comprehensive summary of anemia and will be helpful for readers interested in this field.

I hope that this book, with its visionary approach, will be a valuable addition and will promote interest among readers. Each of the authors has provided their extraordinary competence in their specific fields by providing different perspectives as they come from diverse nations and regions. I thank them for their contributions.

Editor

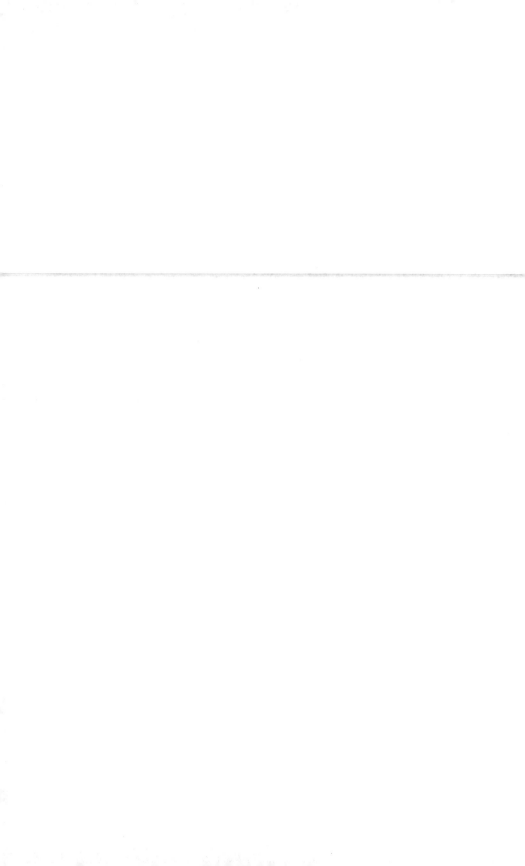

Management of Anaemia in Pregnancy

Ezechi Oliver[1] and Kalejaiye Olufunto[2]
[1]Chief Research Fellow and Consultant Obstetrician and Gynaecologist
Coordinator, Sexual, Reproductive and Childhood Diseases Research Programme
Head of Division, Clinical Sciences Division,
Nigerian Institute of Medical Research, Yaba Lagos
[2]Senior Research Fellow and Haematologist
Unit Head, Laboratory Services Unit ,
Clinical Sciences Division, Nigerian Institute of Medical Research, Yaba Lagos
Nigeria

1. Introduction

Obstetric practice in developing countries is known for unacceptably high maternal morbidity , mortality and perinatal deaths. Factors contributory to these include poor health care delivery system, cultural beliefs, poor nutrition, illiteracy, gender inequality, teenage pregnancies and high parity. Other factors such as infections and infestations ultimately cause anaemia and increase morbidity and mortality in pregnant women and their offspring. Anaemia during pregnancy is a well-known risk for unfavourable pregnancy outcomes.

Globally, anaemia has been found to be the most common complication in pregnancy. The World Health Organization (WHO) estimates that more than 40% of non-pregnant and over 50% of pregnant women in developing countries are affected. The majority of the cases occur in sub-Saharan Africa and South East Asia. In 1993, the World Bank ranked anaemia as the 8th leading cause of disease in girls and women in the developing world. Apart from maternal morbidity and mortality, neonatal mortality is high among the babies of anaemic mothers.

2. Hematological changes in pregnancy

Pregnancy is associated with normal physiological changes that assist fetal survival and prepares the mother for labour, delivery and breastfeeding. The changes start as early as 4 weeks of gestation and are largely as a result of progesterone and oestrogen. The total blood volume increases steadily from as early as 4 weeks of pregnancy to reach a maximum of 35-45 % above the non-pregnant level at 28 to 32 weeks. The plasma volume increases by 40-45 % (1000mls). Red blood cell mass increases by 30- 33 % (approximately 300mg) as a result of the increase in the production of erythropoietin. Erythropoietin levels increase throughout pregnancy, reaching approximately 150% of their prepregnancy levels at term.

The increase is steady until term. The greater increase in plasma volume than the increase in red blood cell mass results in a modest reduction in haematocrit, with peak haemodilution occurring at 24-26 weeks. This is termed physiological anaemia of pregnancy (see Fig 1). This dilution picture is often normochromic and normocytic. Occasionally physiologic anaemia can also be associated with a physiologic macrocytosis, MCV increases to 120fl although average at term is 104 fl.

In pregnancy, there is an additional demand of about 1000 mg iron equivalent to 60 mg elemental iron or 300 mg ferrous sulphate daily. While the transferrin and total iron binding capacity rises, the serum iron falls . Thus women who enter pregnancy in an iron deficient state are then unable to meet the demands of pregnancy by diet alone and require supplementation. It takes approximately 2-3 weeks after delivery for these haematologic changes to revert to pre-pregnancy status.

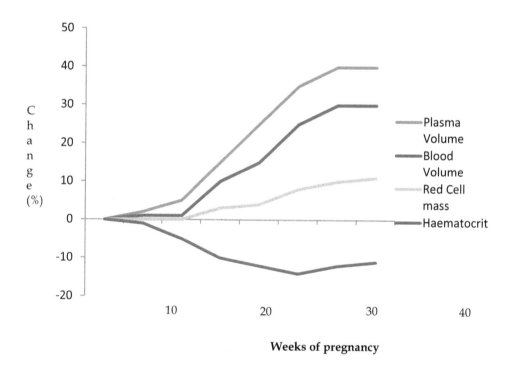

Fig. 1. Graphical representation of haematological changes in pregnancy.

3. Epidemiology of anaemia in pregnancy

Anaemia has been found to be associated with poverty and underdevelopment and is one of the most common disorders globally. The incidence of anaemia varies from place to place even within the same country and depends on the socioeconomic status and level of development. The World Health Organization reports anaemia among the top ten most important contributors to global ill health and deaths. It estimated that about a third of the world's population of 7 billion have haemoglobin levels below the WHO criteria for diagnosis of anaemia. The majority of these persons reside in Sub-Saharan Africa and South East Asia.

Pregnant women are particularly considered to be the most vulnerable group because of the additional demands that are made on maternal stores during pregnancy. The average global prevalence of anaemia in pregnancy is reported to be 51%. Like anaemia in the general population the prevalence of anaemia in pregnancy varies from 17% in Europe to 52 % and 60% respectively in Africa and Asia. In sub-Saharan Africa it is estimated that 20% of maternal deaths are associated with anaemia. It is also a major risk factor for infant iron deficiency which has been shown to be associated with adverse behavioural and cognitive development of children and low birth weight, which is one of the main risk factors for infant mortality.

4. Definition of anaemia

The term anaemia refers to the reduction in the oxygen-carrying capacity of the blood due to fewer circulating red blood cells than normal or a reduction in the concentration of haemoglobin. The deficiency may occur as a result of a reduction in the production or an increased loss of erythrocytes.

Anaemia is said to occur when the haemoglobin content of blood is below the normal range expected for the age and sex of the individual, provided that the presence of pregnancy, the state of hydration of the individual and the altitude have been taken into account. While several authorities and experts accepts the lower limits of normal haemoglobin concentration as 12g/dl in women and 14g/dl in men, WHO accepts up to 11gm percent as the normal haemoglobin level in pregnancy. Thus any haemoglobin level below 11gm in pregnancy by WHO standard should be considered as anaemia. However in most of the developing countries the lower limit is often accepted as 10 g/dl because a large percentage of pregnant women in this setting with haemoglobin level of 10 g/dl tolerate pregnancy, labour and delivery very well and with good outcome.

The centre for disease control, USA defined anaemia as a hemoglobin (Hgb) or hematocrit (Hct) value less than the fifth percentile of the distribution of Hgb or Hct in a healthy reference population.

5. Classification of anaemia

Anaemia can be classified as physiological (eg pregnancy), according to the aetiology (Table 1) and red blood cell morphology (Table 2).

Classification based on red cell morphology classifies anaemia based on the size and shape of the red blood cell,(normocytic MCV80-90fl, macrocytic MCV>100fl, microcytic MCV<80fl), as well as .pigmentation (hypochromic, normochromic, hypochromic) (Table 2).

Blood loss
    a.   Acute
        i.   Antepartum haemorrhage (eg placenta praevia , abruptio placenta)
        ii. Intrapartum haemorrhage
    b.   Chronic
        i.   Hookworm infestation
        ii. Bleeding hemorrhoids
        iii. Peptic Ulcer Disease

B.   Nutritional Anaemia
        i.   Iron deficiency
        ii. Folate deficiency
        iii. B12 deficiency

C.   Bone marrow failure
    a.   Aplastic anaemia
    b.   Isolated secondary failure of erythropoiesis
    c.   Drugs (eg Chloramphenicol, Zidovudine)

D.   Haemolytic
    a.   Inherited
        i.   Haemoglobinopathies (eg Sickle cell disorders, Thalassemia)
        ii. Red cell Membrane defects (eg Hereditary spherocytosis, elliptocytosis)
        iii. Enzyme deficiencies (eg G6PD deficiency, Pyruvate kinase defeciency)
    b.   Acquired
        i.   Immune Haemolytic anaemias (eg autoimmune, alloimmune, drug induced)
        ii. Non- Immune Haemolytic anaemias
                a.   Acquired membrane defects (eg Paroxysmal nocturnal Haemoglobinuria)
b.Mechanical damage (eg Microangiopathic haemolytic anaemia)
iii Secondary to systemic disease (eg renal diseases, liver disease)
iv.Infections (Malaria, Sepsis, HIV)

Table 1. Classification of anaemia based on aetiology.

A. **Hypochromic Microcytic**
- Iron deficiency
- Thalassemia
- Sideroblastic anemia
- Anaemia of chronic disorders
- Lead poisoning

B. **Macrocytic**
- Folic acid deficiency
- Vitamin B12 deficiency
- Liver disease
- Myxoedema
- Chronic Obstructive Pulmonary Disease
- Myelodysplastic syndromes
- Blood loss anemia

C. **Normocytic Normochromic**
- Autoimmune haemolytic anaemia
- Systemic Lupus Erythomatosis
- Collagen vascular disorders
- Hereditary spherocytosis
- Haemoglobinopathies
- Bone marrow failure
- Malignancies
- Myelodysplasia
- Blood loss anemia
- Anemia of chronic disease

Table 2. Morphological Classification of Anemia and causes.

The classifications are not necessarily independent of each other as the cause of the anaemia could be multifactorial.

Anaemia can be classified according to severity as mild, moderate, severe and very severe (Table 3). Following the diagnosis and possible cause(s) of anaemia in the pregnant woman, management as regards the need for blood transfusions or not will depend on the severity as well as rapidity of development of anaemia.

Degree of Severity	Haemoglobin level (g/dl)
Normal haemoglobin level	>11g/dl
Mild Anaemia	9-11g/dl
Moderate	7-9g/dl
Severe	4-7g/dl
Very severe	<4g/dl

Table 3. Classification of Anaemia by degree of severity.

6. Aetiology

The causes of anaemia in the general population are generally same for anaemia in pregnancy. The causes of anaemia in pregnancy are often multifactorial. In developing countries, the major causes of anaemia in pregnancy are nutritional deficiencies, infections and infestations, haemorrhage and haemoglobinathies. Anaemia is also seen also in some chronic medical disorders like renal and hepatic diseases.

6.1 Nutrition

In many regions of the world nutritional deficiency is the major cause of anaemia in pregnancy. The World health Organization ((WHO) estimates that about half of all pregnant women globally suffer from nutritional anaemia. Nutritional anaemia is mainly due iron and folate deficiency in diet. Diseases that cause poor dietary intake or malabsorption of these nutrients will also result in nutritional anaemia.

Iron deficiency is the commonest cause of nutritional anaemia in both developing and industrialized countries and is usually as a result of poor diet. Sources of iron include meat(liver in particular) vegetables and dairy products. The demand for iron increases in pregnancy as it is required by both mother and fetus for growth and development. In developing countries the already depleted iron stores as a result of poor diet, too early, too many and too frequent pregnancies are unable to cope with the requirement of 1000mg of iron required during a normal pregnancy. The resultant effect is iron deficiency anaemia. Hook worm infestation is another cause of iron deficiency anaemia in the tropics.

The folic acid requirement is also increased two fold in pregnancy. Normal body stores can only last for 3- 4 months. Folate deficiency in pregnancy often develops as a result of poor dietary intake which is often the case in developing countries as well as excess utilization. Sources of folate include liver, egg yolk, and leafy green vegetables. Folate deficiency results in ineffective erythropoesis.

Folate deficiency can be further exacerbated in pregnant women with hemoglobinopathies as well as in those residing in areas of high malaria endemicity as increased haemolysis leads to high red cell turnover and increased folate demand.

Vitamin B12 is rare during pregnancy as the daily requirement is as low as 3- 5μg and liver stores last for as long as 2 years.

6.2 Infections

Pregnant women are more prone to infections as a result of depressed immunity. Anaemia due to infections is usually as a result of products from the infecting organisms causing ill health, fever, red cell destruction and/ or reduced red cell production. Bacterial infections used to be a leading cause of anaemia, however in the tropics and developing countries, malaria and more recently, HIV/AIDS are leading contributors to anaemia in pregnancy.

6.3 Malaria

Malaria infection is a leading cause of anemia in the tropics both in pregnant and non-pregnant individuals. Malaria induced anaemia is more profound in pregnancy as the susceptibility to malaria is greater in the primigravidae. Anaemia resulting from malarial infection is caused by the destruction of infected and uninfected red blood cells as well as bone marrow suppression. Red blood cells infected with malaria parasites also accumulate and sequester in the placenta. Macrophages and cytokines(e.g.Tumor necrosis factor α, Interferon γ and interleukin 1),enhance red cell destruction, splenic clearance capacity,and depress bone marrow erythropoesis. Concurrent micronutrient deficiencies, infection with HIV , hookworm infestation or other chronic inflammatory states will worsen anaemia in these persons.

6.4 HIV/AIDS

Anaemia is the most common haematological complication of the Human Immunodeficiency Virus (HIV) infection and may be consequent upon the effects of the virus itself or treatment with various drugs. The mechanisms of HIV induced anaemia occur through three mechanisms of decreased red blood cell production, increased red cell destruction and ineffective production of red blood cells. The aetiology of HIV associated anaemia is multifactorial and may include the infiltration of the bone marrow by tumour or infection, bone marrow suppression by the virus itself, the use of myelosuppressive drugs like Zidovudine or drugs that prevent the utilization of folate like cotrimoxazole. Other aetiologies include decreased production of erythropoietin , red cell destruction as a result of autoantibodies to red blood cells, and nutritional deficiencies. Nutritional deficiencies could occur as a result of reduced intake due to difficult in swallowing as a result of oropharnygeal thrush, malabsorption or increased catabolism as a result of ill health and associated fever from various infections. Apart from iron and folate deficiency, other reported vitamin deficiencies in HIV infection include vitamin B12, vitamin B6 and vitamin A.

6.5 Haemoglobinopathies

Haemoglobinopathies are inherited disorders affecting haemoglobin structure (Sickle cell disorders) or synthesis (thalassemias). They are usually seen in individuals from Africa, the Middle East, the Mediterranean, Asia and the Far East. The haemoglobinopathies that cause anaemia in pregnancy are sickle cell disorders- HbSS, HbSC and HBS-β thalassemia. Haemoglobinopathies cause a chronic haemolytic anaemia. In sickle cell disorders, the abnormal haemoglobin S sickles in hypoxic states, predisposing the structurally damaged cells to early destruction hence affected persons are chronically anaemic. Folate demands are increased and concurrent infections will worsen anaemia.

6.6 Haemorrhage

Acute blood loss as result of ectopic pregnancy, antepartum haemorrhage and abortions are common causes of anaemia in pregnancy. Chronic blood loss from worm infestations, gastrointestinal ulcers and hemorrhoids results in depletion of iron stores and ineffective erythropoesis.

6.7 Red cell aplasia

This is a rare cause of anaemia in pregnancy and results from a selective failure of erythropoesis. In most cases, the cause is unknown The identified causes of pure red cell aplasia include autoimmune diseases (e.g. SLE,) drugs, and infection with parvovirus B19.

7. Risk factors for anaemia in pregnancy

Pregnant women in developing countries of sub-Saharan Africa, South America and South East Asia are at particular risk of anaemia in pregnancy as a result of poverty, malnutrition and depleted iron stores from too early, too many and too frequent pregnancies. Irrespective of race and economic situation, the prevalence of anemia in pregnancy is highest amongst teenage mothers. A recent report by Scholl estimates that in a low income setting, rates of iron deficiency anemia are 1.8% in the first trimester, 8.2% in the second trimester, and 27.4% in the third trimester.

In all regions of the world, the risk factors for iron deficiency anemia include a diet poor in iron-rich foods, a diet poor in iron absorption enhancers, a diet rich in foods that diminish iron absorption, gastrointestinal disease affecting absorption, heavy menstrual bleeding and postpartum bleeding.

8. Consequences of anemia in pregnancy

8.1 Fetal

The fetal consequences of anaemia in pregnancy are well established and depend not only on the severity of anaemia but also on the duration of the anaemic state. A fall in maternal haemoglobin below 11.0 g/dl is associated with a significant rise in perinatal mortality rates. The rate of perinatal mortality triples at maternal haemoglobin levels below 8.0 g/dl and increase by ten fold when anaemia is very severe. Similar findings have also been noted for both infant birth weight and preterm delivery rates. A significant fall in birth weight as a result of increase in preterm rate and intrauterine growth restriction has been reported with maternal haemoglobin levels below 8.0 g/dl .

8.2 Maternal

The presence of, severity and duration of anaemia affect maternal as well as fetal well being. Women whose means of livelihood involve manual labour may find it difficult to earn a living as tolerance and capacity for exercise is reduced. This is worse if the onset of anaemia is acute. When anaemia is of gradual onset and is chronic, adequate compensatory mechanisms enable the women to go through pregnancy and labour without any adverse consequences.

Where anaemia is moderate, there is a substantial reduction in work capacity and she may be unable to cope with household chores and child care. Women with moderate anaemia tend to experience higher rates of morbidity during pregnancy as compared to those with mild anaemia. Evidence has shown that a large percentage of maternal deaths due to antepartum haemorrhage, pre-eclampsia and infections occur in women with moderate anaemia.

The maternal outcomes in severe anaemia depend on level of decompensation. If not recognized early and corrected, the heart is unable to compensate for the severity of anaemia and eventual circulatory failure occurs leading to pulmonary oedema and death. The women are unable to tolerate third stage of labour and blood losses associated with delivery. When the anaemia is very severe, there is a steep rise in maternal deaths.

9. Clinical features

The clinical features of anaemia in pregnant or non pregnant states are dependent on rapidity of onset and severity of anaemia. In general, symptoms occur with moderate to severe anaemia and are more severe when anaemia has been rapidly progressive. In presence of anaemia the body initiates a number of compensatory mechanisms. The symptom (s) that is subsequently felt by the individual is dependent on whether the compensation is sufficient or insufficient. As such, a pregnant woman with anaemia may be asymptomatic body systems adjust to reduced haemoglobin mass. Where the patient is symptomatic, symptoms may be those of vague ill health, headaches, light headedness, tinnitus, intermittent claudication, or symptoms of angina. However, as decomposition ensues, there may be palpitations, easy fatigability and patients can present in heart failure.

The signs of anaemia can be general or specific. General signs of anaemia include pallor of the mucous membranes, hyperdynamic circulation with tachycardia, a bounding pulse, cardiomegaly and a apical systolic flow mummur (haemic mummur) . The specific signs are associated with particular types of anaemia e.g painless glossitis, angular stomatitis,ridged or spoon shaped nails, unusual dietary cravings for non-food substances(pica) in iron deficiency, jaundice in haemolytic and megaloblastic anaemias, neuropathy, widespread melanin pigmentation in B12 deficiency. Hepatoslenomegaly (may be difficult to elicit when pregnancy is advanced) may be features of chronic hemolytic disorders, megaloblastic anaemia, or other haematologic pathologies. The findings of anaemia with fever and spontaneous bruising may be indicative of bone marrow failure.

10. Diagnosis of cause(s) of anaemia

A detailed history, physical examination and appropriate investigations are necessary for the identification of the cause(s) of anaemia. Except in very severe anaemia where there is an urgent need to treat the pregnant woman to avoid death, the cardinal rule is to establish the cause of anemia before commencing treatment.

10.1 History

A detailed history including diet, gynaecological, obstetric,drug and social history should be taken. As nutritional anaemia is common in developing countries, a detailed enquiry into the person's and diet and feeding habits should be made. Knowledge of the dietary and food habits will be necessary to plan strategies to prevent reoccurrence after management of the present anaemic state. It is also important to enquire in detail about duration and symptoms of anaemia (if any), symptoms of decompensation and possible predisposing factors. Other specific symptoms like a beefy red painful tongue, discoloured nails, parasthesias can also be sought. Previous history of postpartum haemorrhage or abortion, drug ingestion should be sought. Ideally, the history should address all possible aetiology of anaemia, features and its complications.

10.2 Physical examination

A good physical examination should confirm the presence of anaemia, possible aetiology and signs of decompensation. Where anaemia has been chronic, physical examination may reveal cardiomegaly, bounding pulses and a systolic flow murmur (hemic murmur). In acute blood loss the patient can present in shock. On examination the presence of pallor, jaundice, spleen and liver size should be documented.

10.3 Investigations

Investigations for anaemia are general and specific. A full blood count is required as part of the general investigation and includes the haemoglobin levels, packed cell volume, white cell and platelet counts. Red cell indices include mean corpuscular volume (MCV), mean corpuscular haemoglobin (MCH) and mean corpuscular haemoglobin concentration (MCHC). These indices will in the classify anaemia into either microcytic (MCV <80 fL), macrocytic (MCV >100fL) and normocytic (MCV80-100fL) or hypochromic or normochromic (MCH and MCHC)., A peripheral blood smear and reticulocyte count are also mandatory. While peripheral blood smear provides information about red cell morphology , variations in size, and shape, the reticulocyte count provides information on the marrow response. In the presence of anaemia a reticulocyte count less than 2-3 times normal indicates inadequate bone marrow response. Elevated neutrophil counts may suggest an infection.and peripheral smears that reveal a pancytopenia is suggestive of marrow failure. Stools should also be examined for colour, consistency, occult blood, ova and parasites. It is also important to note that in the tropics most of the causes may coexist. Other specific tests are often dictated by suspected cause of the anaemia. In the tropics, it is usual to screen for malaria as it is a well documented cause of anaemia in pregnancy. Some specific tests necessary to confirm some common causes and features of anemia is shown in Table 4.

1.	**Iron deficiency**
	  a. **Serum ferritin**
	  b. **Total iron binding capacity**
	  c. **Transferrin saturation**
	  d. **Marrow iron stain**
		2.
		
		3.
			Haemoglobinopathies
			  a. **Hb electrophoresis**
			HIV infection
			  a. Detection of antibody to HIV using ELISA or Western blot assays.	

4.	**Chronic medical disorders**
	  a. **Liver function tests**
	  b. **Serum electrolyte, urea and creatinine**
	  c. **Screening for autoimmune diseases**
		5.	**Antepartum haemorrhage**
			  a. Ultrasonography	

Table 4. Specific investigations for some common causes of anaemia.

11. Treatment

It is of utmost importance to establish the cause of anaemia prior to definitive management. However, features of decompensation, very severe anaemia and acute blood loss require immediate red cell transfusion as soon as the required samples have been collected. The only caveat is that we must ensure that all necessary samples have been collected before transfusion.

The goal of treatment of anaemia in pregnancy is therefore to maintain wellbeing, identify and correct the underlying cause(s) and correct anemia within shortest time possible and improve patient quality of life and survival.

The definitive management of anaemia depends on the cause. The identified causes must be treated appropriately otherwise the anaemia becomes recurrent.

By and large, the management of anaemia in a pregnant woman depends on the duration of pregnancy, severity of the anaemia and complication (obstetric, medical or both).

Mild and moderate anaemia in pregnancy as a result of iron deficiency should be carefully assessed for the cause and the patient placed on iron therapy apart from the treatment of the aetiology. The preferred route of iron replacement is oral route as there is no benefit in giving parenteral iron as opposed to oral iron. Ferrous sulphate (200mg per tablet containing 67mg elemental iron) is the least expensive and best absorbed form of Iron. Ferrous glutamate (300mg per tablet containing 37mg elemental iron) and fumarate can also be used where iron sulphate is not tolerated. The optimal doses are 120-200mg daily of elemental iron in divided doses. Oral iron should be given for long enough to correct the anaemia and to replenish iron stores which usually means for at least 6 months. Haemoglobin should rise at the rate of approximately 2g/dl every 3 weeks. Side effects of oral iron include gastrointestinal symptoms such as diarrhea, nausea, constipation, abdominal pain.

Parenteral iron may be indicated in cases of poor adherence, intolerable side effects or malabsorption of oral iron. In such situation parenteral iron such as iron dextran or sorbitol may be administered by the intravenous or intramuscular route. The hematological response to parenteral iron is not faster than adequate dosage of oral iron but the stores are replenished faster. Ferric hydroxide –sucrose (Venofer) is the safest form and is administered by slow intravenous injection or infusion usually 200mg in each infusion. Iron dextran (Cosmofer) can be given as slow injection or infusion in small doses or as a total dose infusion given in one day.

Total dose Intravenous infusion of iron with iron dextran in pregnancy (50mg iron per ml) Dose (mL) = 0.0442 (Desired Hb - Observed Hb) x Lean Body Weight (45.5 kg + 2.3 kg for each inch of patient's height over 5 feet.) + (0.26 x LBW) + 1g.

The total dose of iron dextran is added to 500ml normal saline and infused over a period of 4 hours. The major drawback of parenteral iron is anaphylaxis which can occur within 30 mins of commencing the infusion and may prove rapidly fatal.

Intramuscular iron therapy can be given as iron sorbitol (Jectofer)(50mg/ml). Injections should be given deep into the gluteal muscle. The drawbacks of intramuscular iron include pain and staining of the skin at the injection site,myalgia, athralgia and injection abscess

Severe or very severe anaemia requires the immediate hospitalization of the woman, management of heart failure and transfusion of packed cells. Once the emergency is averted, the iron replacement is as in mild to moderate anaemia.

Treatment of anaemia from folate deficiency is with folic acid 5mg daily for 4 months and is usually given throughout pregnancy. Vitamin B12 deficiency is rare in pregnancy and is treated with intramuscular injections of hydroxocobalamin 1000ug . Initial doses are 6 injections over 2-3 weeks then 100ug every 3 months.

Erythropoietin is beneficial in patients -with marrow suppression . 100-200U/Kg 3times a week until normalization of the red cell and then once a weekly to maintain haemoglobin of approximately 12g/dl.

Treatment of malaria with artemisin combination therapy, bacterial infections with appropriate antibiotics, hookworm infestation with mebendazole or Albendazole and use of highly active antiretroviral therapy according to treatment guidelines in HIV infection. Other co-morbidities e.g. diabetes, hypertension should also be managed.

12. Prevention

Approximately 1g of iron is required during a normal pregnancy. Up to 600mg of iron is required for the increase in maternal red cell mass, and a further 300mg for the foetus. These requirements exceed the iron storage of most young women and often cannot be met by the diet. Therefore, few women avoid depletion of iron reserves by the end of pregnancy. Folate requirements are increased approximately twofold in pregnancy (800ug/day vs 400ug/day because of transfer of folate to the growing fetus and if diet is insufficient, may exceed the body's stores of folate(5-10mg).

To prevent anaemia in pregnancy the following are necessary. Routine screening for anaemia in adolescence, nutritional education about foods rich in iron(meat, liver, leafy green vegetables, legumes) and folate (liver, egg yolk, yeast and leafy green vegetables) to encourage consumption, early as well as regular antenatal clinic attendances, iron, folate supplementation in pregnancy and early treatment of concomitant infections. In areas of high malaria endemicity, intermittent prophylactic therapy with pyrimethamine-sulphodoxine for malaria should also be given at 16-17 weeks and 4 weeks later. A third dose is given in HIV infection.

13. Conclusion

Anaemia in pregnancy is a major public health problem in developing countries and is associated with an increased risk of maternal and perinatal morbidity and mortality. Fortification of foods with iron and folate, routine screening for anaemia from adolescence, health education, and prompt treatment of infections and attendance of antenatal facilities by pregnant women can reduce this burden.

14. References

Agarwal KN, Agarwal DK, Mishra KP. Impact of anaemia prophylaxis in pregnancy on maternal hemoglobin, serum ferritin and birth weight. Indian J Med Res 1991;94:277–8

Aimakhu CO, Olayemi O. Maternal haematocrit and pregnancy outcome in Nigerian women. West Afr J Med. 2003;22(1):18–21.

Blanc B, Finch CA, Hallberg L, et al. Nutritional anaemias. Report of a WHO Scientific Group. WHO Tech Rep Ser. 1968;405:1-40.

Beutler E, West C. Hematologic differences between African-Americans and whites: the roles of iron deficiency and α_-thalassemia on hemoglobin levels and mean corpuscular volume. Blood.2005;106:740-745.

Breymann C, Iron Deficiency and Anaemia in Pregnancy: Modern Aspects of Diagnosis and Therapy. Blood Cells, Molecules, and Diseases. 2002; 29(3) Nov/Dec: 506–516

Centers of Disease Control . CDC Criteria for Anemia in Children and Childbearing-Aged Women. Morbidity and Mortality Weekly Report 1989; 38(22: 400–404.

Ezzati M, Lopez D, Rodgers A, Murray CJL, eds. Comparative quantification of health risk: Global and regional burden of disease attributable to selected major risk factors. Vol 1. Geneva: World Health Organization; 2004:163–208.

Harrison KA. Anaemia in pregnancy. In: Lawson JB, Harrison KA, Bergstrom S, editors. Maternity care in developing countries. RCOG Press. 2001:112–128.

Hemminki E, Rimpela U. Iron supplementation, maternal packed cell volume, and fetal growth. Arch Dis Child 1991;66:422–5.

Hisano M, Suzuki R, Sago H, Murashima A, Yamaguchi K. Vit B6 deficiency and anaemia in pregnancy. Eur J Clin Nutr. 2010;64:221–223.

Hoque M, Hader SB, Hoque E. Prevalence of anaemia in pregnancy in th uthungulu health district of KwaZulu- NatalSouth Africa. SAFamPract2007:49(6)16-16d.

Hoque M, Hoque E, Kader SB. Risk factors for anaemia in pregnancy in rural KwaZulu-Natal, South Africa: Implication for health education and health promotion SA Fam Pract 2009;51(1):68-72

Ilobachie GC, Meniru GI. The increasing incidence of anaemia in pregnancy in Nigeria. Orient J Med. 1990;2:194–198.

International Nutritional Anaemia consultative group. The INACG Symposium, "Integrating programs to move Iron Deficiency and Anaemia Control Forward". Marrakech, Morocco, International life Science Institute; 2003.

Iron dextran dosing calculator. Total dose infusion –iron deficiency anaemia. http://www.globalrph.com/irondextran.htm

Komolafe JO, Kuti O, Oni O, Egbewale BE. Sociodemographic characteristics of anaemic gravidae at booking: A preliminary study at Ilesha, western Nigeria. Nig J Med. 2005;14(2):151–154.

Lone FW, Qureshi RN, Emanuel F Maternal anaemia and its impact on perinatal outcome. Trop Med Int Health. 2004 Apr;9(4):486-90.

Massawe SN, Urassa En, Nystrom L, Lindmark G. Effectiveness of primary level care in decreasing anemia at term in Tanzania. Acta Obstet Gynecol Scand. 1999;78:573–579.

Martha P. Mims, Josef T. Prchal.Haematology during pregnancy. In Lichtman MA, Beutler E, Kipps TJ, Seligsohn U, KaushanskyK, Prchal JT editors.Williams Haematology 7thed 2006 Mcgraw-Hill publishers pp101-106.

McMullin MF, White R, Lappin T et al. Haemoglobin during pregnancy :Relationship to erythropoietin and haematinic status. Eur J Haematol 71:44,2003

Nduka N, Aneke C, Maxwell Ochukwu S. Comparison of some haematological indices of Africans and Caucasians resident in the same Nigerian environment. Haematologica budap. 1988;21 (1) 57-63

Nokes C, Van Den Bosch C, Bundy DAP. The effect of iron deficiency and anemia on mental and motor performance, educational achievement and behavior in children: An annotated bibliography. Washington,DC, International Nutritional Anaemia Consultative Group; 1998.

Nyuke RB, Letsky EA. Etiology of anaemia in pregnancy in South Malawi. Am J Clin Nutr. 2000;72:247–256

Ogbeide O, Wagbatsoma V, Orhue A. Anaemia in pregnancy. East Afr Med J 1994;71:671–3.

Ogunbode O. Anaemia in Pregnancy. In: Okonofua F, Odunsi K, editors. Contemporary Obstetrics and Gynaecology For Developing Countries. Benin City, Nigeria: Women's Health and Action Research Center; 2003. pp. 514–529.

Omigbodun AO. Recent trends in the management of anaemia inpregnancy. *Trop J Obstet Gynaecol.* 2004;21(1):1–3.

Ross J, Thomas EL. Iron deficiency anaemia and maternal mortality. Profiles 3. Working Notes Series No3.WashingtonDC;Academy for Educational Development;1996.

Rusia U, Madan Sikka M, Sood S. N Effect of maternal iron deficiency anaemia on foetal outcome. Indian J Pathol Microbiol 1995;38:273-9

Sarin AR. Severe anaemia of pregnancy – recent experience. Int J Gynae col Obstet 1995;50:S45–S49.

Scholl TO. Iron status during pregnancy: setting the stage for mother and infant. Am J Clin Nutr 2005;81: 1218S–22S. (Level III)

Singla PN, Tyagi M, Kumar A, Dash D, Shankar R. Fetal growth in maternal anemia. J Trop Pediatr 1997;43:89–92.Stoltzfus RJ. Update on issues related to iron deficiency and anaemia control. Report of the 2003

Sharma A, Patnaik R, Garg S, Ramachandran P. Detection & management of anaemia in pregnancy in an urban primary health care institution. *Indian J Med Res 2008; 128 :* 45-51

Society for Gynaecology and Obstetrics of Nigeria (SOGON). Report of the maternal mortality situation in six (6) tertiary hospitals in Nigeria. Needs assessment. 2004:1–65

Uneke CJ, Sunday-Adeoye I, Iyare FE, Ugwuja EI, Duhlinska DD. Impact of maternal Plasmodium falciparum malaria and haematological parameters on pregnancy and its outcome in Southeastern Nigeria. *J Vector Borne Dis.* 2007;44:285–290.

World Health Organization. The prevalence of anaemia in women: A tabulation of available information. Geneva, World Health Organization; 1992 (unpublished document WHO/MCH/MSM/92.2; available upon request from Division of Reproductive Health, World Health Organization, 1211 Geneva 27, Switzerland).

World Health Organization (WHO) The prevalence of Anaemia in women: a tabulation of available information. Geneva, Switzerland: WHO; 1992. WHO/MCH/MSM/92.2 .

World Health Organization (WHO) Prevention and Management of Severe Anaemia in Pregnancy: Report of a Technical Working Group. Geneva, Switzerland: WHO; 1993. WHO/FNE/MSM/93.5.

World Health Organization. Prevention and management of severe anaemia in pregnancy. WHO; 1993

Severe Malaria Anaemia in Children

Ayodotun Olutola and Olugbenga Mokuolu
University of Maryland/Institute of Human Virology
Nigeria

1. Introduction

Severe malaria anaemia is defined as haemoglobin concentration <5g/dl associated with Plasmodium falciparum parasitaemia.(WHO, 1986) Other causes of anaemia have to be excluded as asymptomatic falciparum parasitaemia is common in endemic areas.(Salako et al,1990) Severe anaemia may exist alone or in combination with other complications particularly cerebral malaria and respiratory distress in which it portends worse prognosis.(WHO, 2004)

It is a significant cause of morbidity and mortality in children below five years of age. Children below 3 years are predominantly affected with a mean age of 1.8 years.(Krause,2000) Available data suggests that severe malaria anaemia is the commonest complication of malaria in areas subjected to high inoculation rates throughout the year.(Newton & Krishna, 1998). It accounts for between 26 and 62% of severe malaria admissions in malaria endemic countries (Satpathy et al,2004, Mockenhaupt et al,2004) and up to 29% of total hospital admissions as reported in Ilorin(Ernest,2002) and Kenya.(Lackritz et al,1992). Hospital based data of deaths from anaemia ranges between 11.2% in Sierra Leone and 14% in Kenya for children below 5 years.(Brabin et al,2002). Most deaths occur within 2 days of admission underscoring the importance of adequate blood banking facilities in our primary health care centres. (Newton &Krishna, 1998, Lackritz et al,1992).

2. Pathogenesis of severe malaria anaemia

Multiple mechanisms may account for anaemia in children infected with malaria. Host factors, associations with parasitic infections, nutritional deficiencies of iron, Vitamins B12, Vitamin E, and folate, in addition to drug associated causes are important considerations. Children under 5 years are more prone to severe malaria anaemia. The following are some of the key pathogenetic mechanisms:

2.1 Host factors

Age: Malaria affects all age groups and congenital malaria is relatively uncommon.(Stephen et al,1996, Falade et al,2007)) There is no sex predilection. It is relatively uncommon in the first few months of life due to the high concentration of haemoglobin F which is not favorable for parasite growth, presence of maternal immunoglobulins (Falade et al,2007) and selective shielding of infants from parasite. Exclusively breastfed infants are also deficient in paraaminobenzoic acid which the parasite thrives upon.(Gilles, 1957)

Immune status: Natural immunity occurs in subjects that are heterozygous for Haemoglobin S, thalassaemia, G6PD deficiency, Human Leucocyte Antigen classes I and II alleles, Band 3, Spectrin, Lewis, Kid Js red cell types.(Luzatto, 1974, Miller et al,1976, Allison 1954, Marsh, 2002) They are believed to be a protective mutation representing a balanced genetic polymorphism that occurred over the years in response to the threat of malaria. Individuals that are duffy negative also lack the receptor for vivax merozoites on their red cells and are resistant to vivax infection. (Miller et al, 1976) Although new evidence is beginning to contradict this age long position and there are increasing reports of P vivax infection in Duffy negative individuals.(Mercereau-Puijalon &Menard, 2010) Acquired immunity which may be passive as in transplacental transfer of maternal IgG to babies(Falade et al, 2007, Marsh,2002) or active immunity following repeated exposure to the parasite determine incidence and severity of infection. IgM and IgG immunoglobulin response to malaria particularly IgG protects against invasion of red cells by merozoites.(Anonymous, 1975) These immunoglobulins also promote phagocytosis of erythrocytes containing maturing schizonts.

Blood group type: Parasite virulence has been found to be reduced in blood group O erythrocytes compared with groups A, B and AB suggesting that Blood group O may confer some resistance to severe falciparum malaria. A matched case-control study of 567 Malian children found that group O was present in only 21% of severe malaria cases compared with 44–45% of uncomplicated malaria controls and healthy controls. Group O was associated with a 66% reduction in the odds of developing severe malaria compared with the non-O blood groups.(Rowe et al, 2007) Others have confirmed that blood group A is a co receptor for plasmodium falciparum rossetting, a mechanism by which the parasite potentiates its virulence causing severe malaria.(Barragan et al, 2000)

Nutritional status: Nutritional status of the host also plays a role as severe malaria has been reported to be uncommon in marasmic and kwarshiokor patients.(Goyal, 1991) Malnutrition is thought to contribute to 53% of under-5 mortality in the developing world.(Caulfield et al, 2004) The global distribution of malnutrition overlaps with that of malaria. However the relationship between malnutrition and malaria is unclear. The pathology of malaria is partly immune mediated requiring both cellular and humoral mechanisms for its evolution.(Jhaveri et al, 1997, Turrini et al, 2003, Sandau,2001) This partly explains why under-nutrition is widely believed to be protective for severe malaria.(Goyal, 1991)

Genetic disorders: Haemoglobinopathies, membranopathies and inherited enzyme deficiencies particularly G6PD all contribute to the anaemia in affected children. In each case multiple mechanisms are at work though one or two mechanisms predominate. (Wickramasinghe & Abdallah,2000) Generally severe malaria anaemia is characterized by a low reticulocyte response and high erythropoietin levels.(Roberts et al, 2005)

2.2 Lysis of parasitized erythrocytes

As part of the malaria life cycle, rupture of erythrocytes to release merozoites result in cell lysis. The merozoites destroy the red blood cell by its own protease enzyme. The released merozoites attack other red cells and through the repeated cycles of red cell lysis, anaemia ensues. This is particularly important for falciparum as it has the propensity to invade large cell populations of all age groups.(Miller, 1976) This also partly accounts for the reticulocytopenia as the reticulocytes are not spared of the direct invasion in addition to other mechanisms that suppress regeneration of red cell precursors in the bone marrow (dyserythropoeisis) In contrast p vivax invades only the young and large cells with less severity of anaemia (Miller et al, 1976) Severe anaemia develops rapidly in children and the rate is directly proportional to the degree of parasitaemia in many cases.(WHO, 2004, Afolabi et al, 2002) However, parasitaemia is not a very reliable indicator of severity as a large number of parasitized red cells may be sequestered in capillaries and venules of vital organs and hence not detected in the peripheral blood film.(Silamut & While, 1993) Prior treatment and continuous immune lysis after parasitic clearance also impair the reliability of parasitaemia as a reliable indicator of severity of anaemia.

2.3 Immune mediated lysis

There is evidence for immune mediated lysis of both parasitized and non parasitized red cells as specific antibodies are produced against them. Increased clearance of red blood cells still occur even after parasitic clearance.(Ouma et al, 2008, Edington & Gilles, 1976, Warell et al, 2002, Stouti et al, 2002) This occurs as a result production of antibodies to non parasitized cell, binding of soluble malaria antigens to the red cells, binding of immune complexes to red cell surface with subsequent removal by immune lysis and the erythrophagocytosis. (Warell et al, 2002) The observation of reduced complement particularly C3 during acute attacks, increased destruction of transfused cells in malaria patients also support the possibility of an immune mediated lysis. Complement mediated lysis is increased due to loss of complement regulatory protein CD-55 and CD -59 associated with malaria which protects inadvertent complement mediated lysis. (Stouti et al, 2003) In addition to this the increased production of immune complexes including malaria antigen and drug associated complexes increase complement activation. Non specific polyclonal activation of B cell is a common finding in malaria and may cause production of autoantibodies some of which could conceivably be directed at red cell antigens.(Jhaveri et al, 1997) Transfusion of malaria antigens alone in the absence of infection in animals giving rise to adverse effects on the red cells further strengthen the evidences for immune lysis. (Satpathy et al, 2004)

2.4 Removal by the reticuloendothelial system

Removal, particularly in the spleen, of deformed, parasitized red cells and immune sensitized red cells appears to be the most significant mechanism and explains why majority of patients do not present with overt signs of hemolysis such as jaundice and dark colored urine as is commonly found in other causes of intravascular hemolysis. Cytokine dysregulation and increased Tumor Necrosis Factor α (TNF - α) can activate macrophages which in a hyperactive stage may even reduce its threshold for amount of antibody coating needed for phagocytosis i.e. minimally sensitized red cells which otherwise would not have been phagocytosed now are actively phagocytosed due to activation of the monocytes and macrophages.(Turrini et al, 2003)

2.5 Bone marrow suppression

Anaemia due to malaria is hyporegenerative along with mild to moderate shortening of red cell life span. It is characterized either by normochromic normocytic or hypochromic microcytic features and associated with hypoferinaemia, low total iron binding capacity, transferring, low reticulocyte count and raised levels of inflammatory proteins like fibrinogen.(Abdalla, 1990) These are all features of anaemia of chronic disorder. So long as the insult persists, administration of iron does not correct the anaemia. Interleukins (IL-1 and IL-6) and TNF - α have been found to be significantly elevated in patients with severe anaemia due to malaria and they have an inverse relationship to the degree of anaemia found in such patients.(Issifou et al, 2003, McDevitt et al, 2004) The bone marrow shows a non specific suppression of all cell lines and there is a sequestration of young erythrocytes and reticulocytes.(Edington & Gilles, 1976)

2.6 Iron shunting for parasite use
The hypoferrinaemia discussed above can be explained by three mechanisms (Ghosh, 2007)
1. Locking of iron in macrophage stores
2. Synthesis of iron binding proteins with higher affinity for iron than transferrin by inflammatory cells leading to a mop up of available iron
3. Reduction in transferrin synthesis by the hepatocytes

The overall effect is a reduction in iron (a growth promoting nutrient) available to the parasites and the other cells that require iron for their metabolism. This contributes to reduced erythropoiesis. Malaria parasite has an enormous need for iron for its life cycle and extracts iron from host by inserting parasite specific transferring - like receptors on the host red cell membrane. This significantly contributes to the picture of iron deficiency anaemia seen particularly in children with borderline or low iron stores.(Oppenheimer, 1989)

2.7 Hypersplenism
Intense stimulation of monocyte macrophage system associated with malaria and hypersplenism persists 4 -6 weeks after parasitic clearance.(Looaressuwan et al, 1997)2 Some non parasitized red blood cells are removed as a result of changes in the membrane and increased osmotic fragility as a result of the changes in the chemical and immunological constituents of plasma.(Ghosh, 2007) Tropical splenomegaly syndrome following repeated or chronic falciparum malaria infection and may contribute to increased red cell removal by the reticulo -endothelial system.

2.8 Dyserythropoiesis
High levels of erythropoietin and suppressed marrow response are paradoxically associated with malaria anaemia. The high erythropoietin levels is caused by high levels of hypoxia inducing factor (HIF) induced by a combination of high levels of TNF- α.(Sandau et al 2001) Deficiency of IL -12 and IL - 10 have been found to correlate to the marrow suppression seen in malaria.(Weatherall et al 2002) Erythroid precursors like BFU – E (Burst forming colonies) and CFU –E (Colony Forming colonies) are inhibited. It is believed that therapeutic application of IL-10 and IL-12 provides prospects for correcting severe malaria anaemia. The inability of young children to maintain IL-10 production in response to inflammatory processes contributes to the anaemia. This cytokine is a growth factor that stimulates the differentiation of haemopoietic progenitor cells in response to anaemia.(Angela O'Donnell et al 2007). Ouma et al investigated the polymorphic variability in innate immune response genes, susceptibility to malaria and circulating inflammatory mediator levels (i.e., IL-10, TNF-alpha, IL-6 and IL-12) in 375 Kenyan children. Results demonstrated that common IL-10 promoter haplotypes modulate susceptibility to severe malaria anaemia and functional changes in circulating IL-10, TNF-alpha, and IL-12 levels in children with falciparum malaria. The expression of these haplotypes have been found to be age dependent and may account for less erythropoeitic response to anaemia in the younger child.

2.9 Role of nitric oxide

Acute malaria is associated with increases in Nitric oxide (NO) production.(Clark et al, 1991) High levels of nitric oxide inhibit Na+/K+ ATPase in the red cell membrane and oxidizes the membrane lipids through generation of peroxiynitrate causing poor deformability of red cells. Overactivation of poly-ADP ribose polymerase-1 (PARP-1) by nitric oxide and other proinflammaotry cytokines causes rapid depletion of nicotinamide adenine dinucleotide (NAD) and adenosine triphosphate (ATP) from red cells.(Clark & Cowden,2003) Hence it can inhibit red cell glycolysis. Membrane-damaged red cells are removed by the spleen. Nitric Oxide also suppresses erythropoiesis by mitochondrial damage to erythroid progenitors and early erythroid.(Xie & Wolin, 1996)

2.10 Role of haemozoin

Haemozoin, a product of catabolism of haemoglobin by malaria parasite contains iron in the ferrous state which catalyzes the production of free radicals. This leads to increased production of 15-hydroxy-eicosatetraenoic acid (15-HETE) and 4-Hydroxy Nonenal (4HNE) from red cell membrane lipids. These products increase red cell stiffness and shorten red cell life span.(Arese & Schwarzwer, 1997)

2.11 Pitting of parasitized red cell

Spherocytes have been found in high prevalence in peripheral blood in malaria endemic areas, and a detailed study of mechanism of whole parasitized red cell removal versus pitting out the parasite from red cell along with some amount of red cell membrane (leading to spherocyte formation) proved that the later mechanism appears to be preferred by the human body.(Anyona et al, 2006) Pitting as one of the major parasite mechanisms is also suggested by high levels of parasite-related antigens on the unaffected spherocytic red cells in malarial infection.(Anyona et al, 2006) Spherocytosis in malarial infection can be caused by several mechanisms. Spherocytes are less compliant than normal red cells and are easily removed by the spleen.

2.12 Tropical splenomegaly syndrome (hyperactive malarial splenomegaly)

In some patients with chronic exposure to malaria, P. falciparum leads to chronic and intense stimulation of splenic macrophages leading to gross splenomegaly, low levels of parasitaemia and very high levels of IgM in the serum. These patients have a defect in immunoglobulin class switching and a genetic predisposition to develop this condition. Clonal B cell proliferation in this syndrome has also been recognized.(Bates et al, 1991) Huge spleen and hyperactive reticulo-endothelial system chronically can cause significant anemia by red cell pooling. A small proportion of these patients develop non-Hodgkin lymphoma, which adds to the existent causes of anemia in this infection as a future consequence.

2.13 Endothelial injury

Parasitized red cell develops special receptors to stick to endothelial cells. This property is seen particularly with P. falciparum infection. Attachment of these parasites can take place through CD-36 ligand (Gamain et al, 2001) or through interaction with endothelial cell chondroition sulphate-like molecule. Cytokine dysregulation could up regulate endothelial adhesion molecules and converts the anti-coagulant endothelium to a procoagulant surface.

Hence combination of these two mechanisms may cause intense red cell sequestration in deeper capillaries and disseminated intravascular coagulation (DIC) with hemorrhage. Both conditions can contribute to acute anemia in P. falciparum infection. A proportion of patients can also develop microangiopathic hemolysis.

3. Clinical features

The features of severe malaria anaemia are those of malaria with or without features of cardio respiratory decompensation. The signs and symptoms of uncomplicated malaria are non specific and there exists a wide range of differential diagnosis for malaria in an endemic region. Many children with malaria parasitemia are asymptomatic particularly in malaria endemic regions. Threshold values of parasitemia based on epidemiological surveys are established for various regions of endemicity to be able to ascribe the clinical features to malaria in the presence of malaria parasitemia.(Salako et al, 1990, Krause, 2000) In malaria endemic regions, a threshold of 5,000 -10,000 parasites/ml is commonly quoted.(Snow et al, 2002) However clinical malaria can occur in the absence of detectable parasite in the blood particularly in falciparum malaria during the process of deep tissue schizogony where the maturing schizonts are sequestered in the capillaries of deep tissues like the muscle and bone marrow.(Taylor & Molyneux, 2002)

Malaria is a febrile illness and majority of patients present with fever.(Ehrhardt et al, 2006) The fever may be of any pattern, the classical intermittent description of fever, within every 48 hours in falciparum, ovale, and vivax and within every 72 hours in malariae is seen if only one brood of parasite causes infection so that the cyclical rupture of erythrocytic schizonts are synchronous with the clinical symptomatology, otherwise fever may be continuous, high or low grade in nature. In cases unmodified by treatment, it starts with malaise, myalgia, anorexia, headache followed by an intense feeling of cold associated with shivering called the cold phase, core temperature is high and tachycardia is common. This lasts for about 15-30 minutes and followed by a rapid rise in temperature to as high as 410C, vomiting, headache, convulsion and delirium may occur while splenomegaly may be detected at this phase. This hot phase lasts 2-4 hours after which is the wet or defervescence where the child sweats profusely and feels better this lasts 2-4 hours. The whole cycle is repeated within 48 hours in falciparum, vivax and ovale malaria and within 72 hours in p. malariae. In the infant and younger child, symptoms are less specific and include irritability, refusal to feed, diarrhea cough and fever of any pattern predominating. (Ehrhardt et al, 2006) Vomiting, diarrhea, cough may occur and confuse the diagnosis with gastroenteritis or an acute upper respiratory tract infection. Anaemia, tachypnea, hepatosplenomegaly and dehydration are common in uncomplicated cases.(Grobusch & Kremsner, 2005) Altered consciousness, repeated convulsions, severe pallor, shock, jaundice, dark or coke colored urine, oliguria, prostration, respiratory distress and hyperpyrexia put patients at a high risk of dying and in addition to laboratory findings of hypoglycemia and hyperparasitemia are classified as forms of severe malaria.(WHO, 2004)

The features of severe malaria anaemia are those enumerated above in addition to symptoms and signs of cardiorespiratory compromise in decompensated children, however many children have severe malarial anaemia with few or no life threatening symptoms (Lackritz et al, 1992, English et al, 2002) and this usually follows when anaemia has developed slowly. Other children with systemic organ diseases particularly cardiac, respiratory, renal diseases and sepsis may present with signs of decompensation at higher haematocrit levels. If anaemia occurs rapidly or when these compensatory mechanisms are overwhelmed, anaerobic metabolism commences with the generation of acids and development of the signs and symptoms of decompensation. The cardinal signs of decompensation are respiratory distress (tachypnea, chest in-drawing, acidotic breathing)(WHO, 2004, English et al, 1996) tachycardia with or without gallop rhythm and tender hepatomegaly. These signs are also those of congestive cardiac failure.(Afolabi et al, 2002) Others include features of hypovolemic shock, (English et al, 1996a,1996b) cold clammy extremities, weak thready pulses, delayed capillary refill time.(Pamba & Maitland, 2004) An overlap commonly occurs with severe anaemia coexisting with cerebral malaria, respiratory distress and other forms of severe malaria in which it portends worse prognosis.(WHO, 2004)

Pathophysiology of Some Clinical Features of Severe Malaria

Clinical Features	Pathophysiology
Fever	Cytokine mediated
Gastrointestinal symptoms (Nausea, Diarrhea)	Mechanism unclear Intestinal dysfunction secondary to hypoxia from parasitic sequestration in splanchnic bed
Jaundice and Dark urine	Hemolysis Dehydration
Difficulty in breathing	Hypoxia Low pH Lactic acidosis Pyrexia
Tachypnea	Hypoxia, Low pH Lactic acidosis Pyrexia
Tachycardia	Hypoxia Pyrexia
Hepatosplenomegaly	Parasitic sequestration Reticuloendothelial hyperactivity Increased preload from right sided heart failure
Loss of consciousness	Cerebral hypoxia and ischaemia, Sludging as a result of parasitic sequestration Micro circulatory obstruction Increased capillary permeability Cerebral oedema

4. Biochemical and laboratory changes

Anaemia is a common finding in malaria and the degree correlates with severity of parasitaemia. (Grobusch & Kremsner, 2005) In severe anaemia, haematocrit is less than 15% or haemoglobin concentration less than 5g/dL. Anaemia is usually haemolytic normochromic and normocytic though macrocytic picture is seen if there is folate deficiency or with marked reticulocytosis. Mean corpuscular volume, however, varies with age in children and its interpretation has to be related to the expected for age. Leucopenia with a left shift is a common finding though leucocytosis may occur in the early stage of infection or when a concomitant bacterial infection coexists. Monocytosis and malaria pigments in form of granules are found in large monocytes.(Edington & Gilles, 1976, Warrell et al, 2002) Thrombocytopenia (Grobusch & Kremsner, 2005) with some degree of depletion of clotting factors and accumulation of fibrinogen degradation products is seen though disseminated intravascular coagulopathy is very rare.(Warrell et al, 2002) This is as a result of consumption coagulopathy triggered by parasite products, phagocytosis of platelets by the reticuloendothelial system and an inappropriate bone marrow response. The activation of the coagulation cascade is via the intrinsic pathway and has been found to be proportional to disease severity and is least severe in uncomplicated malaria cases.(Clemens et al, 1994)

The peripheral blood film shows parasitized red cells, polychromasia, anisocytosis, poikilocytosis, target cells and in severe cases nucleated red blood cells. The presence of schizont and gametocytes in the peripheral blood film indicates severity of infection. Blood film may show few parasites as a result of deep tissue sequestration or following prior treatment with antimalarial drugs. The bone marrow shows erythroblastic hyperplasia with large eosinophilic normoblastic cells. Erythrocyte sedimentation rate (ESR) is increased in malaria cases and variation due to the intensity of infection can be expected.(Viroj, 2008, Karunaweera et al, 1998) It has been found that an increase in the mass of individual red cell due to inclusion bodies reduce the time for sedimentation.(Viroj, 2008) Malarial parasites act as inclusion bodies thereby increasing red cell mass (weight) and ESR. However ESR is a non specific hematological parameter that cannot be reliably used for diagnosis of malaria or monitoring of response to treatment.

Oxygen delivery is determined by tissue blood flow and the arterial oxygen content.(Moroff & Dend, 1983) While tissue blood flow is dependent on the cardiac output (function of the stroke volume and the heart rate), the arterial oxygen content is a function of haemoglobin concentration and saturation and minimally the amount of oxygen dissolved in plasma. Stroke volume is determined by the preload (venous return), myocardial contractility and the afterload (resistance to flow). All these parameters are delicately regulated by a host of local autoregulatory, hormonal and neural mechanisms to maintain optimal oxygen delivery even in the face of disease. (William, 1997) In anaemic states the arterial partial oxygen pressure (pO_2) reduces and pCO_2 is elevated. These factors in addition to low pH, fever, lactate, potassium and a host of others are potent stimuli for arteriolar vasodilation increasing tissue blood flow in vital organs like the brain and the heart. (William, 1997b) Autonomic discharges from the sympathetic system results in generalized vasoconstriction and venoconstriction, increase in blood pressure and a reduction in blood pool in the capacitance vessels culminating in an increase in venous return. More importantly in children the sympathetic discharge increases the heart rate by a direct stimulatory effect on the sinoatrial node and a reduction in the vagal inhibitory pulses. Additional effect of the sympathetic discharge on the renal vessels result in increased production of renin by the juxtaglomerular apparatus with subsequent activation of the Renin-Angiotensin-Aldosterone system resulting in water and salt retention further accentuating the preload.(William, 1997b)

Blood viscosity which is a function of the haematocrit drops with a progressive reduction in haematocrit such that resistance to flow further reduces in the blood vessels contributing to the increase in tissue blood flow and the venous return.67 Children in contrast to adults have a greater capacity to increase cardiac output by increasing heart rate than by increasing stroke volume; therefore tachycardia is a more prominent feature in children. Oxygen extraction from the arterial circulation is enhanced by the higher concentration of 2,3 diphosphoglycerate in children particularly in high oxygen consumption and supply dependent organs which include the brain and the heart(Marsh, 2002) while more is synthesized within 24-36hours of onset of anaemia.(Card & Brain, 1973) This results in a wider arteriovenous oxygen differential across the tissues. Depending on how rapid the anaemia develops in children, these mechanisms are brought to play so that a 50% reduction in oxygen carrying capacity results in less than 25% reduction in tissue oxygen availability.(Moroff & Dend,1983)

5. Treatment

Blood transfusion with 10ml/kg of packed cells should be given over 2-4 hours with diuretic therapy to prevent volume overload (Newton et al, 1992) while whole blood transfusion is advocated for patients with proven hypovolemia. There is an increasing tendency towards whole blood transfusion based on evidence that many patients with severe malaria anaemia are actually hypovolemic with hypotension, delayed capillary refill time and low central venous pressures.(Maitland et al, 2003) Based on these findings, this school of thought postulates that cardiac failure does not occur and its features are rather those of a compensated hypovolemic shock,(WHO, 2004) thus they advocate whole blood transfusion or initial volume expansion with colloid to improve tissue perfusion and correct acidosis while awaiting blood transfusion.(Maitland et al, 2003) Severe malaria has been found to be associated with about 6.7% reduction in total body water, a loss slightly more than mild dehydration such that overzealous volume expansion may be detrimental.(Planche et al, 2004)

Blood transfusion is fraught with many risks of immediate and long term complications which must be weighed against their potential benefits. Such risks include transmission of infections including HIV, Hepatitis, Ebstein Barr, cytomegalovirus and other pathogens in screened and unscreened blood. (Halim et al, 1999, Anderson & Weinstein, 1990) Risk of transmitting HIV via transfusion of screened blood in the window period has been estimated to be 1 in 3 x 105 – 2 x 106 while hepatitis is 1 in 1 x 105 transfusions in the USA. (Anderson & Weinstein, 1990) Others include volume overload, electrolyte abnormalities, transfusion reactions, alloimmunization in females and graft vs host disease rarely in immunocompetent hosts. (Anderson & Weinstein, 1990)

Various studies have been done with the aim of increasing the threshold for blood transfusion to limit transfusion to only those at the risk of dying while advocating conservative management for the others with potent anti malarial agents with or without haematinics. (Holzer et al, 1993, Bojang et al, 1997) These studies defined decompensation as respiratory distress or a combination of tachycardia and tachypnea in addition to tender hepatomegaly. Cochrane review of 2 of 42 such studies involving 230 children found no significant tendency towards dying among 2 groups of patients randomized for transfusion and non transfusion. (Meremikwu & Smith, 2004) In one study in Gambia with severe anaemia, those with haematocrit <12 and all those with severe anaemia in association with respiratory distress and cardiac failure were transfused while others were randomized for transfusion and conservative management with antimalarial medication and iron therapy. No stastistical significance in mortality was found and haematologic restoration viz a viz haematocrit at 28 days was better in those treated conservatively.(Bojang et al, 1997) However the need for close monitoring was reduced as well as shortened hospital stay. A study in Tanzania recruited patients with similar criteria and conservative management was with antimalarial alone. They achieved similar result except that haematocrit at 28 days was not significantly different in both groups probably due to the omission of haematinics in their treatment protocol. (Holzer et al, 1993)

Antimalarial drug of choice are Quinine and Artemether. Artemether has a faster parasitic clearance than quinine and the additional advantage of less potential side effects.(Taylor et al, 1998) In comparison to sulphadoxine/pyrimethamine it has both a shorter parasite and fever clearance time but high recrudescence rate.(Salako et al, 1994) Artemisinin based combination therapy is being advocated as a result of this and are now available. However they are expensive, mostly come in oral preparations and may not be easily applicable in emergency situations.(WHO, 2002)

6. Findings from a clinical study on severe malaria anaemia in Ilorin, Nigeria

A cross sectional study was carried out in the Emergency Paediatric Unit of the University of Ilorin Teaching Hospital over a ten month period from February to November 2006 to document the clinical profile and haematological indices of children with severe anaemia due to malaria. The study attempted to determine the:

1. Hospital prevalence of severe anaemia in children.
2. Clinical presentation of children with severe anaemia due to malaria
3. Haematological indices (Hb, PCV,MCV,MCH, MCHC), Genotype, and Blood group of children with severe anaemia due to malaria.
4. Factors associated with risk of cardiac decompensation in children with severe anaemia due to malaria

Children between 6 months and 12 years of age with suspected malaria anemia were enrolled into a case control study at the University of Ilorin Teaching Hospital from February to November 2006.

Severe malaria anaemia was defined as haemoglobin concentration <5g/dl associated with Plasmodium falciparum parasitaemia in the absence of other identifiable cause of anaemia. The controls were age and sex matched children with similar characteristics above who had malaria without severe anaemia (Haematocrit >15%).

Detailed history and physical examination were done on all recruited subjects. Venous samples were collected for haematocrit check, haemoglobin electrophoresis, Mean Corpuscular Volume (MCV), Mean Corpuscular Haemoglobin(MCH) and blood film analysis for malaria parasite prior to blood transfusion. Investigations were done using Sysmex 18 auto analyzer and Volkam SAE 2761 electrophoretic tank. Presence of malaria parasitaemia was noted while specie of parasite is detected on the thin film. Parasite count was determined by calculating the number of parasitized red blood cells corresponding to 200 white blood cells multiplied by the total white cell count divided by 200.

All the subjects in the study received blood transfusion. Intravenous fluids and sodium bicarbonate were used as required. Artemether or quinine was administered at the appropriate dose.

Data analysis was done using Epi-info 2004 software package on a microcomputer. For simple proportion, frequency tables were generated. Chi square test and student's 't' test was used to test for significance of the difference between categorical and continuous variable respectively. Yates correction of Chi-square and Fisher's exact were used when appropriate. A p-value of <0.05 was regarded as significant.

7. Results

A total of nine hundred and eighty one (981) children were admitted into the Emergency Paediatric Unit from February to November 2006 of which 209 (21.3%) were cases of severe malaria. Among the children admitted with severe malaria, 96 (45.9%) had severe anaemia; thus severe anaemia due to malaria accounted for 9.8% of total admissions in the emergency paediatric unit. One hundred and eighty six children were recruited for the study, 93 each in the subject and control groups. There were 49 males and 44 females in each group with a male to female ratio of 1.1:1. (Table 1) The mean age for the subjects was 24.03 + 14.2 onths (range 6 – 60 onths) compared to 23.97 ± 14.3 onths in the controls and both were comparable (p = 0.91) About a third (32.3%) of the subjects were infants less than 12 months of age while 5.4% were children older than 48 months.

19.4% of the subjects presented to the hospital less within 3 days of onset of illness. A significantly higher proportion of the subjects presented later than 3 days compared to the controls ($\chi 2$ = 21.24; p = 0.001).

Parameter	Subjects		Controls		
	n	%	n	%	P
Sex					
Male	49	52.3	49	52.3	
Female	44	47.7	44	47.7	
Age in months					
6 -12months	30	32.3	30	32.3	
13-24months	25	26.9	27	29.0	
24-36months	18	19.4	17	18.3	
37-48months	15	16.1	14	15.1	
49-60 months	5	5.4	5	5.4	
Duration of illness					
<3 days	18	19.4	48	51.6	
≥3 days	75	80.6	45	47.4	0.01
Mean age (months)	24.01 ± 14.2		23.97 ± 14.3		

Table 1. Sex and age distribution of the subjects and controls.

Figure 1 shows that forty five (45%) percent of the subjects were within social class IV-V while thirty two (32%) percent were in social class III using the Oyedeji Social classification Scheme.110 A statistically higher proportion of the subjects were in the lower socio economic classes IV – V compared to the controls. ($\chi 2$ - 9.16; p = 0.002)

The predominant symptoms in both subjects and controls groups were fever, vomiting and refusal of feeds with comparable proportions as shown in Table 2. Breathlessness and convulsion were significantly prominent among the subjects than controls while easy fatigability, abdominal swelling and loss of consciousness were seen only among the subjects.

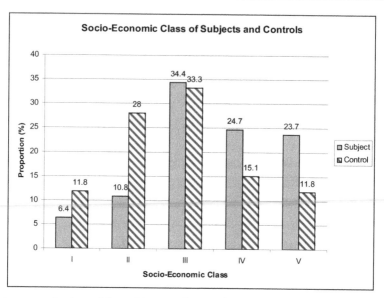

Fig. 1. Socioeconomic class of the subjects and controls.

Symptom	Subjects		Controls				
	n	%	n	%	χ^2	p	OR(CI)
Fever	91	97.8	86	92.5	2.90	0.088	1.6(1.1 -2.3)
Vomiting	51	54.8	43	46.2	1.38	0.241	1.18(0.89-1.6)
Refusal of feeds	68	73.1	56	60.2	3.48	0.062	1.32(1.0 -1.8)
Diarrhea	20	21.5	18	19.4	0.13	0.72	1.07(0.74 -1.5)
Cough	22	23.7	17	18.3	0.88	0.35	1.19(0.8 -1.8)
Breathlessness	25	26.9	4	4.3	18.0	0.001	4.1(1.6 -10.3)
Convulsion	26	30.0	3	3.2	21.6	0.001	5.5(1.88 -16.3)
Easy fatigability	3	3.2	0	0	3.05	0.81	0.42(0.42 -0.6)
Abdominal swelling	6	6.5	0	0	6.2	0.03	0.48(0.4 -0.6)
Loss of consciousness	13	14.0	0	0	13.9	0.01	0.46(0.39 -0.5)

Table 2. Symptoms among subjects and controls.

A combination of tachycardia and tachypnea was found in 33.3% of the subjects and 19.4% of the controls and the difference was statistically significant (χ^2 = 4.22; p = 0.04). Among the subjects, 28% had a combination of tachycardia, tachypnea and tender hepatomegaly while 5.4% of the controls demonstrated similar signs and the difference was statistically significant.(χ^2 = 17.07; p = 0.001) (Table 3).

Sign	Subject		Control		χ^2	p	OR(CI)
	n	%	n	%			
Temperature							
<37.5⁰C	19	20.4	14	15.1	0.92	0.33	1.45 (0.64 – 43.31)
37.5-38.5⁰C	41	44.1	43	46.2	0.09	0.76	0.92 (0.49 – 1.70)
>38.5⁰C	33	35.5	33	38.7	0.02	0.88	1.00 (0.52 – 1.91)
Hydration Status							
Normal	62	66.7	74	79.6	3.74	0.06	0.51 (0.25 – 1.05)
Mild – Moderate Dehydration	27	29	19	20.4	1.85	0.17	1.59 (0.77 – 3.30)
Severe Dehydration	4	4.3	0	0	4.09	0.04	2.04 (1.76 – 2.37)
Weight(% of expected							
<60%	1	1.1	0	0	1.01	0.31	-
60-80%	27	29	20	21.5	1.40	0.24	1.49 (0.73 – 3.07)
>80%	65	69.9	73	78.5	1.80	0.18	0.64 (0.31 – 1.02)
Acidotic breathing	18	19.4	7	7.5	5.6	0.01	2.95(1.1-8.3)
Tachypnea	33	35.5	17	18.3	7.0	0.01	2.46(1.2-5.1)
Tachycardia	37	39.8	30	32.3	1.14	0.28	1.39(0.73 -2.65)
Gallop rhythm	15	16.1	2	2.2	9.32	0.001	8.75(1.83 -57.2)
Blood pressure for age							
Hypotension	2/31	6.5	0/42	0	-		-
Normal	29/31	93.5	42/42	100	0.89	0.4	-
Hepatomegaly	87	93.5	54	58.1	31.92	0.001	2.3(1.8 -2.9)
Splenomegaly	58	62.4	43	46.2	4.87	0.03	1.4(1.03-1.1.84)
Glasgow Coma Score							
≤ 10	5	5.4	0	0	3.29	0.06	
11-14	8	8.7	0	0	6.4	0.01	-
15	80	85.9	93	100	13.98	0.001	-
Tachycardia + Tachypnea							
	31	33.3	18	19.4	4.68	0.03	2.1(1.0- 4.3)
Tachycardia+Tachypnea+Tender hepatomegaly							
	26	28	5	5.4	17.07	0.001	3.52(1.56 -7.9)

Table 3. Physical findings in the subjects and controls at presentation.

Table 4 shows the relationship between selected features and signs of decompensation defined as a combination of tachycardia, tachypnea and tender hepatomegaly among the subjects.

Parameter		Compensated n (%)	Decompensated n (%)	χ^2	p	OR(CI)
Age	<36 months	48(71.6%)	19(28.4%)			
	≥36months	19(73.1%)	7(26.9%)	0.02	0.89	1.1(0.50-2.21)
Sex	Male	36(84.7%)	13(15.3%)			
	Female	31(82.9%)	13(17.1%)	0.10	0.75	1.04(0.8-1.34)
Social Class	I-II	13(81.3%)	3(18.8%)	0.08	0.77	1.5(0.35-7.53)
	III	23(71.9%)	9(28.1%)	0.3	0.58	0.76(0.26-2.25)
	IV-V	34(75.6%)	11(24.4%)	0.01	0.95	1.03(0.36-2.93)
Duration of illness	≤3days	32(71.1%)	13(28.9%)			
	>3days	35(72.9%)	13(27.1%)	0.04	0.03	1.1(0.56-2.0)
Weight for age	<80%	47(72.3%)	18(27.7%)			
	≥80%	20(71.4%)	8(28.6%)	0.01	0.93	0.97(0.48-2.0)
Hydration Status						
Normal		48(75.0%)	14(25.0%)	2.09	0.14	1.93(0.72-5.19)
Mild to Moderate dehydration		17(65.5%)	10(34.5%)	0.44	0.51	0.73(0.26 -2.05)
Severe dehydration		1(25.0%)	3(75.0%)	1.79	0.18	0.11(0.1-1.27)
Temperature	≥38.9	30(45.5%)	36(54.5%)			
	<38.9	8(29.6%)	19(70.4%)	1.99	0.16	0.76(0.56-1.1)
PCV	≤12%	41(68.3%)	19(31.7%)			
	>12%	26(78.8%)	7(21.2%)	1.16	0.28	1.5(0.70-3.2)
PCV	<15%	67(72%)	26(28%)			
(Controls)	15 -20%	26(96.3%)	1(3.7%)	2.41	0.01	0.1(0.00-0.72)

Table 4. Factors associated with features of decompensation among the subjects.

Cardiac decompensation was not significantly affected by age, sex and social class. However children older than 36 months (OR 1.1(0.5-2.21) and male sex (OR 1.2 (0.5 -2.9) demonstrated an increased risk for decompensation though these were not statistically significant. Though approximately half (49.5%) of the subjects had PCV less than 12%, a higher proportion (31.7%) of the children in this group decompensated compared to 21.2% who decompensated in those with PCV greater than 12%. The difference however was not statistically significant. (p = 0.28 OR 1.5 CI 0.7 -3.2)). A statistically significant relationship was seen between duration of illness and risk of cardiac decompensation.(p = 0.03 OR – 1.1 CI 0.56 – 2.0)

Fifty percent of the subjects had PCV equal or greater than 12% while 36.6% and 12.9% had PCV of 9-11%.and less than 9% respectively. Among the controls, 70.3% had PCV 21-30% while approximately equal proportions had PCV 16-20% and greater than 30%. (Figure 2)

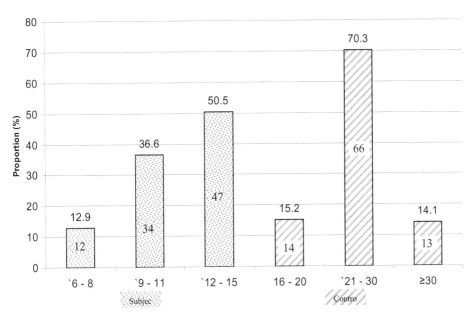

Fig. 2. PCV among subjects and controls.

About a fifth (21.5%) of the patients in both groups had comparable MCV values less than normal for age. However a significantly higher proportion of the subject group had high MCV values for age when compared with those with normal MCV ($\chi 2$ = 5.59; p = 0.02). (Table 5)

A significantly higher proportion of the subjects had low MCH values with 26.8% and 11.8% of subjects and controls respectively demonstrating low MCH values for age. ($\chi 2$ = 7.92; p = 0.004).

Leucocytosis was prominent in 53.7% of the subjects and 41.2% of the controls and a significantly lower proportion of the subjects (4.4%) had WBC less than 4000/mm3 compared to the 17.2% among the controls.($\chi 2$= 8.07;p = 0.01)

Thrombobocytopenia was significantly found in 76.4% of the subjects ($\chi2$ = 6.30; p =0.01).

Parameter	Subject	Controls	p	χ^2	t
MCV					
Low	20(21.5%)	18(19.3%)	0.72	0.13	
Normal	55(59.1%)	68(73.2%)	0.04	4.06	
Elevated	18(19.4%)	7(7.5%)	0.02	5.59	
MCH					
Low	25(26.8%)	10(11.8%)	0.004	7.92	
Normal	66(71%)	82(88.2%)	0.003	8.47	
Elevated	2(2.2%)	1(1.1%)	0.50	0.34	
WBC Count(cells/mm³)					
<4000	4(4.4%)	16(17.2%)	0.001	8.07	
4-11000	39(41.9%)	35(37.6%)	0.55	0.36	
>11000	50(53.7%)	42(41.2%)	0.24	1.38	
Platelet Count (cells/mm³)					
< 150,000	71(76.4%)	55(59.2%)	0.01	6.30	
150-450000	20(21.5)	37(38.7%)	0.006	7.31	
>450000	2(2.2%)	1(1.1%)	1.0	0.34	
Blood Group					
A	28(30.1%)	33(35.5%)	0.43	0.61	
B	30(32.3%)	27(29%)	0.63	0.23	
O	33(35.5%)	32(34.4%)	0.88	0.02	
AB	2(2.2%)	1(1.1%)	0.56	0.34	
HbGenotype					
AA	78(83.8%)	73(78.5%)	0.35	0.88	
AS	14(15.1%)	20(21.5%)	0.26	1.30	
AC	1(1.1%)	0	0.32	1.01	
Mean Values					
PCV(%)	11.2 ± 2.24	25.6 ± 5.01	0.00		25.0
MCV(µm³)	79.3 ± 10.28	81.5 ± 6 .92	0.06		1.9
MCH(pg/cell)	26.5 ± 4.08	28.4 ± 3.64	0.001		3.44
MCHC(%Hb/cell)	31.0 ± 3.68	31.4 ± 2.84	0.6		0.59
WBC Count (cells/mm³)	15.1 ±1 2.93	10.9 ± 6.94	0.03		3.1
Platelet Count(cells/mm³)	112.8 ± 89.47	151.6 ± 86.94	0.01		3.5

Table 5. Haematological Indices.

Fifty three percent (53%) of the subjeects and 18(19.4%) of the controls had parasite count greater than 250,000. (Figure 3)
The mean parasite count for children in the subject group was 499,450.43 ± 449,018.98 parasites/ml (range 8000 – 3,100,000) while for controls was 283,646 ± 357,224 parasites/ml (range 23000 -730000). Mean parasite count was significantly higher among subjects compared to the controls.($\chi 2$ = 2.52; p = 0.014).

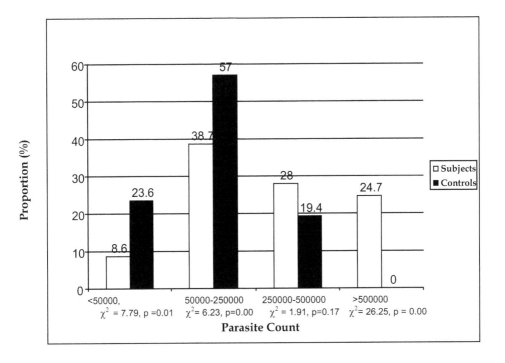

Fig. 3. Parasite Count in the subjects and controls

Table 6 shows the distribution of subjects and controls based on their parasite density across all age bands. Parasite count greater than 250,000 parasites/ml was significantly prominent among children less than 24 months. Sixty percent and forty eight percent of children in age bands 6 -12 months and 12-24 months respectively had parasite density higher than 250,000 parasites/ml (p = 0.01). Among older children the proportions with parasite density higher than 250,000 parasites/ml were comparable with controls.

Age Range (months)		Parasite density		χ^2	p
		<250,000 n(/%)	>250,000 n(%)		
6-12	Subjects	12(40%)	18(60%)		
	Controls	22(73%)	89(27%)	6.79	0.01
13-24	Subjects	13(52%)	12(48%)		
	Controls	23(85%)	4(15%)	6.71	0.01
25-36	Subjects	10(56%)	8(44%)		
	Controls	14(82%)	3(18%)	2.91	0.09
37-28	Subjects	8(53%)	7(47%)		
	Controls	13(93%)	1(7%)	6.77	0.05
49-61	Subjects	3(43%)	4(57%)		
	Controls	3(60%)	2(40%)	0.00	1.00

Table 6. Parasite count and age distribution among subjects and controls.

8. Discussion

Severe anaemia due to malaria accounted for 9% of all admissions into the Emergency Paediatric Unit (EPU) of the University of Ilorin Teaching Hospital similar to earlier reports of 5.2% in the same facility. (Ernest SK et al) This is comparable to 11.3% reported from Ibadan, Western Nigeria. (Orimadegun et al,2007) and 9.5% from Zambia (Biemba et al, 2000) Several studies in holoendemic regions have documented severe anaemia as the predominant presentation of severe malaria including this study where it accounted for 45.9% of all cases of severe malaria.(Orimadegun et al,2007, Biemba et al, 2000) This is similar to the WHO report of a multicentre study that attributed a 51.2% contribution of severe anaemia to severe malaria burden in Ibadan.(WHO Report 2002) However Schellenberg et al in Tanzania and Modiano et al in Burkina Faso reported 24 and 21% prevalence of severe anaemia among severe malaria cases respectively. The huge burden of severe malaria and particularly severe malaria anaemia in malaria endemic region may be underestimated as a result of limited access to hospitals in developing countries.

Sixty percent (60%) of the children in the study were less than 24 months of age. This finding supports previous evidence that severe malaria anaemia is seen more frequently below 3 years with a mean age of 1.8 years.(WHO 2004) A reduction in the frequency of severe anaemia beyond 24 months of life with a two fold increase in prevalence of cerebral malaria across same age band had earlier been reported in Ghana and Mali.(Oduro et al, 2007, Ranque et al, 2008) The fact that most cases of severe anaemia are seen in children less than 2years of age is attributable to the smaller red cell mass and the relatively lower immunity to the malaria parasite compared to the older children.(Newton & Krishna, 1998) This study demonstrated a progressive and consistent reduction in proportion of severe malaria anaemia with increasing age supporting the assertion that repeated exposure to malaria with advancing age increased acquired immunity to the parasite with a reduction in severity of malaria presentation. There was a slight male preponderance among children with severe anaemia with a male to female ratio of 1.1:1. This simulates the pattern among general hospital admissions as has been reported in most studies on severe malaria.(Berkley et al, 1999, Chessebrough, 1998) More than half of the children were from the lower socioeconomic classes III-V. Hedberg et al in Kinshasha found low socioeconomic status to be independently associated with anaemia. The children of parents with high socioeconomic status are likely to be relatively shielded from mosquitoes, live in environments with little or no breeding grounds for mosquitoes, have access to malaria prevention methods, early diagnosis and treatment. Poor nutrition, high cost and or unavailability of health services contribute to poor health seeking behaviour in this group of children of parents who belong to low socio economic classes.

Severe malaria anaemia in many cases presents as an acute illness as found in this study with 48% of the patients presenting to the hospital within 3 days after onset of illness. The mean duration of illness of the subjects was 4.3 days. Studies in The Gambia and Burkina Faso reported mean duration of illness of 2 and 3.1 days respectively for children with severe malaria.(Jaff et al, 1997, Modiano et al, 1999) It has been established that severe malaria is rapidly progressive in children with most deaths occurring within 24 hours thus definitive intervention must be undertaken within first 24 -48 hours of the illness if mortality is to be prevented. (Ernest et al, 2002, Greenwood, 1997) Fever was the commonest symptom reported in 97% of patients and pyrexia was documented at presentation in 77.4% of the children with severe malaria anaemia. Vomiting and refusals of feeds were equally prominent symptoms in this study. These are largely nonspecific symptoms and are found in most febrile illnesses in children. In this study, fast breathing and convulsion were more prominent in the patients with severe anaemia than controls. A third of the children in this study were underweight while Kwashiokor and Marasmic Kwashiokor were not common findings. The low weight for age may be related to the socio economic status of the study group and suggests an interplay between nutritional anaemia and malaria amongst them. Several studies have however reported a high incidence of severe anaemia due to malaria among children with low weight for age.(Oduro et al, 2007, Hedberg et al, 1993) The rarity of Marasmus and Marasmic Kwashiokor further confirms earlier findings that severe malaria particularly cerebral malaria is not commonly seen in children with severe malnutrition. Severe malaria anaemia is partly immune mediated requiring both cellular and humoral mechanisms for its evolution.(Turrini et al, 2003, Sandau et al, 2001) Immunosuppression depresses this mechanism and account for the uncommon presentation of severe malaria among children with severe malnutrition. Hepatomegaly, splenomegaly, pyrexia and tachycardia were the most prominent signs. Hepatomegaly and splenomegaly occurred in 94% and 58% of children respectively. A strong correlation between parasitaemia and organ enlargement has been reported.(Hedberg et al, 1993, Mongensen et al, 2006) This is explained by the congestion of parasite infested red cells, hypertrophy and erythrophagocytosis in the reticuloendothelial system particularly the spleen and liver.(Taylor & Molyneux, 2002) The higher preponderance of hepatomegaly over splenomegaly suggests additional mechanism for organ enlargement particularly fluid retention as may occur following anaemic heart failure in decompensated children.

Tachycardia was more prominent among children with severe malaria anaemia (40%) than controls (32%) though this was not found to be statistically significant. The pathophysiology of tachycardia in severe malaria is multifactorial particularly with in the presence of fever, dehydration and anaemia. Therefore tachycardia in isolation may not necessarily imply cardiac decompensation. Slow decline in haematocrit allows for effective adaptation to anaemic states and may reduce the severity of tachycardia seen among the children with severe malaria anaemia who presented late for treatment. (Moroff & Dend, 1983, Card & Brabin, 1973)

Less than a third of the children in both groups had signs of dehydration. Gastrointestinal symptoms (diarrhea, vomiting, anorexia) and late presentation contribute to dehydration. The reduced body water and intravascular space also contribute to tachycardia. In one study, severe malaria was found to be associated with about 6.7% reduction in total body water, a loss, marginally greater than values for mild dehydration such that overzealous volume expansion may be detrimental (Planche et al, 2004) Increased insensible loss from pyrexia, sweating and tachypnea are contributory factors to fluid loss in the study population. Despite the longer duration of illness and prominence of tachypnea, many of the children with severe malaria anaemia showed no or minimal signs of dehydration. We postulate that activation of the renin angiotensin aldosterone system secondary to hypoxia and hypovolemia result in compensatory fluid retention.

Decompensation occurs as a result of a breakdown in maintenance of tissue oxygenation and manifests as signs of cardiorespiratory decompensation or cardiac failure. These signs are tachycardia tachypnea and tender hepatomegaly with or without cardiomegaly. (Orimadegun et al, 2007(A combination of tachycardia, tachypnea and tender hepatomegaly was seen in 28% of the children while the majority of children in the study (72%) were stable. Therefore it may be possible to avoid blood transfusion with its attendant risks among majority of children with SMA if facilities for close observation and early identification of need for transfusion are available. This has been severally reported that many children with severe malaria anaemia remain stable.(Mulenga M et al, 2005, Lackritz et al, 1992, English et al, 2002) The mean PCV of the subjects was 11.2% and half of the children had PCV less than 12%. Signs of cardiac decompensation were demonstrated by similar proportions of subjects with PCV $\leq$ 12% and those with higher PCV however, among the 26 children who decompensated, seven (27%) had haematocrit levels higher than 12% while 73% had levels $\leq$ 12%. A study found no difference in mortality among children with a mean of PCV 14.1% randomized for blood transfusion or a more conservative management.(Holzer et al,1993) Mortality was significantly higher in children who had a combination of Hb < 4.7g/dL and clinical findings of respiratory distress. (Lackritz et al, 1992) Similar findings of high mortality in children with PCV < 14% with or without respiratory distress was documented in a study by English et al in 1996. A strict PCV threshold may be insufficient for instituting blood transfusion across board. This study has shown that signs of decompensation become more prominent when PCV declines below 15% compared to higher levels of PCV among controls. However other factors contribute to the risk of decompensation as majority of children remain stable irrespective of haematocrit.

Presentation at a health facility later than 3 days after onset of illness significantly reduced the risk of decompensation (p = 0.03). Decompensation occurred within first 72 hours of onset of illness in many cases. This can be attributed to the sudden onset of illness before compensatory mechanisms were well established. Lackritz et al reported that blood transfusion given after a delay of 2 days did not significantly affect mortality suggesting that deaths due to anaemia may be considerably greater in the communities than in hospitals where prompt treatment is administered.(Lacritz et al, 1992) In Ilorin, North Central Nigeria a reduction in mortality in children with severe anaemia who did not receive blood transfusion when they survived longer than 24 hours was found.(Ernest et al, 2002) All these confirm that severe malaria is a rapidly progressing disease and early intervention is required within the first 48hours of illness if mortality is to be limited.(Greenwood, 1997) This also accounts for the relative stability observed in the majority of the study subjects as majority presented later than 72 hours to the facility. Less occurrence of features of decompensation in the children who presented later than 3 days after onset of illness may also be attributed to the possible slower decline in haematocrit during the course of the illness and the gradual deployment of compensatory mechanisms particularly synthesis of 2, 3 diphosphoglycerate which allows for increased oxygen extraction from haemoglobin. (Tuman, 1990)

Age at presentation did not significantly contribute to the risk of decompensation when comparing children younger or older than 36 months. This contrasts with previous works that younger children tolerate anemia better. (Ehrhardt et al, 2006, Tuman,1990) A conclusion however can not be made on the protective value of age as no comparison was made with older children and adults. Dehydration was not significantly associated with decompensation in this study. Ranque et al in Mali reported that SMA was less associated with dehydration than cerebral malaria. (Ranque et al, 1990) Conversely in another study, volume contraction and reduced central venous pressure were found in decompensated children advocating for volume expansion or whole blood transfusion for children presenting with severe anaemia due to malaria.(Marsh et al, 1995) The degree of dehydration is variable and may also be affected by other factors including reduced intake, vomiting and hyperpyrexia. It is therefore difficult to give general recommendations for fluid therapy in severe malaria anaemia cases without individual assessment of hydration status. Other factors that showed no relationship with decompensation include sex, socio economic status and temperature at presentation. High grade pyrexia was seen in 29% of the children, among whom 70.4% were observed to have decompensated compared to 55% that decompensated among children with low grade pyrexia. However this finding was not statistically significant and may be as a result of the small number of children in the category with high grade pyrexia. It does however suggests the contribution of temperature to degree of tachycardia as it is known that heart rate increases by 2.44 beats for every 0.6oC rise above normal temperature.(Mackowaik et al, 1992) The management of pyrexia is therefore of utmost importance not only in prevention of febrile convulsions but also to reduce its contribution to cardiac decompensation.

Hyperparasitaemia was a common laboratory finding in children with severe anaemia in this study as 24.7% and 52.7% of children with severe malaria anaemia had parasite densities greater than 500,000parasites/mL and 250,000parasites/mL respectively. Sowunmi et al in Ibadan, South western Nigeria found age less than 5 years to be an independent risk factor for hyperparasitaemia. (Sowunmi et al, 2004) Hyperparasitaemia was significantly prominent in children with severe malaria anaemia who were less than 24 months compared with the controls. This finding can be explained by the waning of maternal antibody protection and increased exposure to the mosquito as the child becomes more ambulant. The prominence of hyperparasitemia in this age range reiterates the need for appropriate chemotherapy for malaria parasitaemia to prevent severe malaria. Leucocytosis was the predominant finding among children with severe anaemia. The possibility of superimposed bacterial sepsis may explain the prominence of leucocytosis in these children as over half of the subjects presented later than 3 days after onset of illness. Researchers have documented 7.8 – 15.6% prevalence of bacteraemia complicating severe malaria particularly in children under 3 years. (Berkley et al, 1999, Enwere et al, 1998) A great overlap exists between severe malaria and the incidence of bacteremia as the two conditions are commoner in younger children.(Newton et al, 1997) Severe malaria potentiates this by reducing splanchnic perfusion and causing intestinal and hepatic hypoxia. This effect is brought about by sequestration of parasites in splanchnic beds and the shunting of blood away from the gastrointestinal tract to essential organs as a compensation for hypoxia associated with severe anaemia. Entry of gram negative organisms and endotoxins from the gut lumen is thus enhanced coupled with the reduction in normal hepatic filtration of these toxins and bacteria.(Usawattanahul et al, 1985) Reduced gastric acidity and immaturity of the gut lymphoid tissue in young children contribute to this.(Miller et al, 1995) Gram negative organisms particularly Non Typhoidal Salmonella sp have been reported in association with severe malaria.(Ayoola et al, 2005) They also found Escherichia coli as the commonest organism isolated in association with malaria parasitaemia. The predisposition to bacteraemia may be related to low socioeconomic status of the study group with associated poor living conditions particularly as enteral organisms have been commonly reported by many studies. WHO recommends that, threshold for administration of broad spectrum antibiotics should be low in severe malaria because of the diagnostic overlap between severe malaria and septicaemia.(WHO Library, 2006) The use of antibiotics for children with severe malaria who demonstrate poor response to potent anti malaria chemotherapy is justified to reduce mortality. Thrombocytopenia was found in 76.4% of the children, however none presented with features of disseminated coagulopathy such as bleeding diathesis. This has been reported to be a feature of falciparum malaria and is more profound in severe forms.(Viroj, 2008) Reasons for thrombocytopenia include reduced platelet survival, bone marrow suppression, destruction by anti platelet antibodies and most significantly sequestration of platelets and removal by the spleen. Disseminated intravascular hemolysis is uncommon and if present suggests an additional pathology in most instances particularly gram negative septicaemia. Normocytic normochromic anaemia with normal MCV and MCH for age was found in majority of the children with severe malaria anaemia. A fifth (21.5%) of the children had microcytic anaemia with low MCV for age. A similar proportion had low MCH values. Isolated SMA presents as normocytic normochromic anaemia however co morbidities like nutritional deficiencies and parasitic infections particularly hook worm infestations may complicate the picture with microcytic or macrocytic features. Iron deficiency anaemia, a common consequence of nutritional deficiency of iron may not be unexpected as a third of children had low weight for age while majority of the children were from low socio economic class. Premji et al reported that majority of children infected with P. falciparum were iron deficient. (Premji et al, 1995) In a randomized study in Tanzania, children given iron supplementation had low incidence of severe anaemia than those who had placebo.(Menendez et al, 1997) These findings support the multifactorial aetiology of severe anaemia and the use of iron supplementation to reduce incidence of severe anaemia in children living in malaria endemic regions. In this study

Children with SMA had a significantly higher incidence of microcytic anaemia than controls with 19.4% presenting with high MCV for age. A co morbid state of megaloblastic anaemia or reticulocytosis following rapid bone marrow response to hemolysis may account for these findings.

AS genotype was found in a smaller proportion (15.1%) of children with severe malaria anaemia compared to controls (22%) though the difference showed no statistical significance. Traditional knowledge AS genotype has been established to protect against the progression to severe forms of malaria. The mechanisms by which mutant haemoglobins protect against severe malaria have not been definitively established and are likely multifactorial. In vitro culture experiments have shown that parasitized AS erythrocytes are more likely to sickle and support reduced parasite growth rates than their non parsitized counterparts under conditions of low oxygen tension.(Pasvol, 1980) The protection is however at the expense of early clearance of parasitized red blood cell by the spleen and contributes to some degree of anemia seen among children with AS genotype in malaria endemic regions. In this study, the lesser proportion of AS genotype found among the children with severe malaria anaemia strengthens the assertion. The ABO blood group also demonstrated no protection against severe malaria anaemia as a similar blood group distribution in the general population was found among children with severe anaemia due to malaria. This is at variance with the findings of other workers who found that parasite virulence is reduced in blood group O erythrocytes compared with groups A, B and AB suggesting that Blood group O may confer resistance to severe falciparum malaria. A matched case-control study of 567 Malian children found that group O was present in only 21% of severe malaria cases compared with 44–45% of uncomplicated malaria controls and healthy controls. Group O was associated with a 66% reduction in the odds of developing severe malaria compared with the non-O blood groups.(Mercereau & Menard, 2010) Others have confirmed that blood group A is a co receptor for plasmodium falciparum rossetting, a mechanism by which the parasite potentiates its virulence causing severe malaria.(Barragan et al, 2000) The sample size may be too small to demonstrate this effect in the study in addition to other findings that suggest the multifactorial aetiology of severe anaemia in children with malaria.

9. Conclusion

This study has demonstrated the clinical burden of severe malaria anaemia as a common indication for admission of young children into emergency units particularly children less than 24 months of age. The common clinical and laboratory presentation of this disease were also highlighted.

This study suggests a multifactorial aetiology for SMA and also confirming that majority of affected children are clinically stable without signs of decompensation. Clinical stealth needs to be applied in determining need for transfusion in the current era of blood borne morbidities particularly HIV and hepatitis in malaria prone regions. A larger randomized study with alternative therapies needs to be conducted to prescribe clinical and laboratory guides for transfusion interventions.

But in the interim, a higher threshold has been sensitized particularly in 3 situations;

a. clinical stable children with severe malaria anaemia with PCV >12%,

b. presence of capacity for close monitoring of patient's clinical profile for emergency transfusion while undergoing conservative management
c. availability of potent appropriate anti malaria interventions.

Appropriate preventive strategies should focus on early recognition and prompt treatment of malaria to prevent progression to severe malaria, provision of free or cheap anti malaria medications to reduce progression of malaria to severe forms and improvement in the living conditions particularly appropriate feeding practices to reduce incidence of malaria and anaemia associated with iron deficiency.

10. Acknowledgement

We acknowledge the contributions of individuals, paediatricians who have contributed to the body of knowledge on severe malaria and haematological conditions in children. We thank all those whose active or passive participation enriched the process particularly the published works on severe malaria.

11. References

Abdalla SH. Hematopoiesis in human malaria. Blood Cells 1990; 16: 401–416.

Afolabi BM, Salako LA, Mafe AG, Ovwigbo UB, Rabiu KA, Sanyaolu NO et al. Malaria in the first six months of life in urban African infants with anaemia. Am J Trop Med Hyg 2002; 65: 822-827.

Allen SJ, O'Donnell A, Alexander ND, Alpers MP, Peto TE, Clegg JB et al. thalassaemia protects children against disease caused by other infections as well as malaria. Proceedings of the National Academy of sciences of the USA. 1997; 94: 14736-14741.

Allison AC. Protection afforded by sickle cell trait against sub tertian malaria infection.Br Med J 1954; 1: 290-294.

Angela O'Donnell, Premawardhena A, Arambepola M, Allen SJ, Peto EA, Fisher CA et al. Age related changes in adaptation to severe anaemia in childhood in developing countries. Proc Natl Acad Sci USA 2007;104:9440-9444.

Anderson KC, Weinstein HS. Transfusion associated graft vs host disease. N Eng J Med 1990; 323: 315-321.

Anonymous: Developments in malaria immunology. WHO Technical Report Series, 1975; 579:1-45.

Anyona SB, Schrier SL, Gichuki CW, Waitumbi JN. Pitting of malaria parasites and spherocytes formation. Malaria Journal 2006; 5: 64-65.

Arese P, Schwarzwer E. Malarial pigment (haemozoin): a very active "inert" substance. Ann Trop Med Parasitol 1997; 91:501–516.

Ayoola OO, Adeyemo AA, Osinusi K. Concurrent bacteraemia and malaria in febrile Nigerian infants. Trop Doct 2005; 35: 34 -36.

Barragan A, Kremsner PG, Wahlgren M, Carlson J. Blood group A antigen is a coreceptor in Plasmodium falciparum rosetting. Infect Immun 2000; 68: 2971-2975.

Bates I, Bedu Addo G, Bevan DH. Use of immunoglobin gene rearrangement to show clonal lymphoproliferative is hypereactive malarial splenomegaly. Lancet 1991; 337:505–507.

Berkley J, Nwarumba S, Bramham K, Lowe B, Marsh K. Bacteraemia complicating severe malaria in children. Trans R Soc Trop Med Hyg 1999; 93: 283-286.

Biemba G, Dolmans D, Thuma PE, Weiss G, Gordeuk VR. Severe anaemia in Zambian children with Plasmodium falciparum malaria. Trop Med Int Health. 2000; 5: 9-16.

Bojang KA, Palmer A, Boelevan Hensbroek M, Banya WA, Greenwood BM.Management of severe malarial anaemia in Gambian children. Trans R Soc Trop Med Hyg 1997; 91: 557-561.

Brabin BJ, Premji Z, Verhoeff F. An analysis of anaemia and child mortality. J Nutr 2002; 131: 636-645.

Card R, Brain M. The "anaemia" of childhood, evidence for physiologic response to hyperphosphatemia. N Eng J Med 1973; 28: 388-392.

Caulfield LE, Richard SA, Black RE: Undernutrition as an underlying cause of malaria morbidity and mortality in children less than five years old. Am J Trop Med Hyg 2004; 71:55-63.

Cheesebrough M. Haematological tests. In Cheesbrough M (eds). District Laboratory Practice in Tropical countries. Cambridge: University Press UK; 1998. pg 320-329..

Clark IA, Cowden WB. The pathophysiology of falciparum malaria. Pharmacol Ther 2003; 99: 221–260.

Clark IA, Rockett KA, Cowden WB. Proposed link between cytokines, nitric acid and human cerebral malaria. Parasitol Today 1991; 7:205–207.

Clemens R, Pramoolsinaap C, Lorenz R, Pukrittayakamee S, Bock HL, white NJ. Activation of the coagulation cascade in severe falciparum malaria through the intrinsic pathway. Bri J Haem 1994; 87:100-105.

Edington GM, Gilles HM. Malaria. In: Pathology in tropics. 2nded. London: Edward Arnold Ltd; 1976. pg 10-34.

Ehrhardt S, Burchard GD, Mantel C, Cramer JP, Kaiser S, Kubo M et al. Malaria, anemia, and malnutrition in african children - defining intervention priorities. J Infect Dis. 2006; 194: 108-114.

English M, Waruiru C, Amukoye E, Murph S, Crawley J, Mwangi I et al. Deep acidotic breathing in children with severe anaemia: Indicator of metabolic acidosis and poor outcome. Am J Trop Med Hyg 1996; 55: 521-524.

English M, Waruiru C, Marsh K. Transfusion for life threatening respiratory distress in severe childhood malaria. Am J Trop Med Hyg 1996; 55: 525-530.

English M, Ahmed M, Ngando C, Berkley J, Ross A. Blood transfusion for severe anaemia in children in a Kenyan hospital. Lancet 2002; 359: 494-5Ernest SK, Anunobi NE, Adeniyi A. Correlates of emergency response and mortality from severe anaemia in childhood. West Afr J Med 2002; 21: 177-179.

Enwere G, Hensbroek MBV, Adegbola R, Palmer A. Bacteraemia in cerebral malaria. Ann Trop Paediatr 1998; 18: 275-278.

Falade C, Mokuolu O, Okafor H, Orogade A, Falade A, Adedoyin O et al. Epidemiology of congenital malaria in Nigeria: a multi-centre study. Trop Med Int Health. 2007; 12 :1279-1287.

Gamain B, Smith JD, Miller LH, Baruch OI. Modification of CD 36 binding domain of P. falciparum variant antigen are responsible for the inability of chondrointin sulphate adherent parasites to bond CD 36. Blood 2001; 97: 3268–3274.

Ghosh K. Pathogenesis of anaemia in malaria, a concise review Parasitol Res. 2007; 101:1463-1469.

Gilles HM. The development of malaria infection in breastfed Gambian infants. Ann Trop Med Parasitol 1957; 51: 58-59.

Grobusch MP, Kremsner PG. Uncomplicated Malaria. Currr Top Microbiol Immunol 2005; 295: 83-104.

Guidelines for red blood cell and plasma transfusion for adults and children. Can Med Ass J 2004; 156: 121-134.

Halim NKD, Offor E, Ajayi OI. Epidemiological study of seroprevalence of Hepatitis B surface antigen and HIV 1 in blood donors. Niger J Clin Pract 1999; 2: 1-34.

Hedberg K, Shaffer N, Davachi F, Hightower A, Lyamba B, Paluku KM et al. Plasmodium falciparum-associated anemia in children at a large urban hospital in Zaire. Am J Trop Med Hyg. 1993; 48: 365-371.

Holzer B, Egger M, Teuscher T. Chidhood anaemia in Africa: To transfuse or not transfuse. Acta Trop 1993; 5: 47-51.

Issifou S, Mavoungou E, Borrmann S, Bouyou-Akotet Mk, Matsiegui PI, Kremsner PG, et al. Severe malarial anaemia associated with increased soluble Fas ligand concentrations in Gabonese children. Eur Cytokine Netw 2003; 14: 238-41.

Jaff S, Hensbroek MBV, Palmer A, Schneider G, Greenwood B. Predictors of a fatal outcome following cerebral malaria. Am J Trop Med Hyg 1997; 57: 20-24.

Jhaveri KN, Ghosh K, Mohanty D, Parmar BD, Surati RR, Camoens HM, Joshi SH et al. Autoantibodies immunoglobulins, complement and circulating immune complexes in acute malaria. Natl Med J India 1997; 54: 23–29.

Karunaweera ND, Carter R, Grau GE, Mendis KN. Demonstration of anti-disease immunity to Plasmodium vivax malaria in Sri Lanka using a quantitative method to assess clinical disease. Am J Trop Med Hyg 1998; 58: 204-210.

Krause PJ. Malaria. In: Behrman RE, Kligman RM, Jenson HB (eds). Nelson textbook of Paediatrics, 18th Ed. Philadelphia: WB Saunders; 2000. pg 1477-1484.

Lackritz EM, Campbell CC, Ruebush TK, Hightower AW, Wakube W, Steketee RW et al. Effect of blood transfusion on survival among children in a Kenyan hospital. Lancet.1992; 340: 524-528.

Looareesuwan S, Ho M, Wattanagoon Y, White NJ, Warrell DA, Bunnaq D et al. Dynamic alterations in splenic function during acute falciparum malaria. N Engl J Med 1997; 317: 678–681.

Luzzattto L. Genetic factors in malaria. Bull WHO 1974; 50: 195-202.

Maitland K, Pamba A, Newton CR, Levin M. Response to volume resuscitation in children with severe anaemia. Paedtr Crit Care Med 2003; 4: 426-431.

Mackowaik PA, Wasseman SS, Levine MM. A critical appraisal of 98.6F, the upper limit of the normal body temperature and other legacies of Carl Reinhold August Wunderlich. JAMA. 1992;268:1578-1580.

Marsh K. Immunology of malaria. In: Warell DA, Gilles HM(ed). Essential Malariology 4th Ed. London: Arnold Publications; 2002. pg 252 – 267.

Marsh K, Forster D, Waruiru C, Mwangi I, Wistanley M, Marsh V et al. Life threatening malaria in African children; clinical spectrum and simplified prognostic criteria. N Eng J Med 1995; 322: 1399-1404.

McDevitt MA, Xie J, Gordeuk V, Bucala R. The anaemia of malaria infection: role of inflammatory cytokines. Curr Haematol Rep 2004; 3: 97-106.

Menendez C, Kahigwa E, Hirt R, Vounatsou P, Aponte JJ, Font F et a. Randomised placebo-controlled trial of iron supplementation and malaria chemoprophylaxis for prevention of severe anaemia and malaria in Tanzanian infants. Lancet. 1997; 350: 844-850.

Mercereau-Puijalon O, Ménard D Plasmodium vivax and the Duffy antigen: a paradigm revisited Transfus Clin Biol. 2010 Sep;17(3):176-83. Epub 2010 Jul 23.

Meremikwu M, Smith HJ. Blood transfusion for treating malarial anaemia. In: The Cochrane Library, 2004; 3:1-76.

Miller SI, Hohmann EL, Pegues DA. Salmonella (including Salmonella typhi). In: Mandell GL, Bennett JE, Dolin R. (eds). Mandell, Douglas and Bennett's principles and practice of infectious diseases, 4th edn. New York, Churchill Livingstone,1995: 2013

Miller LH, Mason SJ, Clyde DF, McGinniss MH. Innate resistance in malaria. Exp Parasitol 1976; 40: 132-146.

Miller LH, Mason SJ, Clyde DF, McGinniss MH. The resistance factor to plasmodium vivax in blacks. The Duffy-blood-group genotype, Fy Fy. N Engl J Med 1976; 295: 302-304.

Mockenhaupt FP, Eghardt S, Buckhardt J, Bosomtwe SY, Laryea S, Anemana SD, et al. Manifestations and outcome of severe malaria in children in Northern Ghana: Am J Trop Med Hyg 2004; 71: 167-72.

Modiano D, Sirima BS, Sawadogo A, Sanou I,Pare J,Konate A et al. Severe malaria in Burkina Faso: urban and rural environment. Parasitologia 1999; 41: 251-254.

Mongensen CB, Soerensen J, Bjorkman A, Montgomery SM. Algorithm for the diagnosis of anaemia without laboratory facilities among small children in a malaria endemic of rural Tanzania. Acta Trop 2006; 99: 119-125.

Moroff G, Dend D. Characterization of biochemical changes occurring with storage of red cells; comparative studies with CPD and CPDA-1. Transfusion 1983; 23: 484-489.

Mulenga M, Malunga P, Bennett S, Thuma PE, Shulman C, Fielding K et al. Factors associated with severe anaemia in Zambian children admitted with Plasmodium falciparum malarial anaemia. Ann Trop Paediatr 2005; 25: 87-90.

Newton CR, Krishna S. Severe falciparum malaria in children. Current understanding of pathophysiology and supportive treatment. Pharmacol Ther 1998; 79: 1-53.

Newton CR, Marsh K, Peshu N, Mwayi I. Blood transfusion For severe anaemia in African children. Lancet 1992; 340: 917-918.

Newton CR, Warn PA, Winstanley PA, Peshu N, Snow RW, Pasvol G et al. Severe anaemia in children living in a malaria endemic area of Kenya. Trop Med Int Health. 1997; 2: 165-178.

Oduro AR, Koram KA, Rogers W, Atuguba F, Ansah P, Anyorigiya T et al. Severe falciparum malaria in young children of the Kassena-Nankana district of northern Ghana. Malar J. 2007; 6: 96-97.

Okiro EA, Al-Taiar A, Reyburn H, Idro R, Berkley JA, Snow RW. Age patterns of severe paediatric malaria and their relationship to plasmodium falciparum intensity. Malar J. 2009; 8: 4 -5.

Oppenheimer SJ. Iron and malaria. Parasitol Today 1989; 5:77–82.

Orimadegun AE, Fawole O, Okereke JO, Akinbami FO, Sodeinde. Increasing burden of childhood severe malaria in a Nigerian tertiary hospital: implication for control. J Trop Pediatr. 2007; 53: 185-189.WHO Malaria action programme; severe and complicated malaria. Trans R Soc Trop Med & Hyg 1986; 80:1-76.

Ouma C, Davenport GC, Awandare GA, Keller CC, Were T, Otieno MF et al. Polymorphic variability in the interleukin (IL)-1beta promoter conditions susceptibility to severe malaria anaemia and functional changes in IL-1 beta susceptibility. J Infect Dis. 2008;198:1219-1226.

Pamba A, Maitland K. Capillary refill: Prognostic value in Kenyan children. Arch Dis Child 2004; 89: 950-955.

Pasvol G. the interaction between sickle haemoglobin and the malaria parsite. Trans R Soc Trop Med Hyg 1980; 74:701-750.

Planche T, Onanga M, Schwnk A, Dzeing A, Borrman S, Faucher J et al. Assessment of volume depletion in children with malaria. Plos Med 2004; 1:18-20.

Premji Z, Hamisi Y, Shiff C, Minjas J, Lubega P, Makwaya C. Anaemia and Plasmodium falciparum infections among young children in an holoendemic area, Bagamoyo, Tanzania. Acta Trop. 1995; 59: 55-64.

Ranque S, Poudiougou B, Traoré A, Keita M, Oumar AA, Safeukui I et al. Life-threatening malaria in African children: a prospective study in a mesoendemic urban setting: Pediatr Infect Dis J. 2008; 27: 130-135.

Roberts DJ, Casals-Pascul C, Weatherall DJ The clinical and pathophysiological features of malarial anemia. Curr Trop Microbiol Immunol 2005; 295:137–167.

Ronald G. Strauss. Blood and blood component transfusion. In: Behrman RE, Kligman RM, Jenson HB(editors). Nelson textbook of paediatrics 18th Ed. Philadelphia: WB Saunders; 2000. pg 2055 – 2056.

Rowe JA, Handel IG, Thera MA, Deans AM, Lyke KE, Koné A et al. Blood group O protects against severe Plasmodium falciparum malaria through the mechanism of reduced resetting. Proc Natl Acad Sci U S A 2007; 104: 17471-17476

Salako LA, Ajayi FO, Sowunmi A, Walker O. Malaria in Nigeria: a revisit. Ann Trop Med Parasitol 1990; 84: 435-45.

Salako LA, Walker O, Sowunmi A, Omokhodion SJ, Adio R, Oduola AM. Artemether in moderately severe and cerebral malaria in Nigerian children. Trans R Soc Trop Med Hyg 1994; 88: 13-15.

Sandau KB, Zhou J, Kietzmann T, Brune B. Regulation of hypoxia-inducible factoralpha by the inflammatory mediators nitric oxide and tumor necrosis, factor alpha in contrast to desferroxamine and phenylarsine oxide. J Biol Chem 2001; 276: 39805–39811.

Satpathy SK, Mohanby N, Naida P, Samal G. Severe falciparum malaria. Indian J Pediatr 2004; 71: 133-5.

Schellenberg D, Menendez C, Kahigwa E, Font F, Galindo C, Acosta C. African Children with Malaria in Area of Intense Plasmodium Falciparum Transmission : Features on admission to the hospital and risk factors for death. Ann. J Trop Med Hyg 1999; 61: 431-438.

Severe falciparum malaria(WHO).communicable diseases cluster. Trans R Soc Trop Med Hyg 2004; 94:1-90.

Silamut K, White NJ. Relation of the stage of parasite development in the peripheral blood to prognosis in severe falciparum malaria. Trans Roy Soc Trop Med Hyg 1993; 87: 436-443.

Snow RW, Gilles HM. Sinden RE, Gilles HM. The malaria parasite, In: Warell DA, Gilles HM(ed). Essential Malariology 4th Ed. London: Arnold Publications; 2002. pg 85-106.

Sowunmi A, Adedeji AA, Fateye BA, Babalola CP. Plasmodium falciparum hyperparasitaemia in children. Risk factors, treatment outcomes, and gametocytaemia following treatment. Parasite 2004; 11: 317-323.

Stephen CR, Wirima JJ, Steketee RW. Transplacental transmission of p. falciparum in rural Malawi. Am J Trop Med Hyg 1996; 55: 57-60.

Stouti JA, Odindo AO, Owuor BO, Mibei EK, Opollo MO, Waitumbi JN et al. Loss of red blood cell compliment regulatory proteins and susceptibility to severe malarial anemia. J Infect Dis 2003; 187:522-525.

Taylor TE, Molyneux ME. Clinical features of malaria in children. In: Warell DA, Gilles HM(ed). Essential Malariology 4th Ed. London: Arnold Publications; 2002. pg 206-218.

Taylor TE, Willis BA, Courval JK, Molyneux ME. Intramuscular artemether vs intravenous quinine: an open randomized trial in Malawian children with cerebral malaria. Trop Med Int Health 1998; 3: 3-8.

Tuman KJ. Tissue oxygen delivery. The physiology of anaemia\a. Anaesthesiol Clin North Am 1990; 9: 451-469.

Turrini F, Giribaldi G, Carta F, Mannu F, Arese P. Mechanism of band-3 oxidation and clustering in the phagocytosis of Plasmodium falciparum-infected erythrocytes. Rodex Report 2003; 8: 300-303.

Usawattanakulb W, Tharavanij S, Warrell DA, Looareesuwan S, White NJ, Supvej S et al. Factors contributing to the development of cerebral malaria II Endotoxin. Clin Exp Immun 1985; 61:562-568.

Viroj Wiwanitkit. Malarial parasite infection and increase of erythrocyte sedimentation rate. Irn J Med Hypotheses Ideas 2008; 2: 20-23.

Warell DA, Turner GDH, Francis N. Pathology and pathophysiology of human malaria. In: Warell DA, Gilles HM(ed). Essential Malariology 4th Ed. London: Arnold Publications; 2002. pg 236-251.

Weatherall DJ, Miller LH, Barruch DI, Marsh K, Doumbo OK, Casals-Pasual C et al. Malaria and red cell. In "Hematology: ASH education programme book" 2002; 35:1-25.

Wickramasinghe SN, Abdalla SH. Blood and bone marrow changes in malaria. Clin Haematol 2000; 13:277-299.

William F. G.. Cardiovascular regulatory mechanisms. In: Review of medical physiology. 18th ed. Norwalk: Appleton and Lange; 1997. pg 553-566.

William F. G. Endocrine functions of the kidney, heart and pineal gland. . In: Review of medical physiology. 18th ed. Norwalk: Appleton and Lange; 1997. pg 425-434.

World Health Organization. Antimalarial Drug Combination Therapy. Report of a WHO Technical Consultation(document WHO 2002).

WHO Library. WHO guidelines for treatment of malaria. 2006.

WHO Report. Clinical, Behavioral and Socioeconomic factors related to severe malaria. A multicenter study in African Region. 2002.

World Health Organization. Severe falciparum malaria. Trans Roy Soc Trop Med Hyg 2004; 94 : 1-90.

Xie YW, Wolin MS. Role of nitric oxide and its interaction with superoxide in the suppression of cardiac muscle mitochondrial respiration. Involvement in response to hypoxia/ reoxygenation. Circulation 1996; 94: 2580–2586.

3

The Effect of Retinol Supplement on Blood Cytokine Concentrations in Children with Non-Severe Malaria Vivax

Viviana Taylor, Rosa Uscátegui, Adriana Correa,
Amanda Maestre and Jaime Carmona
*Universidad de Antioquia/Grupo de Investigación en
Alimentación and Nutrición Humana and Grupo Salud y comunidad*
Colombia

1. Introduction

Malaria, malnutrition, low concentrations of retinol and intestinal parasitism coexist among the habitants of tropical regions of the world (Nacher, 2002). The Turbo municipality is one of the highly endemic malaria regions of Colombia. During 2006, 5.674 cases of malaria were reported in Turbo, corresponding to annual parasite index >10 (number of malaria cases per 1,000 persons per year). From these, 85% were caused by *Plasmodium vivax* (Eventos de interes en salud Pública, 2006). Also, the Urabá region, where Turbo is a major urban area, is one of the regions of Colombia with more cases of malnutrition in children under 15 years; 53.3% of children under 10 years presented chronic malnutrition risk (T/E<-1Unit Z) and 14.9% acute malnutrition (P/T<-1Unit Z), whereas 33.8% of the adolescents had weight deficit according to the Body Mass Index (Alvarez et al., 2005). Furthermore, 85% of children aged 4 to 10 years with malaria had intestinal parasitism (Carmona et al., 2009).

Previous studies in Colombian children with malaria reported low retinol values during the acute phase, which recovered to normal values > 0.7 mmol/l (20 µg/dL) (WHO, 2009) once malaria receded. Within the children with malaria, 85% had anemia, and their haemoglobin values increased after one month of antimalarial treatment, although anemia persisted in 51% of them (Uscátegui & Correa, 2007).

During malaria, TH1 cytokines like interferon gamma (IFN - γ) and tumor necrosis factor alpha (TNF-α), are required to control the primary parasitemia. Nevertheless antinflammatory cytokines or TH2 cytokines, such as interleukin 10 (IL-10) and transforming growth factor beta (TGF-β), that modulate the proinflammatory effect, must be present along with those of the TH1 type, in order to prevent emergence of immune pathology (Schofield et al., 2005). Some in vitro studies revealed that retinol had an effect on the TH1/TH2 balance, as evidenced by reduction of IFN -γ and TNF -α secretion by TH1 cells or by promoting TH2 cells growth and differentiation to produce larger quantities of the IL-10 (Cantorna et al., 1994; Iwata et al., 2003). Vitamin A deficiency has been associated with an increase in TH1 response, intestinal parasitism and malnutrition (Jason et al., 2002; Azevedo et al., 2005). Furthermore, the prevalence of TH1 cytokines in children with malaria has been associated with severe anemia (Kurtzhals et al., 1999).

1.1 Anemia and relationship with cytokines TH1 and TH2, in patients with malaria

Ferritin deficiency is defined basically as the reduction of iron in the body and its diagnosis when not associated with anemia is based on quantification of serum ferritin. However, determinations of serum levels of this protein, which are performed systematically to determine the iron status, ferritin acts as a positive acute phase reactant in the presence of inflammatory/infectious disease clinics and subclinics (Aleo et al., 2004) as happens during malaria.

This explains why this protein is not useful tool for evaluating iron stores, and in contrast, constitutes a good indicator of inflammatory status along with the C reactive protein (CRP). CRP is produced by the liver, is also known as a positive acute phase reactant during malaria and main function is to join the organism, acting as an opsonin, with activation of the classical complement pathway, which is responsible for recruitment of inflammatory cells, opsonization and dead direct of the pathogen (Marsh & Kinyanjui, 2006).

Unlike ferritin, hemoglobin is not considered a reactant acute phase and the low concentrations of blood, result in anemia, which is a public health problem in many regions around the world with a high prevalence in economically dependent countries, especially among children and resulting from the interaction between biological, nutritional and cultural factors (Blair et al., 1999). The Anemia is a common complication of malaria and the mechanisms originally involved have not yet been fully defined. The cause is multifactorial and includes aspects related to the increase destruction of parasitized and non-parasitized cells and other factors causing a decreased production of erythrocytes, by alteration in the maturation of erythroid precursors or lack on response of bone marrow to erythropoietin (EPO). Additionally, there are others conditioning agents of anemia related with the characteristics of the parasite and host as resistance to *Plasmodium* or some disease in the host as well as thalassemia or sickle cell anemia, which enhances the severity of anemia, as well as deficiencies of iron and other micronutrients (Llanos et al., 2004).

In adults living in Kenya with acute malaria by *P. falciparum* found that TNF-α, interleukin 1 (IL-1) and IL-6, cytokines produced by monocytes, suppresses the synthesis of erythropoietin (Vedovato et al., 1999). Similar results were seen in children in Ghana (Kurtzhals et al., 1999). In Uganda, children 1 to 10 years who had acute uncomplicated malaria by *P. falciparum*, the authors found that age, high concentrations of erythropoietin, low concentrations of α-1 glycoprotein, and IL-10/TNF-α high proportion were associated with significantly increased hemoglobin concentrations. These data indicate that children younger with malaria do not maintain the production of IL-10 in response to inflammatory process, a mechanism that may contribute to the severity of the anemia (Nussenblatt et al., 2001). A study in Kenya in children with malaria revealed that the TNF-α and IL-10 were significantly higher in those subjects with high parasitemia and anemia, compared with control group, the same age and sex, but without malaria (Othoro et al., 1999). In children Colombians living in El Bagre (Colombia), aged from 4 to 9 years old who had acute uncomplicated malaria, 67% *P. vivax*, 29% *P. falciparum* and 4% mixed infection was found average of IL-10 of 266.18 ± 47.9 pg/ml, highly significant and higher than in children with the same age, but not malaria, which was 8.52 ± 1.17 pg/ml (P <0,001); the values of IL-10 in children with malaria correlated with parasitaemia and body temperature. Conversely, TNF-α was only detected in 12% of study subjects, no significant differences between average children malaria and those without the disease. In children with moderate or high parasitemia but not anemia, the proportion was IL-10/TNF-α significantly higher compared with those who did have anemia, indicating that high values of this proportion can prevent development of anemia with control of excessive inflammatory activity TNF-α (Grencis et al., 1996). The evidence presented shows that high values in the proportion of TH2/TH1 cytokines (IL-10/TNF-α) protect to development severe anemia malaria in children (17). It is proposed that the pathways by which IL-10 exerts its beneficial effects on malaria could be: 1) activating cytotoxic T lymphocytes, with the elimination of cells infected, 2) stimulating the production of antibodies directed against the parasite and 3) inhibiting or blocking the production of cytokines proinflammatory response characteristics TH1 (Blair et al., 1999). According to the studies presented is clear that, in children with acute malaria, the severity of the anemia is determined by the balance in the production of proinflammatory cytokines such as anti-and IL-10 and TNF-α respectively, which therefore are related to the change in hematological and contribute or not to increase hemoglobin and erythropoietin. Although there is no information linking the paper simultaneously TH1/TH2 response modulator by supplements of vitamin A, with hematological values in children with malaria, there may be this interrelationship, it is clear that supplementation with vitamin A improve hemoglobin levels and erythropoietin and favor mobilization of iron deposits, and also is known its immunomodulatory role, as evidenced by the reduction of proinflammatory cytokines, which are also associated with the severity of anemia, and present during acute malaria. For this reason, further research is required to clarify the relationship between the simultaneous retinol, the immune response and iron metabolism in the population children with acute malaria, especially that produced by *P. vivax* that is more prevalent in Colombia.

2. Materials and methods

2.1 Study type and sample

A Pilot study balanced, nonblind, with random allocation of the "exposure factor" (retinol supplement) was carried out. Two groups, each of 25 children with nonsevere *P. vivax* malaria were compared according to WHO criteria (Lopez & Schmunis, 1998) and matched according the sex, age and place of residence. One of the group received retinol supplements (200.000 U.I. retinol palmitate, Retiblan®, Procaps laboratories, Colombia), for one year every 3 months, the final dose was administered between one week and six months before the *P. vivax* episode. Te other group did not receive supplement. The "final effect" in each child was the cytokines levels, and nutritional, biochemical and inflammatory indicators.

This project was approved by the committee of ethics of the Centro de Investigaciones Médicas de la Facultad de Medicina, Universidad de Antioquia. A written informed consent was obtained from each patient. The resolution N° 008430 of 1993 of the Ministerio de Salud de Colombia was considered.

2.2 Inclusion criteria

It required the following requirements: a) Reside on a regular basis in El Tres, Antioquia, Colombia b) Have not chronic (diabetes) or infectious disease (such as tuberculosis or leprosy) at the time of admission, c) Be free from trauma, accident or poisoning, known and judged as serious by the medical examination; d) A number of 25 children must have participated in research in which they received supplementation with retinol and 25 should not have received such a supplement; e) Have uncomplicated malaria by *P. vivax*; f) Agreeing to participate in the study by signing for his guardian, written informed consent.

2.3 Exclusion criteria
Participants were excluded if: a) Occurre done of those events in subparagraphs b) and c) inclusion criteria; b) Withdrawal of informed consent or for any reason of the study.

2.4 Diagnosis and treatment of malaria
The parasitological diagnosis of malaria was carried out as recommended by PAHO/WHO (López & Schmunis, 1988) with respect to sampling, processing and reading it. Antimalarial treatment was carried out orally, according to the schemes of the Ministry of Health of Colombia and the Regional Health Direction of Antioquia (drug and dose by age), the drugs are accompanied with water and food as well:
a. Chloroquine: total dose of 25 mg/kg body weight, which is split into three days: day 1 was given 10 mg/kg, days 2 and 3 are supplied 7.5 mg/kg in each.
b. Primaquine at 0.25 mg/kg/day for 14 days, given from day 4 (after completion of chloroquine).

The treatments were obtained in the DSSA-Ministry of Health and were delivered as monitored by the researchers observing the patient during the first half hour, in case of vomiting; the full dose was repeated, with new supervision for 30 minutes. If the patient vomited again, it was excluded from the study and transferred to the municipal hospital.

2.5 Anthropometric evaluation
Weight was measured on the children in an standing position, few clothing and without shoes; with an electronic scale of 100 kg capacity and 0.01 kg sensitivity. Height was measured with a flexible estadiometer fixed on the wall, of 2 m capacity and 1 mm sensitivity. Each measurement was evaluated and registered. The mean reading was recorded. The age was calculated as the difference between date of birth and date of evaluation. The height for age index (T/E) was constructed and those who had values <-1 of Z unit were classified as with chronic malnutrition risk and those with equal or greater values to -1 of Z unit as without risk. The population of the National Center of Statistics of Health of the United States (NCHS) was used as reference as accepted by the WHO for international comparisons (WHO, 1995).

Since reference values for weight and height are not available for men higher than 145 cm and children higher than 137 cm, it was not possible to evaluate acute malnutrition with the indicator P/T, hence Body Mass Index (BMI, weight / height ^{2}) was used, which is accepted by the WHO for evaluation of children up to 15 years, using as reference values the proposed by the same organization. Those children below percentile 15 (p<15) were classified as low weight.

2.6 Laboratory examinations
The procedure followed for each of the laboratory tests was as follows:

2.6.1Testing for malaria
The parasitological diagnosis of malaria to detect the presence of *Plasmodium* parasites by thick film was confirmed in the extended, in the manner provided by the OMS (López & Schmunis, 1988). The spread thin and thick were stained with Field and Giemsa, respectively. The thick smear was observed with 100X magnification and the search for parasites was done in 200 consecutive microscopic fields. The parasitemia was calculated based on 200 leukocytes and a

standard of 8,000 cells /mL and expressed in rings/µL. A thick smear was diagnosed as negative when there was no asexually in 200 microscopic fields.

2.6.2 Stool

The stool test was conducted on one single sample, once the patient was admitted to the study.

We established the presence of helminths, the eggs were quantified and trophozoites and cysts of protozoa were identified. To do this we proceeded as follows: 3 g of feces was added formaldehyde 10% to cover the sample, which was stored in 4-7days, as was reviewed, consisting of "direct examination "and, if the parasites were not passed to "concentration examination". Treatment with 10% formalin well preserved helminths eggs and protozoan cysts. Direct stool examination with saline-iodine and examination by formalin-ether concentration as Ritchie were made according to the usual procedure only when the second evaluation was negative as declared such to the sample (Botero & Restrepo, 2003). Stool analysis was performed by professional staff of the Laboratory of Intestinal Parasites of the Faculty of Medicine of the University of Antioquia.

2.6.3 Determination of biochemical parameters

2.6.3.1 C-reactive protein

Serum was measured by a kit BioSystems (CRP) Latex. C-reactive protein serum causes agglutination of latex particles coated with anti-human C-reactive protein. The agglutination of latex particles is proportional to the concentration of CRP and can be measured by turbidimetry (Rice et al., 1987). Inflammation was considered when the concentration of CRP was 8 mg/L or higher, recommended by the Clinical Laboratory of the IPS at the University of Antioquia, where they processed these samples.

2.6.3.2 Ferritin

The ferritin was measured in serum with Abbott AxSYM kit ® Sistem (reference 7A58-20B7A583 56-4324/R12, Abbott Laboratories, USA). The AxSYM Ferritin assay was based on microparticle enzyme immunoassay technology (MEIA). The determinations were made in Clinical Laboratory of the IPS at the University of Antioquia.

2.6.3.3 Plasma retinol

Chemical analysis was done by affinity high performance liquid chromatography (HPLC) (Talwar et al., 1998), with a team scores Waters, using a manual injection system Reodyne 77251, a solvent delivery system 660E, a UV-VIS detector 400 and a spine C-18 Simetry, using the Millennium software for management. 0.5 mL of plasma were measured and denatured with 0.5 mL of absolute ethanol with BHT (1.0 g/L) as antioxidant and 0.5 mg/mL of ethyl-β-apo-8-carotenoato and 0.5 mg/mL retinol acetate as internal standards. The mixture was extracted five times with 5 mL of hexane.

The separated hexane was evaporated with N2 and the residue was reconstituted with 200 mL of methanol, an aliquot of 50 mL was injected into the HPLC system, the mobile phase used was methanol, acetonitrile in a proportion 70: 30. There were three chromatograms for each sample to evaluate. It was considered subclinical deficiency of vitamin A, when plasma levels were <20µg/dL. Measurements were made at the Laboratory of the National Institute of Health in Bogotá.

2.6.4 Hemoleucogram (cyanmethaemoglobin (g/dL) and Leucogram)

Hemoleucogram became type III-V in automated equipment in the clinical laboratory of hospital Francisco Valderrama of Turbo, Antioquia, Colombia, when it was not possible, was performed manually. The method used was that of the cyanmethaemoglobin recommended by WHO. The reference values for classifying anemia were those recommended by WHO as the concentration of hemoglobin (Hb) as follows: for children 2-4 years <11.0g/dL and the 5 years and older <12 g/dL (WHO, 2001).

Hemoglobin values were not corrected for altitude because Turbo is located less than 200 meters above sea level.

2.6.5 Determination of serum cytokines

The cytokines IFNγ, TNFα, IL-10 and TGF-β1 were determined by sandwich ELISA using the Duo Set kit developed by ELISA (R&D systems), the basis and procedure are described below:

2.6.5.1 Fundament

This assay used an ELISA (Enzyme Linked Immuno sorbent Assay) quantitative sandwich, which was based on the detection of cytokines that bind to an immobilized antibody (capture antibody) on a solid phase antibody which directly or indirectly produced a reaction whose product could be measured by spectrophotometry.

2.6.5.2 Reagents and samples required

Were used: a) Polystyrene microplates with 96 wells previously sensitized or attached to a polyclonal antibody capture (From mouse)-specific cytokine (IL-10, IFN-γ, TNF-α and TGF-β1). b) Standard, 1 vial of lyophilized cytokine (IL-10, IFN-γ, TNF-α and TGF-β1) recombinant in a buffered protein base. c) Sample from human serum (approximately alliquotes of 600 mL) and stored in liquid nitrogen or at -70° C. d) 21 mL of concentrated buffer solution mixed with condoms (wash buffer solution). e) Conjugate is 21 mL of polyclonal antibody specific for each cytokine detection coupled with horseradish peroxidase with preservatives. f) Substrate solution de12.5 made mL stabilized hydrogen peroxide (reagent color A) and 12.5 mL of stabilized chromogen (color reagent B). g) 6 mL of 2 N sulfuric acid (stop solution) h) Diluent of standard and diluents of sample RD1-51.

2.6.5.3 Procedure

In the commercial kits used in this procedure microplates were previously coated with a capture antibody polyclonal-specific cytokine (IL-10, IFN-γ, TNF-α and TGF-β1). The standards and samples were added to the wells contained each plate (96 wells per plate) in the amount stated and corresponding cytokine (contained in the standard and samples) are joined to the capture antibody. After the corresponding washes to remove nonspecific binding, was added the respective conjugate (polyclonal antibody specific for each cytokine, together with an enzyme). Subsequently was it washed to remove nonspecific binding to conjugate. Substrate solution was added to the plates, and development color (corresponding to the product) was proportional to the amount of cytokine bound in the initial step of the procedure. After time estimated to measure the color reaction, the development of this stopped with stop solution and the color intensity was measured by a spectrophotometer at the wavelength indicated.

2.7 Statistical analysis

For variables exhibiting a normal distribution, the mean values between the groups were compared using the T test for matched groups. For variables lacking a normal distribution, median values were compared using the Mann Whitney test. To explore intragroup relations was applied spearman correlation coefficient. The comparison between the groups of the categorical variables was made using Chi square. The programs Prism, Epi info version 6.4D and SPSS version 15.0 were used and unilateral values of $P<0.05$ were set up as significative.

3. Results

In total 17 boys and 8 girls in each treatment group were included, they were aged 2.8 -15.7 years old in the supplemented group, and 3.2 - 15.7 years old in the non-supplemented group. The weight, height and parasitemia values were similar in both groups (Table 1).

Variable	Group with retinol	Group without retinol	p
Weight in kg (X±SD)	28±10	30±13	0.621[a]
Height in cm (X±SD)	127±20	131±20	0.567[a]
Parasitemia (P/µl)	5557±4350	5830±3901	0.574[a]
With chronic under nutrition risk (T/E) (yes/no)	17/8	15/10	0.384[b]
Low weight for BMI (yes/no)	6/19	4/21	0.363[b]
Coprologic positive (yes/no)	19/4	20/4	0.625[b]
Helminths (yes/no)	10/13	17/7	0.054[b]
Protozoa (yes/no)	17/6	17/7	0.536[b]

X= average, SD= Standard deviation, P/µl= parasites/microlitre, T/E= indicator height for age,
BMI= Body Mass Index
a U de Mann-Whitney test p<0.05.
b Chi square p<0.05.

Table 1. Characteristics of the children according to treatment group.

All children were tested for parasitaemia, ferritin, retinol and C reactive protein, 40 of them were tested for cytokines and 47 for haemoglobin and stool tests.

The risk of chronic malnutrition (T/E) in the group with retinol supplement was 68% in contrast to 60% in the non-supplemented group. Prevalence of low weight (IMC) was 24% in the supplemented children versus 16% in the non-supplemented.

Prevalence of intestinal parasites in children was high in both groups; overall 83% of the children had a positive stool test. The group supplemented with retinol exhibited infection in 74% and 43% with protozoa and helminths, respectively; while 71% of the non-supplemented group had protozoa and helminths (Table 1). There was no significant diference in the presence of intestinal parasitism among the groups. With exception of the haemoglobin and retinol, the remaining variables did not exhibit a normal distribution. The cytokines, C reactive protein, ferritin, haemoglobin and retinol, were similar among the groups and only the C reactive protein and haemoglobin values showed significance with the lower concentrations. The TNF- α median values were zero in the non-supplemented group, which means that at least in 50% of the children, this cytokine was not detected (Table 2). For IL-10, the highest concentration for both groups was 677pg/ml, and only 25% of the children from the group supplemented with retinol and 15% of the children from the non-supplemented group reached that value. With the technique used, no TGF-β1 values were detected in any sample tested.

The frequency of inflammation, anemia and subclinic deficiency of vitamin A was similar in both groups (Table 3).

Variable	With retinol			Without retinol			p
	n	X±SD	Median	n	X±SD	Median	
IL-10 (pg/ml)	20	275±283	112	20	233±253	125	0.989
TNF-α (pg/ml)	20	32.2±66.3	5.5	20	16.2±49.2	0.0	0.162
IFN-γ (pg/ml)	20	49.1±60.2	29.3	20	68.5±80.3	31.1	0.473
C reactive protein (mg/l)	25	29±25	24	25	48±39	36	0.070
Haemoglobin (g/dl)	23	10.5±1.5	10.3	24	11.2±1.8	11.1	0.054
Ferritin (µg/l)	25	143±191	105	25	154±108	113	0.160
Retinol (mmol/l)	25	0.59±0.06	0.57	25	0.61±0.08	0.59	0.786

IL-10=interleukyne 10, TNF-α=tumor necrosis factor alpha, IFN-γ=interferon gamma, SD= Standard desviation.
U de Mann-Whitney test, except haemoglobin and retinol that one became for T pared test p<0.05.

Table 2. Comparison of the concentrations of cytokines and nutritional biochemical indicators in children according to treatment group.

Category	With retinol	Without retinol	p
Inflamation (yes/no)	21/4	23/2	0,334
Anemia (yes/no)	22/1	19/5	0,104
Subclinic deficiency of vitamin A	23/2	23/2	1

Inflamation = PCR values ≥ 8 mg/L, Subclinic deficiency of vitamin A = retinol values<20 µg/dL, anemia= haemoglobin in children 2-4 years old <11 g/dL and in children ≥ 5 years old<12 g/dL Chi square p<0.05.

Table 3. Comparison frecuency of Inflamation, anemia and subclinic deficiency of vitamin A according to treatment group

3.1 Stratification by nutritional state and presence of intestinal parasitism

Because intestinal parasitosis and malnutrition affect the variables of our interest, results were analyzed according to: 1) absence of malnutrition risk and parasites, 2) at malnutrition risk and without parasites, 3) absence of malnutrition risk and presence of parasites and 4) malnutrition risk and presence of parasites. From these groups, only the group 4 was adequate for statistical analysis and this included, 13 children in the retinol supplemented group and 14 in the group without retinol supplement.

Subjects with T/E <-1 Unit Z o BMI p < 15 were classified as chronic malnutrition risk or with low weight. Since all children who had chronic malnutrition risk simultaneously presented low weight, the number of children with chronic malnutrition risk or low weight, was identical to that of children with chronic malnutrition risk.

In these children, the concentrations of TNF-α, IFN-γ and IL-10 were similar between both groups. Nevertheless, the group that received retinol exhibited a tendency to have lower values of ferritin and C reactive protein (p=0.058 vs 0.089) (Table 4). The parasite blood count was 6.111±3.801 P/µl in the group receiving retinol versus 7.160±4.046 P/µl in the other (p= 0.332).

Variable	With retinol			Without retinol			p
	n	X±SD	Median	n	X± SD	Median	
IL-10 (pg/ml)	13	283±289	112	8	186±219	119	0.827
TNF-α (pg/ml)	13	43.7±82.7	0.0	8	31.9±74.3	0.5	0.876
IFN-γ (pg/ml)	13	34.5±25.1	24.5	8	85.4±79.7	45.0	0.218
C reactive protein (mg/l)	14	30±25	25	13	47±31	38	0.089
Haemoglobin (g/dl)	12	10.5±1.1	10.7	13	11.6±2.2	11.5	0.120
Ferritin (µg/l)	14	117±72	110	13	184±127	145	0.058
Retinol (mmol/l)	14	0.59±0.07	0.56	13	0.61±0.09	0.59	0.698

X= average, SD= Standard desviation, IL-10=interleukyne 10, TNF-α= tumoral necrosis factor alpha, IFN-γ =interferon gamma.
U de Mann-Whitney test p<0.05.

Table 4. Nutritional comparison of the concentrations of cytokines and biochemical indicators in the stratum of children with chronic malnutrition risk and parasites, according to treatment group.

Among children with chronic malnutrition risk and presence of parasites, no differences were observed when the proportions of inflammation, anemia and subclinical deficiency of retinol were compared, regardless of the group (Table 5). Inflammation was detected in 13 out of 14 children from the group administered retinol versus 13 out of 13 children from the group without retinol. Anemia was detected in 11 out of 12 children from the group that receiving retinol and in 9 out of 13 children from the group without retinol. Finally, 12 out of

14 children supplemented with retinol had subclinical deficiency of retinol, while this was evident in 12 out of 13 from the group without retinol.

Category	With retinol	Without retinol	p
Inflamation (yes/no)	13/1	13/0	0,519
Anemia (yes/no)	11/1	9/4	0,186
Subclinic deficiency of vitamin A	12/2	12/1	0,529

Inflamation = values of PCR ≥ 8 mg/L, Subclinic deficiency of vitamin A = values of retinol <20 μg/dL, anemia= haemoglobin in children of 4 years old <11,0 g/dL and children of 5-10 years old <12 g/dL U Mann-Whitney test, except for hemoglobin and retinol was made by paired t test, p<0.05.

Table 5. Comparison of intensity of inflammation, anemia and deficiency subclinical vitamin A, in the stratum of chronically malnourished children parasites, according to treatment group.

The immunological and biochemical variables studied, which showed correlation among themselves and with parasitemia in one of the two groups of treatment are shown in Table 6. In the group with retinol it is noted that as the parasitemia increased the values of IL-10 and TNF-α were also increased and this was not observed in children of group without retinol. Similarly, in the group receiving retinol, when ferritin increased so did CRP, IL-10, TNF-α and IFN-γ, variables with ferritin which showed positive correlation behavior was not observed in the group without retinol, in which only one ferritin correlated with parasitemia.

The variables that are similarly associated in both groups were IL-10 and TNF-α, which correlated positively with each other and moreover, were those that showed the highest ratios of all the correlations shown in Table 7, with a Rho = 0.786 in group with retinol and 0.751, which received no retinol. This indicated that as it raised one of the two variables, so did the other with the same strength, regardless of having received or not retinol. This same behavior was observed in the supplemented group, between IL-10 and IFN-γ. In the group without supplement there was no correlation of hemoglobin with IFN-γ, which, though unexpected, was one of the highest in this group (Rho = 0.738) (Table 6).

4. Discussion and conclusion

This pilot study answered the need to obtain primary data on the effect of retinol supplements of, on blood concentrations of IL-10, TNF-α, IFN-γ, TGF-β1, C reactive protein, haemoglobin and ferritin, in Colombian children with vivax malaria; as well as the relationships between these variables; aspects rarely addressed .

The prevalence of chronic malnutrition risk (T/E <-1 unit Z) was high (64%), in children with malaria from 6 to 10 years of the same municipality (58.2%) (Uscátegui & Correa, 2007). Similarly, the proportion of children with low weight according to BMI (20%) was higher than in other studies of the region (Alvarez et al., 2005). A common finding within malaria endemic areas is the presence of intestinal parasitism (Nacher, 2002); 83% of our children had a positive stool test, 57.4% with helminths and 73.3% with protozoa, which is similar to previous reports in malaria infected children from the same region (Turbo) (Uscátegui et al., 2008).

Pairs of variables	Measures (1)	With retinol	Without retinol
Parasitemia (P/µL) -IL-10 (pg/mL)	r	0,574	0,643
	p	0,040	0,086
Parasitemia (P/µL)-TNF-α (pg/mL)	r	0,693	0,621
	p	0,009	0,100
Parasitemia (P/µL)-Ferritin (µg/L)	r	0, 330	0,731
	p	0, 108	0,005
Haemoglobin (g/dL)-IFN- γ (pg/mL)	r	-0, 013	0,738
	p	0,954	0,037
Ferritin (µg/L)- CRP (mg/L)	r	0,574	0,330
	p	0,032	0,271
Ferritin (µg/L)-IL-10 (pg/mL)	r	0,696	0,381
	p	0,008	0,108
Ferritin (µg/L)-TNF- α (pg/mL)	r	0,575	0,436
	p	0,006	0,062
Ferritin (µg/L)-IFN- γ (pg/mL)	r	0,580	0,219
	p	0,006	0,367
IL-10 (pg/mL)-TNF- α (pg/mL)	r	0,751	0,786
	p	0,003	0,021
IL-10 (pg/mL)-IFN-γ (pg/mL)	r	0,569	0,068
	p	0,042	0,782

(1) r: Rho spearman coefficient, p probability associated with "r".

It is clear that in our study, the small size sample and the great variability in the data are explained partly because we did not found differences between the groups. In our children the age range was wide, 2-16 years. The age might have contributed to variations in the studied parameters. It is known that when children under 5 years are in contact with a pathogen, they produce a very pronounced TH1 cytokine response but as age increases, they shift towards a TH2 response, as a result of the maturation of the immune system (Kovaiou & Grubeck- Loebenstein, 2006).

In spite of the limited scope of our results, we reached some interesting findings. In the supplemented group, C reactive protein values were lower than in the group not supplemented, this was confirmed in children with chronic malnutrition risk and parasitism. In the later group, lower values of ferritin in the group with retinol (117±72 µg/l) versus the group without retinol were also observed (184±127µg/l). Since C reactive protein and ferritin are acute phase reactants increasing during infections (Gruys et al., 2005), our findings suggest that children that received retinol had less intensity on inflammation, which could be of clinical importance, since a exaggerated inflammatory response during malaria, has been associated with development of complications and death (Riley et al., 2006).

Nevertheless, that tendency to present lower intensity of inflammation associated with the retinol supplement was not reflected in the concentrations of cytokines. We expected that in the group with retinol, concentrations of IL-10 would be higher and TNF-α lower, as it has been found *in vitro* murine models of chronic inflammatory processes (Xu & Drew, 2006), but this effect was not seen in our children, which emphasizes the need to be cautious when extrapolating the results of studies from animal models to humans. In addition, it is important to consider that the dose of retinol supplemented to the cultures did not correlate to blood concentrations reached in humans, even after vitamin A administration (Hamzah et al., 2004).

Although no differences were detected in the concentrations of IL-10 neither among the groups with/without retinol in the children of the study, or in the children with chronic under nutrition risk and parasitism, the values of this cytokine were high; 25% of the children with retinol and 15% without retinol, had values exceeding the maximum limit of detection of the kit (677 pg/ml), concentrations very higher than those found in Turkish subjects with *P. vivax* malaria (Yildiz et al., 2006) . These findings led us to think that our subjects had more ability to modulate the immune response, protecting themselves from later complications, since IL-10 is considered very important in the process of malarial immunopathogenesis due to its anti-inflammatory role, and high serum concentrations of this cytokine have been associated with better prognosis of the disease (Shofield et al., 2005).

Haemoglobin concentrations were lower in the group with retinol in comparison to the group without retinol, when the analysis was unstratified. An increase in the destruction of infected red blood cells, which also increases the anemia might be associated to this result as other authors showed that the main receptor that mediates the phagocytosis of the infected erythrocyte by macrophages is CD36 and that the 9-cis-retinoic acid derived from retinol, stimulated the expression of CD36 and increased phagocytosis of erythrocytes infected with *P. falciparum* (Serghides & Kain, 2001).

Nor was there any difference in the prevalence of deficiency subclinical vitamin A, or retinol values between groups. However, we must take into account that concentrations retinol below 20 mg / dL in most children in this study have not really mean deficiency of vitamin A, due to the retinol binding protein is a reactant negative acute phase (Rosales et al., 2000), which decreases their concentrations during malaria and other infections (Ahmed et al., 1993; Rosales et al., 2000).

As for the correlations seen during the malaria episode, in children with and without retinol in the stratified group, most of these corresponded to what was expected. Correlations between parasitemia, CRP, ferritin, proinflammatory cytokines such as TNF-α and IFN-γ and anti-inflammatory such as IL-10, are adjusted as described during the inflammatory process that causes the early phase *Plasmodium* infection as a strategy to control initial parasitemia, limiting the spread of the parasite, with the subsequent removal of circulating forms (Ansar et al., 2006; Torre et al., 2002; Marsh & Kinyanjui, 2006). Additionally, these results allow us to verify has been seen in other previous studies, including: 1) the important role that TNF-α against asexual stages of *Plasmodium* erythrocytic phase early malaria, with a key role in the immune response protective cell, limiting the rate and contributing to death of *Plasmodium* (Maestre et al, 2002), 2) the behavior of ferritin as acute phase protein positive for malaria, which increases their concentrations in the presence of inflammatory/infectious subclinics clinics and, therefore in this research, and similar to observed in other study (Beard et al., 2006) this protein is not considered an adequate indicator of iron stores during the acute phase infection, and 3) regulation that makes the IL-10 on proinflammatory cytokines, increasing their concentrations simultaneously in to maintain the TH1/TH2 balance, which as mentioned before, important to avoid all the complications associated with immunopathogenesis in malaria (Moormann et al., 2006).

However, an unexpected finding in children in the present study, was the positive correlation between IFN-γ hemoglobin, result which contrasts with other studies that found no association between anemia and iron deficiency in malaria, with high IFN-γ, IL-6, TNF-α and IL-1 (Jason et al., 2002; Kanjaksha et al., 2007; Feelders et al., 1998) situation, although can not be explained, is an interesting finding for further studies.

The undetectable concentrations of TGF-β1 that were found in all subjects might be due to the use of different among the studies (Esmai et al., 2003).

This study is the first one exploring the effect of a supplement of retinol on some immunological parameters in children with *P. vivax* malaria and simultaneous infection with intestinal parasites and at chronic malnutrition risk. Although the results are limited by the small number of the sample and the variability in the data, studies of this type with higher number of subjects and narrower ranges of age, are worthwhile performing to clarify the effect of this supplement on malaria infection. We concluded that: 1) The tendency to have higher values of C reactive protein in the group without retinol and of ferritin in children with chronic malnutrition risk and parasitism of the group without supplement, suggests a possible anti-inflammatory effect of retinol during the acute phase of malaria and 2) A tendency to present lower concentrations of haemoglobin in children of the group that received retinol supplement and 3) The observed positive correlation between IFN-γ and hemoglobin, was a completely unexpected result. These findings could contribute to clarify the issue about the effect of supplemental retinol in children with malaria and relevance of supplementation population, as part of the strategy aimed to control malaria.

5. Acknowledgments

To Colombian Institute for the Development of Science and Technology (COLCIENCIAS Cod. 1115-04-16388 Contract 339-2004), Committee for Development of Research of Universidad de Antioquia (CODI), Sectional Direction of Health of Antioquia (DSSA) and Sustainability Strategy 2009-2010 of the Vicerrectory for Research of Universidad de Antioquia, Colombia, by the financial support of the project and publication of manuscript. To the epidemiologist Alejandro Estrada for data analysis.

6. References

Aleo, E.; Gil, C., González, F.; Martínez, A. & Valverde, F. (2004). Serum transferring receptor in healthy children: Diagnostic yield in ferropenic and infectious anemia. *An Pediatr*. Vol 60, No. 5, pp. 428-35.

Álvarez, M.; Benjumea, M.; Roldán, P.; Maya, M. & Montoya, E. (2005). Perfil alimentario y nutricional de los hogares de la región del Urabá antioqueño. Medellín: Gobernación de Antioquia, Dirección Seccional de Salud, Programa de mejoramiento alimentario y nutricional de Antioquia, Universidad de Antioquia, Escuela de Nutrición y Dietética.

Ansar, W.; Bandyopadhyay, S.; Chowdhury, S.; Habib, S. & Mandal, C. (2006). Role of C-reactive protein in complement-mediated hemolysis in Malaria. *Glycoconj J.* Vol. 23, No. 3-4, pp. 233-240.

Azevedo, Z.; Victal, L.; Fonseca, K.; Camara, F.; Haeffner-Cavaillon, N.; Cavaillon, J. et al. (2005). Increased production of tumor necrosis factor-α in whole blood cultures from children whit primary malnutrition. *Braz J Med Biol Res.* Vol.38, pp.171-183.

Beard, J.; Rosales, F.; Solomons, N. & Angelilli, M. (2006). Interpretation of serum ferritin concentrations as indicators of total-body iron stores in survey populations: the role of biomarkers for the acute phase response. *Am Clin Nutr.* Vol. 84, pp. 1498- 1505.

Botero, D. & Restrepo M. (2003). *Parasitosis humanas* (4th Edition), Corporación para Investigaciones Biológicas, Medellín, Colombia.

Cantorna, M.; Nashold, F. & Hayes, C. (1994). In vitamin A deficiency multiple mechanisms establish a regulatory T helper cell imbalance with excess TH1 and insufficient TH2 function. *J Immunol.* Vol. 152, No. 4, pp. 1515-1522.

Carmona-Fonseca, J.; Uscátegui, R. & Correa, A. (2009). Parasitosis intestinal en niños de zonas palúdicas de Antioquia (Colombia). *Iatreia.* Vol. 22, pp. 27-49.

Esmai, F.; Ernerudh, J.; Janols, H.; Welin, S.; Ekerfelt, C.; Mining, S. & Fosberg, P. (2003). Cerebral Malaria in children: serum and cerebrospinal fluid TNF-α and TGF-beta levels and their relationship to clinical outcome. *J Trop Pediatr.* Vol. 49, No. 4, pp. 216-223.

Eventos de interés en salud publica, Antioquia. (2006). Available from http://www.dssa.gov.co/dowload/EInteresSP-Ver2007.xls.

Feelders, R.; Vreugdenhil, G.; Eggermont, A.; Kuiper-Kramer, P.; van Eijk, H. & Swaak, A. (1998). Regulation of iron metabolism in the acute-phase response: interferon gamma and tumour necrosis factor alpha induce hypoferraemia, ferritin production and a decrease in circulating transferrin receptors in cancer patients. *Eur J Clin Invest.* Vol 28, No.7, pp. 520-527.

Grencis, R. (1996). T cell and cytokine basis of host variability in response to intestinal nematode infections. *Parasitology.* Vol. 112, pp. 31-37.

Gruys, E.; Toussaint, M.; Niewold, T. & Koopmans, J. (2005). Acute phase reaction and acute phase proteins. *J Zhejiang Univ SCI.* Vol. 6, No. 11, pp. 1045-1056.

Hamzah, J.; Davis, T.; Skinner-Adams, T. & Beilby, J. (2004). Characterization of the effect of retinol on *Plasmodium falciparum* in vitro. *Exp Parasitol.* Vol. 107, No. 7, pp. 136-144.

Iwata, M.; Eshima, Y. & Kagenchika, H. (2003). Retinoic acids exert direct effects on T cells to suppress TH1 development and enhance TH2 development via retinoic acid receptors. *International immunology.* Vol. 15, No. 8, pp. 1017-1025.

Jason, J.; Archibald, L.; Nwanyanwu, OC.; Sowell, AL. & Buchanan, I. (2002). Vitamin A levels and immunity in humans. *Clin Diagn Lab Immuno.* Vol. 9, No. 3, pp. 616-621.

Kanjaksha, G. (2007). Pathogenesis of anemia in malaria: a concise review. *Parasitol Res.* Vol. 101, pp. 1463-1469.

Kovaiou, R. & Grubeck- Loebenstein, B. (2006). Age-associated changes within CD4+ T cells. *Immunology Letters.* Vol. 107, pp. 8-14.

Kurtzhals, JA.; Addae, MM. & Akanmori, BD. (1999). Anemia caused by asymptomatic *Plasmodium falciparum* infection in semi-immune African schoolchildren. *Trans R Soc Trop Med Hyg.* Vol. 93, No. 6, pp. 623-627.

Llanos, C.; Flórez, M.; Herrera, M. & Herrera, S. (2004). Mecanismos de generación de anemia en malaria. *Colomb Med.* Vol 35, No.4, pp. 205-214

López, F. & Schmunis, G. (1998). Diagnóstico de malaria. Pub Cient 512. Washington: OPS-OMS.

Marsh, K. & Kinyanjui, S. (2006). Immune effector mechanisms in malaria. *Parasite Immunol.* Vol. 28, No. 1-2, pp. 51-60.

Moormann, A.; John, C.; Sumba, P.; Tisch, D.; Embury, P. & Kazura, J. (2006). Stability of interferon-gamma and interleukin-10 responses to *Plasmodium falciparum* liver stage antigen-1 and thrombospondin-related adhesive protein in residents of a malaria holoendemic area. *Am J Trop Med Hyg.* Vol. 74. No. 4, pp. 585-590.

Nacher, M. (2002). Worms and malaria: noisy nuisances and silent benefits. *Parasite Immunol.* Vol. 24, No. 7, pp. 391-393.

Nussenblatt, V.; Mukasa, G.; Metzger, A.; Ndeezi, G.; Garrett, E. & Semba RD. (2001). Anemia and interleukin-10, tumor necrosis factor alpha, and erythropoietin levels among children with acute, uncomplicated *Plasmodium falciparum* malaria. *Clin Diagn Lab Immunol.* Vol. 8, No. 6, pp. 1164-1170.

Othoro, C.; Lal, A.; Nahlen, B.; Koech, D.; Orago, A. & Udhayakumar V. (1999). A Low Interleukin-10 Tumor Necrosis Factor-α Ratio is associated with Malaria Anemia in Children Residing in a Holoendemic Malaria Region in Western Kenya. *J Infect Dis.* Vol 179, No.1, pp. 279-282.

Rice, C.; Trull, A.; Berry, D. & Gorman, E. (1987). Development and validation of a particle-enhanced turbidimetric immunoassay for C-reactive protein. *J Immunol Methods.* Vol. 99, pp. 205-211.

Riley, E.; Wahl, S.; Perkins, D. & Schofield, L. (2006). Regulating immunity to malaria. *Parasite Immunol.* Vol. 28, No. 1, pp. 35-49.

Schofield, L. & Grau, G. (2005). Immunological processes in malaria pathogenesis. *Nature reviews immunology.* Vol. 5, pp. 722-734.

Serghides, L. & Kain, K. (2001). Peroxisome proliferator-activated receptor gamma-retinoid X receptor agonists increase CD36-dependent phagocytosis of *Plasmodium falciparum*-parasitized erythrocytes and decrease malaria-induced TNF-alpha secretion by monocytes/macrophages. *J Immunol.* Vol. 166, No. 11, pp. 6742-6748.

Talwar, D.; Ha, T.; Cooney, J.; Brownlee, C. & O'Reilly, D. (1998). A routine method for the simultaneous measurement of retinol, alpha-tocopherol and five carotenoids in human plasma by reverse phase HPLC. *Clin Chim Acta.* Vol. 270, No. 2, pp. 85-100.

Torre, D.; Speranza, F. & Martegani, R. (2002). Role of proinflammatory and anti-inflammatory cytokines in the immune response to *Plasmodium falciparum* malaria. *Lancet Infect Dis,* Vol. 2, No. 12, pp. 719-720.

Uscátegui, R.; Correa, A. & Carmona, J. (2008). Efecto de los suplementos de retinol y antiparasitarios intestinales, sobre valores sanguíneos de retinol, hemoglobina, proteína C reactiva y ferritina en niños maláricos y su relación con estado nutricional e inflamación. Memorias quinto premio fundación éxito por la nutrición infantil. Bogotá: Fundación Éxito.

Vedovato, M.; De Paoli Vitali, E.; Dapporto, M. & Salvatorelli, G. (1999). Defective erythropoietin production in the anaemia of malaria. *Nephrol Dial Transplant.* Vol. 14, No. 4, pp. 1043-1044.

WHO/NHD/01.3 I. (2001). Iron deficiency anemia, assessment, prevention, and control a guide for programme managers. United Nations Children's Fund United Nations University, World Health Organization, pp 10.

World Health Organization. (1995). El estado físico: uso e interpretación de la antropometría. Ginebra: OMS. Serie Informes Técnicos: 854

World Health Organization. (2009). Global prevalence of vitamin A deficiency in populations at risk 1995-2005. WHO Global Database on Vitamin A Deficiency. Geneva, World Health Organization. Available from
http://whqlibdoc.who.int/publications/2009/9789241598019_eng.pdf

Xu, J. & Drew, P. (2006). 9-Cis-retinoic acid suppresses inflammatory responses of microglia and astrocytes. *J Neuroimmunol*. Vol. 171, No. 1, pp. 135-144.

Yildiz, F.; Kurcer, M.; Zeyrek, D. & Simsek, Z. (2006). Parasite density and serum cytokine levels in *Plasmodium vivax* malaria in Turkey. *Parasite immunology*. Vol. 28, pp. 201-207

4

The Pathogenesis of Anaemia in African Animal Trypanosomosis

Savino Biryomumaisho* and E. Katunguka-Rwakishaya
Department of Veterinary Medicine, Makerere University, Kampala
Uganda

1. Introduction

The pathogenesis and pathology of animal trypanosomosis has been a subject of numerous investigations and anaemia has long been recognized as a significant pathological feature. It is the consensus that this anaemia is haemolytic in origin, occurring intravascularly in the acute phase and also extravascularly in the subacute and chronic stages of the disease. The cause of this anaemia is multifactorial and includes increase in erythrocyte destruction coupled with shortening of erythrocyte lifespan. The destruction of erythrocytes largely occurs in the liver by erythrophagocytosis. The other mechanism that has been suggested is that trypanosomes may exert a direct haemolytic action on erythrocytes by generating potentially haemolytic factors on autolysis, a phenomenon that was first described by Landsteiner & Raubitscheck (1901) who hypothesized that the haemolytic factor is lipid in nature. Other mechanisms that have been suggested are haemodilution, bone marrow dysfunction (dyshaemopoiesis) and immunologically-mediated destruction of erythrocytes. In this chapter, the roles of biochemical changes particularly the lipid sub-fraction, bone marrow dysfunction and haemodilution in Small East African goats experimentally infected with *Trypanosoma congolense* or *T. brucei brucei* shall be examined. The effect of *T. congolense* on the life span of erythrocytes in sheep, inferred from ^{51}Cr-labelled erythrocytes, will be presented and discussed.

An in-depth knowledge of development of anaemia during trypanosomosis in different animal species is pivotal in instituting appropriate treatment in clinically sick animals and during convalescence. Similarly, the same knowledge can be utilized by animal health workers to manage anaemia derived from causes other than trypanosomosis.

2. Free fatty acids and other blood biochemical changes

The subject of blood biochemical changes and the role of individual biochemicals mainly those derived from the protein and lipid sub-fractions have been investigated over decades with the aim of elucidating the mechanisms by which anaemia in trypanosome-infected animals is induced. Of particular significance in the pathogenesis of anaemia in trypanosome-infected animals are free fatty acids (FFAs). Free fatty acids generated from both *T. congolense* (Tizard & Holmes, 1976) and *T. brucei* (Huan et al., 1975) form potent hemolytic material when permitted to autolyse in saline at 20ºC. This material contains a mixture of FFAs and to a lesser extent lysophospholipids (Tizard et al., 1977). Massive trypanosome destruction as a result of the hosts' immune responses occurs especially during the acute phase of trypanosome infection. Therefore, the rapid decrease of the erythrocyte mass in this phase may among other factors be mediated by the generation of FFAs from autolysing trypanosomes (Biryomumaisho et al., 2003).

Free fatty acids may be saturated and unsaturated; both groups can significantly modify the host immune response (Berken & Benacerraf, 1968) by either blocking lymphocytic reactivity to mitogens (Mertin & Hughes, 1975) or antigens (Field et al., 1974) or through production of potent immunosuppressive prostaglandins (Quagliata et al., 1972). There is remarkable resemblance between the immunological lesions induced by administration of free fatty acids and those observed in trypanosomosis. The question is: what is the significance of variations of FFAs concentrations that are observed during trypanosomosis infections in different animal species? Observations have shown that relatively large quantities of FFA mostly stearic, linoleic, palmitic and oleic acids are generated by autolysing trypanosomes (Tizard et al., 1976; Assoku et al., 1977). These FFAs are potentially cytotoxic and haemolytic *in vitro*. In both *T. congolense* and *T. brucei* infected Small East African goats (Biryomumaisho et al., 2003), FFAs were significantly higher than those of control uninfected animals. However, the other biochemical parameters showed a different pattern: hypoproteinaemia, hypoalbuminaemia, hypocholestraemia, low and high density hypolipidaemia. These changes suggest that growing trypanosomes require some lipids and proteins to support their growth. At the same time, anaemia developed after goats were challenged with trypanosomes; the pattern of increase of FFAs corresponded to the decrease of packet cell volume (PCV), haemoglobin and erythrocyte counts. These observations re-affirm that FFAs generated from autolysing trypanosomes in goats contribute to anaemia development *in vivo*.

The fatty acids of trypanosomes are mainly esterified as phosphoglycerides or as cholesterol esters though they also exist as FFAs (Dixon et al., 1972). Lipids constitute 15-20% of the dry weight of African trypanosomes with total lipid content of the stumpy forms being substantially higher than that of the slender forms (Vankatesan & Ormerod, 1976). On autolysis, *T. congolense* releases a number of haemolytic FFAs of which the most potent is linoleic acid. These fatty acids can lyse washed rat and bovine erythrocytes *in vitro* (Tizard et al., 1978); autolysis will cause increased erythrocyte fragility in whole rat blood but not in whole bovine blood. Observations in Small East African goats during the first 16 days post infection (Biryomumaisho et al., 2003) showed that total serum lipids decreased from 12.88 mg dl^{-1} three days before infection to 8.84 mg ml^{-1} on day 16 post infection in *T. brucei*-infected goats and to 9.46 mg ml^{-1} in *T. congolense*-infected goats respectively. These findings are in agreement with observations made in rats. Although this mechanism of red cell destruction may not be important in cattle, it may be important in small ruminants. In principal, mechanisms of red cell destruction may differ with different animal species; for instance, infections by *T. brucei* in mice (Igbokwe et al., 1994) and sheep (Taiwo et al., 2003) and *Babesia bigemina* in cattle (Saleh, 2009) render to the animals a reduced ability to peroxidation in the erythrocyte membrane. Furthermore, these oxidative changes in the erythrocytes can accelerate the destruction of these cells in the spleen (Morita et al., 1996). Lipid peroxidation studies in rats infected with *T. evansi* (Wolkmer et al., 2009) showed that these oxidative changes reduce the capacity of erythrocytes in rats to prevent oxidative damage in erythrocyte membrane *in vivo* as is the case *in vitro*.

The understanding of the lipid sub-fraction changes in different trypanosomes and animal species is an ongoing process; their effects could be associated with detrimental effects in affected hosts (Adamu et al., 2009). Many studies have observed decline is serum lipids and cholesterol levels in trypanosomosis infections. These phenomena could aggravate the neurological disorders often associated with trypanosomosis since cholesterol is vital in cell signaling in neuronal synapses formation.

3. Dyshaemopoiesis as a mechanism of anaemia development

Studies on the role of dyshaemopoiesis in the pathogenesis of anaemia, done with *T. congolense* infection in cattle (Valli et al., 1978); *T. vivax* infection in calves (Logan et al., 1991); *T. congolense* infection in sheep (Katunguka-Rwakishaya et al., 1992); and in *T. congolense* infection in multimammate rats (Ojok et al., 2001), give conflicting results. In this chapter, the role of dyshaemopoiesis in anaemia development in Small East African goats is presented. Bone marrow biopsies were obtained with a 16-gauge Salah sternal puncture needle positioned at right angles to the bone. All biopsies were collected aseptically after a small sharp incision was made under local analgesia.

Bone marrow function was studied by aspirating bone marrow biopsies once a month lasting four months and determining the myeloid:erythroid ratio (M:E ratio) by making a differential count of a total of 500 cells of nucleated granulocytic precursors divided by the number of precursor cells of the erythrocytic series. Typical bone marrow cells are represented in Figure 1 and the results were recorded in a modified bone marrow tally sheet as described by Schalm et al., (1975). The lowest PCV and mean erythrocyte counts occurred between the 4th and 7th weeks after infection in both groups *T. congolense* and *T. brucei*-infected goats. Concurrently, the M:E ratio progressively decreased as the disease progressed (Table 1).

Days post infection	*T. congolense*	*T. brucei*	Uninfected controls
-5	0.48 ± 0.06	0.46 ± 0.07	0.41 ± 0.07
29	0.33 ± 0.06	0.29 ± 0.03	0.36 ± 0.22
59	0.21 ± 0.04*	0.32 ± 0.05	0.37 ± 0.03
85	0.22 ± 0.05*	0.27 ± 0.05	0.38 ± 0.04
121	0.28 ± 0.04	0.43 ± 0.10	0.44 ± 0.12

*$p < 0.05$.

Table 1. Mean myeloid: erythroid ratios (± standard error of the mean) of goats infected with either *T. congolense* or *T. brucei* and of uninfected controls.

The results from the experiment with goats agree with the findings of Valli et al., (1978) in experimental *T. congolense* TREU 112 infection in Holstein calves: the anaemia was of moderate severity and normochromic and macrocytic in the acute phase changing to normochromic, normocytic with chronicity. At the same time, the anaemia was haemolytic and regenerative as was shown by sharply decreased myeloid: erythroid ratio. In the East African goats, however, the anaemia was severe as shown by a sharp decline of haemoglobin concentration by the 7th week from 9.2 ± 0.2 g dl⁻¹ pre-infection to 5.4 ± g dl⁻¹ in *T. congolense*-infected group and from 9.5 ± 0.2 g dl⁻¹ to 5.9 ± 0.1 g dl⁻¹ in goats challenged with *T. brucei* (Biryomumaisho et al., 2007). At the same time, the anaemia was regenerative, a parameter that was inferred from decreased M:E ratios. For the parameters observed, *T. congolense* produced more severe effects than *T. brucei*.

Panel 1   **Panel 2**

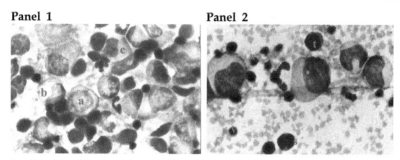

[Micrographs adopted from Biryomumaisho, 2001].

Fig. 1. Giemsa-stained sternal bone marrow biopsies from Small East African goats (x 1,000).
Panel 1. A highly cellular bone marrow micrograph showing precursors of both myelocytic and erythrocytic series at different development stages collected 5 days before infection with trypanosomes in Small East African goats. Cell (a) is progranulocyte; (b) neutrophilic myelocyte; (c) eosinophilic myelocyte and (d) band neutrophil
Panel 2: One month after infection, when animals reached the lowest PCV value, it was more difficult to collect marrow smears without contamination with peripheral blood. (s) dividing metarubricyte; (t) rubricyte and (u) late rubricyte; (v) more late rubricytes can be seen in the micrograph. The large nucleated cells are myelocytic cell line precursors.

Ojok et al., (2001) made similar observations in multimammate rats; but in chronic stages, erythropoietic activity reduced while intra and extra-vascular erythrophagocytic activity increased. Also in agreement is *T. vivax* infection in calves where erythroid hyperplasia, evidenced by decrease in the M:E ratio, was observed (Logan et al., 1991).
The interpretation of results of M:E ratio should be viewed within the framework of the ratio of erythrocytic to granulocytic cell precursors: if the ratio is equal to one, the implication is the rate of manufacture of granulocytic precursors equals that of erythrocytic precursors. A decrease in the ratio means erythrogenesis exceeds granulopoiesis, a phenomenon that was observed in the Small East African goats (Biryomumaisho et al., 2007). The expectation, however, is that if erythrogenesis was increased, anaemia development would be halted. Progressive development of anaemia insinuates that the rate of destruction of erythrocytes exceeds the rate of their replenishment by the bone marrow which results in decrease of all parameters indicative of anaemia *viz.* lowered PCV, hypohaemoglobinaemia and decreased erythrocyte counts in peripheral blood. In the goats in this experiment, increased erythrogenesis did not sufficiently compensate for red cell loss. Similar observations in sheep (Katunguka-Rwakishaya et al., 1992) were made and in both instances erythrogenesis was enhanced but did not sufficiently compensate for the accelerated destruction of erythrocytes. The conclusion here is that anaemia state at those stages of trypanosomosis could be attributed to increased destruction of erythrocytes since there was no evidence of dyshaemopoiesis (as observations in sheep and goats suggest).

4. Reduced red cell lifespan: Erythrokinetic studies

Knowledge of the normal life span of red cells in different animal species is helpful in understanding the dynamics of red cell production and destruction. Life-span studies in animals indicate that erythrocytes of each animal species have a characteristic mean survival time that is the result of both the potential life span and loss of cells from random destruction irrespective of the age of the animal. Early reports of red blood cells (RBC) survival studies were done in canines using a serological technique as reported by Schalm et al., (1975). Serological techniques involve treating the recipient's blood with specific immune serum to cause RBC autoagglutination leaving the donor or transfused cells unagglutinated. For instance, this method estimated RBC life-span to be 90-100 days in the canine; however, a longer (112-133 days) erythrocyte survival period was estimated by Hawkins & Whipple (1938), using bilirubin production as a measure of the length of red cell life. Tagging or labeling erythrocytes with isotopes is considered to be more accurate. Using isotopes, the mean RBC life span in man with ^{15}N is 127 days; 70-133 days in adult sheep by ^{14}C; 125 days in an adult domestic goat by ^{14}C and 150 days in a mature cow by [14]C (Schalm et al., 1975).

4.1 Factors influencing erythrocyte lifespan

Erythrocyte survival may be related to age of the animal; for instance, rapid destruction of erythrocytes has been observed in newborn puppies between birth and 2 weeks of age (Lee et al., 1971). However, erythrocyte survival in new born babies is similar to that of adults (Berlin, 1964) although fetal red cells have a shorter life span of 70 days. Differences in life span (days) with ^{14}C-labeled erythrocytes for sheep at different ages has been shown to be 75 ± 14.8 days for newborn lambs, 46 days for three-month old lambs; 52 days in lambs one year old while adult sheep have an average of 130 days (Schalm et al., 1975).

Diet has been shown to be a factor in erythrocyte survival: *T. congolense*-infected N'Dama 2-5 year old cattle supplemented with 4 kg hay day[-1] of a mixture of rice bran, groundnut cake, milled *Andropogon* hay and common salt developed similar degrees of anaemia as animals which were not supplemented but recovered from the anaemia more rapidly. Ferrokinetic measurement in *T. congolense*-infected Blackface Scottish sheep (Katunguka-Rwakishaya et al., 1997) indicated that plasma iron turnover rates and ^{59}Fe-incorporated rates were higher in the high protein infected group than the low protein infected group. Comparatively, nutritional deficiencies (Vitamin B_{12}, folic acid and iron) in man are reported to result in defective red cells having shortened survival time (Harris & Kellermeyer, 1970). However, in pyridoxine (Vitamin B_6) deficiency, the erythrocyte survival time has been shown to be normal but in folic acid and copper deficiencies, it was decreased in swine (Bush et al., 1956).

4.2 Erythrokinetics during animal trypanosomosis

Studies of animal trypanosomosis have consistently indicated reduced life span of erythrocytes: erythrokinetic studies in N'dama and Zebu cattle experimentally infected with *T. brucei* (Dargie et al., 1979); *T. congolense*-infected calves (Valli et al., 1978; Preston et a., 1979) all showed reduced life span. Erythrokinetic and ferrokinetic studies (Katunguka-Rwakishaya et al., 1992) of sheep after infection with *T. congolense* had lower ^{51}Cr-red cell half lives and lower red cell life spans than control sheep. Similar observations were made by Mamo & Holmes (1975) in *T. congolense*-infected bovines and Ikede et al., (1977) in *T. congolense*-infected mice that was accompanied by progressive increase in osmotic fragility.

5. Blood volume changes and anaemia development

The total volume of circulating blood is a function of lean body weight: in most animals, blood volume occupies approximately 7-8% of the body weight except in the cat (4%) (Radostatis et al., 2000). The blood volume is very important to dynamics of circulation that it is kept relatively constant despite periodic water intake, production of water by metabolism and continuous loss of water through various body organs like the skin, lungs, alimentary tract and kidneys.

5.1 Methods of obtaining blood volume

The earliest methods for estimating blood volume consisted of bleeding animals to death followed by washing out the blood vessels and adding the blood contained in the washings to that collected during bleeding (Schalm et al., 1975). Another early method was by injection of known quantity of isotonic solution (NaCl) into the vascular system and shortly noting the extent of dilution of blood as determined by the change in specific gravity, red cell number or haemoglobin concentration.

At present, the most accurate and reliable method for the determination of plasma volume is by measurement of the intravenous dilution of macromolecules labeled with radioisotopes (Mackie, 1976). However, such animals become unfit for human consumption; coupled with the difficulty of maintaining animals treated with radioactive material and disposal of waste from such animals. Basing on these reasons, Evan's blue dye (T-1824) that binds to albumin component of plasma and can rapidly be removed from the body can be used. Plasma and total blood volume in Small East African goats infected with either *T. congolense* or *T. brucei* (Biryomumaisho, 2001) were determined by injecting a 0.03% solution of T-1824 at a dose rate of 0.4 mg kg^{-1} of the goat in the right jugular vein and after 10 minutes, blood was collected from the left jugular and centrifuged to obtain plasma-tagged dye. By using absorbance of the dye in plasma of the standard against a blank (prepared from plasma of individual goats) in a U-1,000 Hitachi spectrophotometer at a wavelength of 620 nm, the concentration of the dye in plasma was calculated as follows:

$$\frac{\text{[T-1824] in Plasma (mg)}}{\text{[T-1824] in Standard}} = \frac{\textbf{Optical density of diluted Plasma}}{\text{Optical density of the Standard}} \quad (1)$$

$$\text{Plasma volume (mls)} = \frac{\textbf{mg of dye injected}}{\text{mg/ml of dye in Plasma}} \quad (2)$$

$$\text{Blood volume (mls)} = \frac{\textbf{Plasma volume} \times 100}{100\text{-PCV} \times 0.98^*} \quad (3)$$

Trapped plasma after centrifugation was corrected for by including a 2% (0.98) factor.

Plasma volume and total blood volume of individual goats in ml kg^{-1} were determined by dividing the values obtained in (2) and (3) by the body weight of individual goats. Mean values of all 5 measurements taken at 30-day intervals are shown in Table 2 while measurements taken in *T. congolense*-infected Scottish Black Face sheep with ^{125}I-albumin and ^{51}Cr-red cells respectively are shown in Table 3 (Katunguka et al., 1992).

5.1.1 Blood volume changes in trypanosomosis

In trypanosomosis infections, anaemia development has been shown to be mainly haemolytic during the acute phase of the disease. In the sub acute and chronic stages of the disease, however, extravascular mechanisms are thought to play a major role. One such mechanism is thought to involve an abnormal retention of large quantities of fluid within the plasma compartment. Results from T. congolense-infected N'Dama and Zebu cattle (Dargie et al., 1979) showed that both groups developed significant anaemia. Measurement of plasma and red cell volumes showed that the low PCV of infected cattle was due to reductions in red cell volume and not haemodilution.

The implication of increased plasma here can be explained by a normal homeostatic response for maintenance of blood volume and pressure. Studies using ^{51}Cr-red cells, ^{125}I-albumin and ^{59}Fe as ferric citrate 11 weeks after infection revealed that infected sheep had significantly lower mean circulating red cell volumes but higher plasma and blood volumes than control sheep (Katunguka-Rwakishaya et al., 1992). In T. congolense and T. brucei-infected goats (Biryomumaisho, 2001), the mean plasma volume and total blood volume values were higher than those of the controls although the differences were not significant (Table 2).

	T. congolense n = 10	T. brucei n = 10	Controls n = 5	Significance
Plasma volume (mls /kg) ± SEM	58.3 ± 3.0	53.1 ± 6.1	44.7 ± 7.0	P > 0.05
Total blood volume (mls / kg) ± SEM	72.8 ± 3.9	67.9 ± 7.5	58.6 ± 7.4	P > 0.05

[Table adopted from S. Biryomumaisho, 2001].

Table 2. Mean T-1824-plasma and blood volume in trypanosome-infected goats.

	Plasma volume mls kg^{-1} ± SEM	Blood volume mls kg^{-1} ± SEM
Infected, n=5	45.1 ± 1.5	57.9 ± 1.1
Control, n = 5	36.2 ± 1.0	52.9 ± 2.2
Significance	P < 0.01	P < 0.01

Table 3. Blood volumes of sheep infected with T. congolense (mls kg^{-1} ± SEM).

6. Conclusion

Knowledge about the pathogenesis of anaemia can be utilized to manage cases of anaemia caused by trypanosomosis as well as cases of anaemia derived from other causes other than trypanosomosis provided the primary cause is dealt with. The aspects of cross matching the blood of donor and recipient animals and whether to replace whole blood or its components are beyond the scope of this chapter. However, a veterinarian can utilize some aspects of the knowledge of dyshaemopoiesis and blood volume to manage anaemia in routine practice.

Blood volume changes can be estimated at clinical examination: basically, most animals with exception of the cat have blood volumes approximately 7-8% of their body weight. An animal health care worker can estimate the total blood volume of a donor animal that way. However, the amount of blood lost (in the anaemic / recipient animal) can be estimated from measurement of PCV as follows:

$$\text{Blood lost (litres)} \quad = \frac{\textbf{Normal PCV of animal species – patient \ PCV}}{\text{Normal PCV x 0.08 of patient weight in kg}} \quad (4)$$

In our opinion and experience, for blood transfusion to be effective, at least 25% of the deficit should be corrected.

Haemodilution is a state when the fluid content of blood is increased and this results into lowered concentration of the formed elements. For the case of the red cell component, this can result in apparent anaemia. The converse is haemoconcentration, a state in which there is increased concentration of formed elements of blood mainly as a result of loss of water from the body. The clinical importance of both scenarios dictates that the veterinarian should first evaluate the animal as to whether haemoconcentration or haemodilution is pathological or not. In both cases, the primary cause should be dealt with.

The more commonly encountered of the two scenarios is haemoconcentration and subsequent hypovolaemia resulting from loss of fluid such as in diarrhaea / dysentery, vomiting (especially in monogastric animals), skin burns, starvation and thirst, among other causes. In all cases, hypovolaemia leads to reduction in blood plasma and, in severe instances, leads to hypovolaemic shock. A low blood volume leads to multiple organ failure, kidney and brain damage and death. An appropriate fluid for replacement containing electrolytes, metabolic enhancers or plasma expanders should be chosen (selection of suitable fluids for therapy is outside the scope of this chapter).

Basing on presenting clinical signs, the degree of dehydration and hence amount of water lost can be estimated from the percentage of dehydration basing on skin elasticity, demeanor of the animal and sinking of the eyes in the orbit.

7. References

Adamu, S., Barde, N., Abenga, J.N., User, J.N., Ibrahim, N.D.G. & Esievo, K.A.N. (2009). Experimental *Trypanosoma brucei* infection-induced changes in the serum profiles of lipids and cholesterol and the clinical implications in pigs. *Journal of Cell and Animal Biology*. Vol.3, No.2, 15-20.

Assoku, R.K.G., Tizard, I.R. & Nielsen, K.H. Free fatty acids, complement activation and polyclonal B-cell stimulation as factors in the immunopathogenesis of African trypanosomiasis. *Lancet II*, 956-959.

Berken, A. & Benacerraf,B.(1968). Depression of reticuloendothelial system phagocytic function by ingested lipids. *Proceedings of the Society for Experimental Biology and Medicine*, pp. 793-795 (1968), Vol.128. No.3

Berlin, N.I. (1964). Life span of the red cell, In: *The Red Blood Cell*, Bishop, C. & Swigenor, D.M., 423-450, Academic Press, New York.

Biryomumaisho, S. & Katunguka-Rwakishaya, E. (2007). The pathogenesis of anaemia in goats experimentally infected with *Trypanosoma congolense* or *Trypanosoma brucei*: use of the myeloid: erythroid ratio. *Veterinary Parasitology*, Vol.143, 354-357.

Biryomumaisho, S. (2001). Comparative Clinical Pathology of *Trypanosoma congolense* and *Trypanosoma brucei* infection in Small East African goats. M.Sc. Thesis, Makerere University, Uganda, pp. 70-74.

Biryomumaisho, S., Katunguka-Rwakishaya, E. & Rubaire-Akiiki, C. (2003). Serum biochemical changes in experimental *Trypanosoma congolense* and *Trypanosoma brucei* infection in Small East African goats. *Veterinary Archives*, Vol.73, No.3, 167-180.

Radostatis, O.M., Gay, C.C., Blood, D.C. & Hinchcliff, K.W. (2000). Diseases of blood and blood-forming organs, In: *Veterinary Medicine*, pp 399-417, ISBN 0-7020-26042, W.B. Saunders, Saskatoon, Canada.

Bush, J.A., Jensen, W.N., Ashenbrucker, H., Cartwright, G.E. & Wintrobe, M.M. (1956). The kinetics of iron metabolism in swine with various experimentally induced anaemias. *Journal of Experimental Medicine*, Vol.103, 161.

Dargie, J.D., Murray, M., Grimshaw, W.R. & McIntrye, W. I. M. (1979). Bovine trypanosomiasis: red cell kinetics of N'dama and Zebu cattle infected with *Trypanosoma congolense*. *Parasitology*, Vol.78, 271-286.

Dixon, H., Ginger, C.D. & Williamson, J. (1972). Trypanosome sterols and their metabolic origins. *Comparative Biochemical Physiology B*, Vol.41, 1-18.

Field, A. M., Gardner, S. D., Goodbody, R. A., & Wood-House, M. A. (1974). Identity of a newly isolated human polyoma-virus from a patient with progressive multifocal leuko-encephalopathy. *Journal of Clinical Pathology*, Vol. 27, 341–347.

Harris, J.W. & Kellermeyer, R.W. (1970). The red cell, Production, Metabolism, Destruction: Normal and Abnormal. Harvard University Press, Cambridge, Massachusetts, 1970.

Hawkins, W.B. & Whipple, G.H. (1938). The life cycle of the red blood cell in the dog. *American Journal of Physiology*, Vol.122, 418.

Huan, C.N., Webb, L., Lambert, P.H. & Miescher, P.A. (1975). Pathogenesis of the anaemia in African trypanosomiasis: characterization and purification of the haemolytic factor. *Schweizerische Medizinische Wochenschrift*. Vol.105, 1582-1583.

Igbokwe, I.O., Esievo, K.A.N.& Obagaiye, O.K. (1994). Increases susceptibility of erythrocytes to *in vitro* peroxidation in acute *Trypanosoma brucei* infection in mice. *Veterinary Parasitology*, Vol.55, No.4, 279-286.

Ikede, B.O., Lule, M. & Terry, R.J. (1977). Anaemia in trypanosomiasis: mechanisms   of erythrocyte destruction in mice infected with *Trypanosoma congolense* or *T. brucei*. *Acta Tropica*, Vol.34, No.1, 53-60.

Katunguka-Rwakishaya E., McKechnie, D., Parkins, J.J., Murray, M. & Holmes,P.H. (1997). The influence of dietary protein on live bodyweight, degree of anaemia and erythropoietic responses of Scottish blackface sheep infected experimentally with *Trypanosoma congolense*. *Research in Veterinary Science*, Vol.63, No.3, 273-277.

Katunguka-Rwakishaya, E., Murray, M. & Holmes, P.H. (1992). Pathophysiology of ovine trypanosomiasis: ferrokinetics and erythrocyte survival studies. *Research in Veterinary Science*, Vol.53, 80-86.

Landsteiner & Raubitscheck (1901) *as cited in   Firtz Assman (2011).* Beiträge zur Kenntnis pflanzlicher Agglutinine, Pflügers Archiv European Journal of Physiology Volume 137, Numbers 8-10, 489-510, DOI: 10.1007/BF01679970

Lee, P., Brown, M.E. & Hutzler, P.T. (1971). Turnover of red blood cell mass in   new-borne puppies. *Federation Proceedings*, Vol.30, 195.

Logan, L.L., Anosa, V.O. & Shaw, M.K. (1991). Haemopoiesis in Ayrshire-Guarnsey calves infected with Galana stock of *Trypanosoma vivax*. OAU/STRC [1991]. Pp 317-322.

Mackie, W.S. (1976). Plasma volume measurements in sheep using Evan's blue and continuous blood sampling. *Research in Veterinary Science*, Vol.21, 108-109.

Mamo, E. & Holmes, P.H. (1975). The erythrokinetics of zebu cattle infected with *Trypanosoma congolense*. *Research in Veterinary Science*, Vol.18, 105-1

Mertin, J. & Hughes, D. (1975). Specific inhibitory action of polyunsaturated fatty acids on lymphocyte transformation induced by PHA and PPD. International Archives of Allergy and Applied Immunology. Vol. 48, No.2, 203-210.

Morita, T., Saeki, H. & Ishii, T. (1996). Erythrocyte oxidation in artificial *Babesia gibsoni* infection. *Veterinary Parasitology*, Vol.63, Nos.1-2, 1-7.

Ojok, L. & Kaeufer-Weiss, E. (2001). Bone marrow response to acute and chronic *Trypanosoma congolense* infection inmultimammate rats *(Mastomys coucha)*. *Journal of Comparative Pathology*, Vol.124, Nos.2-3, 149-158.

Preston, J.M., Wellde, B.T. & Kovatchi, R.M. (1979). *Trypanosoma congolense*: calf erythrocyte survival. *Experimental Parasitology*, Vol.48, 118-125.

Quagliata, F., Lawrence, V.J.W. & Phillips-Quagliata, J.M. (1972). Prostaglandin E as a regulator of lymphocyte function selective action on B lymphocytes and synergy with procarbazine in depression of immune responses. *Cell Immunology, Vol.6*, 457–465.

Saleh, M.A. (2009). Erythrocytic oxidative damage in crossbred cattle naturally infected with *Babesia bigemina*. *Reseach in Veterinary Science*, Vol. 86, No. 1, 43-48.

Schalm, O.W., Jain, N.C. & Carrol, E.J. (1975). Blood volume and water balance, In: *Veterinary Hematology*, 1-14, Lea and Febiger, IBSN 0-8121-0470-6, Philadelphia.

Schalm, O.W., Jain, N.C. & Carrol, E.J. (1975). The erythrocytes: their production, Function and Destruction, In: *Veterinary Hematology*, 356-404, Lea and Febiger, IBSN 0-8121-0470-6, Philadelphia.

Schalm, O.W., Jain, N.C. & Carrol, E.J. (1975). The Hematopoietic System, In: *Veterinary Hematology*, 301-335, Lea and Febiger, IBSN 0-8121-0470-6, Philadelphia.

Taiwo, V.O., Olaniyi, M.O. & Ogunsanmi, A.O. (2003). Comparative plasma biochemical changes and susceptibility of erythrocytes to *in-vitro* peroxidation during experimental *Trypanosoma congolense* and *T. brucei* infections in sheep. *Israel Journal of Veterinary Medicine*. Vol.58, No.4, 1-7

Tizard, I.R. & Holmes, W.L. (1976). The generation of toxic activity from*Trypanosoma congolense. Experientia*, Vol.32, 1533-1534.

Tizard, I.R., Holmes, W.L., York, DA. & Mellors, A. (1977). The generation and identification of the haemolysin of *Trypanosoma congolense. Experientia*, Vol.33, 901.

Tizard, I.R., Holmes, W.L. & Nielsen, K. (1978). Mechanisms of the anaemia in trypanosomiasis: studies on the role of haemolytic fatty acids derived from *Trypanosoma congolense. Tropenmedicine and Parasitology*, Vol.29, 108-104.

Valli, V.E.O., Forsberg, G.A. & McSherry, B.J. (1978). The pathogenesis of *T. congolense* in calves: Anaemia and erythroid response. *Veterinary Parasitology*, Vol. 15, 733-745.

Vankatesan, S. & Ormerod, W.E. (1976). Lipid content of the slender and stumpy forms of *Trypanosoma brucei rhodesiense*: a comparative study. Comparative Biochemistry and Physiology Part B, Vol. 53, 481-487.

Wolkmer, P., Schafer da Silva, A., Traesel, C.K., Paim, F.C., Cargnelutti, J.F., Pagnoncelli, M., Picada, M.E., Monteiro, S.G. & Terezinha dos Anjos

5

The Mechanisms of Anaemia in Trypanosomosis: A Review

Albert Mbaya[1,*], Hussein Kumshe[2] and Chukwunyere Okwudiri Nwosu[3]
[1]Department of Veterinary Microbiology and Parasitology, University of Maiduguri,
[2]Department of Veterinary Medicine, University of Maiduguri,
[3]Department of Veterinary Parasitology and Entomology, University of Nigeria, Nsukka
Nigeria

1. Introduction

Trypanosomosis is an important disease of both humans and animals commonly found in most parts of Africa and South America (Swallow, 2000). The tsetse fly (*Glossina*) is responsible for biological (cyclical) transmission while haematophagus arthropod vectors of the family, *Tabanidae, Stomoxynae* and *Hippoboscidae* are responsible for its mechanical transmission (Soulsby, 1982). Transplacental transmission has also been recorded in cattle (Ogwu et al., 1992). *Trypanosoma congolense, T. vivax and T. brucei* have been reported to cause nagana in cattle while *T. evansi* caused surra in camels (*Camelus dromedarieus*) (Mbaya et al., 2010). In humans, *Trypanosoma brucei gambiense* and *Trypanosoma brucei rhodeseinse* are responsible for human sleeping sickness in West and East Africa respectively, while *T. cruzi*, transmitted by triatomid bugs (*Triatoma magista*) is responsible for transmitting chagas diseases to humans in South America (Solano et al., 2003). The *T. brucei* group of trypanosomes (*T. brucei, T. b. gambiense, T. b. rhodesianse* and *T. evansi*) mostly invade tissues (humoral) whereas, *T. congolense* and to a lesser extent *T. vivax* and *T. cruzi* predominantly restrict themselves to the blood circulation (haemic) (Igbokwe, 1994; Mbaya et al., 2011).

The mechanism or pathophysiology of anaemia in trypanosomosis is complex and multifactorial in origin (Naessens et al., 2005). It initiates a cascade of events leading to haemolytic anaemia and cardiovascular collapse (Anosa, 1988). In human trypanosomosis, disseminated intravascular coagulation has been reported (Barret-Connor et al., 1973). Among the complex and multifactorial etiologies associated with the anaemia is haemolysin, a sensory/excretory product of living trypanosomes. This product is known to lyse red blood cells in the absence of antibodies (*in-vitro*) and haemodilution (*in-vivo*). This mechanism has been adequately described in gold fish (*Carassius auratus*) infected with *Trypanosoma dahilewskyi* (Nazrul-Islam and Woo, 1991) and in murine models infected with *T. b. rhodesiense* (Naessens et al., 2005).

2. Haemolytic anaemia caused by animal and human trypanosomes

Haemolytic anaemia has been reported in *T. brucei* infection of red fronted gazelles (*Gazella rufifrons*) (Mbaya et al., 2009a), sheep and goats (Edward et al., 1956; Ikede & Losos, 1972), *T.*

congolense infection of sheep and goats (Edwards et al., 1956), *T. vivax* infection of sheep and goats (Anosa, 1977). Similarly, it was reported in vervet monkeys (*Cercopethicus aethiopes*) (Abenga & Anosa, 2006), and baboons (*Papio anubis*) (Mbaya et al., 2009c, b) infected with the West African human sleeping sickness trypanosome; *T.b. gambiense*.

2.1 Various stages of the anaemia in trypanosomosis
Three phases of anaemia have been reported to occur in trypanosomosis. They are, phase I (acute crises), phase II (chronic) and phase III (recovery) (Anosa, 1988).

2.1.1 Phase I: Acute crises
This phase begins with the initial appearance of trypanosomes in peripheral circulation. The parasitaemia in this case is usually high, fluctuating and evident in most days (Maxie & Losos, 1979; Anosa & Isoun, 1980; Anosa, 1988; Abenga & Anosa, 2006; Mbaya et al., 2009a, b, c; 2010; Mbaya & Ibrahim, 2011; Mbaya et al., 2011). During this phase the anaemia is morphologically classified as macrocytic and normochromic (Maxie & Losos, 1979; Anosa & Isoun, 1980). At this stage death commonly occurs due to severe pancytopoenia and other pathologies (Anosa, 1988). Sub-acute cases have been produced experimentally in rodents infected with *T. congolense* (Isoun & Esuroso, 1972) and with *T. brucei* (Mbaya et al., 2007, 2010, 2011).

2.1.2 Phase II: Chronic
This phase follows the acute crises phase and is characterized by low levels of parasitaemia. The low to moderate erythrocyte value at this point persists with minor fluctuations. This period ranges from several weeks to months. With the *T. brucei* group, which mostly invade tissues, this is the aparasitaemic phase when the parasites establish extravascularly and are less numerous in peripheral circulations (Rabo, 1995) or absent (Mbaya et al., 2007, 2009a, d). In this chronic phase, the morphological classification of the anaemia is normochromic and normocytic (Maxie & Losos, 1979).

2.1.3 Phase III: Recovery
This phase is characterized by the low, infrequent or absence of parasitaemia. At this point, declined erythrocyte values begin to return towards pre-infection values and other pathological changes undergo resolution (Anosa, 1988) leading to self-recovery as commonly encountered in trypanotolerant wildlife (Mbaya et al. 2009a).

3. The mechanism of anaemia in trypanosomosis
The interplay of several factors acting either individually or synergistically contributes to the development of haemolytic anaemia in human and animal trypanosomosis (Figure 1).
Most common among these factors are erythrocyte injury caused by lashing action of trypanosome flagella, undulating pyrexia, platelet aggregation, toxins and metabolites from trypanosomes, lipid peroxidation and malnutrition (Murray & Morrison, 1978; Morrison et al., 1981; Saror, 1982; Igbokwe, 1994). Meanwhile, idiopathic (unknown) serum and tumor necrosing factors are responsible for dyserythropoieses (Mabbot & Sternberg, 1995; Lieu & Turner, 1999; Maclean et al., 2001).

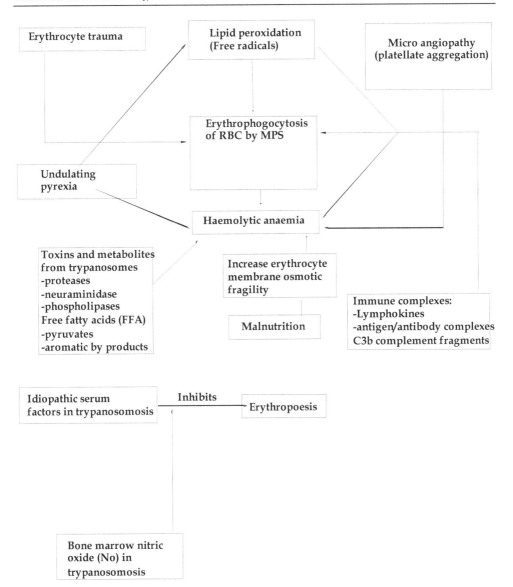

Fig. 1. Pathophysiology of anaemia in African trypanosomosis, Source by Dr. A.W. Mbaya.

4. Anaemia through mechanical injury to erythrocytes

Anaemia caused by mechanical injury to erythrocyte occurs by the lashing action of the powerful locomotory flagella and microtubule reinforced bodies of the millions of the organisms during parasitaemia (Vickerman & Tetley, 1978). Erythrocyte membrane damage has also been associated with adhesion of erythrocytes, platelets and reticulocytes to trypanosome surfaces via sialic acid receptors leading to damages to erythrocyte cell membranes (Bungener & Muller, 1976; Banks, 1980; Anosa & Kaneko, 1983; Shehu et al., 2006). As such, several areas of discontinuity occur along the surface of erythrocyte membranes where they adhere to the trypanosomes. Mechanical damage to vascular endothelium has been reported when tissue-invading trypanosomes such as the *T. brucei* group penetrate tissues via the interstices (Anosa & Kaneko, 1983).

5. Anaemia through undulating pyrexia

In trypanosomosis, a direct relationship exists between undulating pyrexia and fluctuating parasitaemia (Nwosu & Ikeme, 1992; Igbokwe, 1994; Mbaya et al., 2009a, e). Under laboratory conditions, Karle (1974) exposed erythrocytes to temperatures above the normal body temperature and found out that the osmotic fragility and permeability of erythrocytes were greatly enhanced. It was also reported that increased body temperatures decreased erythrocyte plasticity and longevity *in-vivo* (Woodruff et al., 1972). Consequently, temperature elevation increased the rate of immunochemical reactions thereby initiating lipid peroxidation of erythrocytes (Igbokwe, 1994).

6. Anaemia through platelet aggregation (microangiopathy)

Intact trypanosomes or fragments of trypanosomes may cause platelet aggregation commonly called microangiopathy (Davies et al., 1974). This can lead to the release of platelet autoantibodies that in turn releases procoagulants and thereby causing fibrin deposits. Subsequently microthrombi formation or disseminated intravascular coagulation occurs (Igbokwe, 1994). During trypanosomosis, erythrocytes with weak cell membranes become fragmented and lyse as they squeeze through the fibrin deposits of the microthrombi (Anosa & Kaneko, 1983; Murray & Dexter, 1988). Disseminated intravascular coagulation has been reported in *T. b. gambiense* infection of the baboon (*Papio anubis*) (Mbaya et al., 2009b), *T. vivax* infection of cattle (Isoun and Esuroroso, 1972) and in goats (Vanden Inh et al., 1976; Anosa & Isoun, 1983).

7. Anaemia caused by trypanosome toxins and metabolites

Living and dead trypanosomes can produce various forms of active chemical substances, which can elicit erythrocyte injury (Tizzard & Holmes, 1976; 1977; Tizzard et al, 1977; 1978a, b, c; Zwart & Veenendal, 1978; Naessens et al., 2005). Common among these chemical substances are proteases, neuraminidase, phospholipase, free fatty acids, pyruvates and aromatic by-products. Neuraminidase has been generated *in-vitro* by *T. vivax* during periods of parasitaemia, making erythrocytes prone to phagocytosis (Esievo, 1979; 1983). One of the factors that make erythrocytes prone to phagocytosis by the expanded mononuclear phagocytic system (MPS) during trypanosomosis is associated with the activity of neuraminidase. This enzyme cleaves off sialic acids on the surface of erythrocytes and thereby disabling them (Verma & Gautam, 1978; Igbokwe, 1994; Adamu et al., 2009) and by damaging erythropoietin (Igbokwe et al., 1989).

Trypanosomes are capable of releasing proteolytic lysosomal enzymes (proteases) from pockets on their flagella and from damaged or dead trypanosomes (Vickermon & Tetley, 1978; Rautenberg et al., 1982; Londsdale-Eccles & Grab, 1986; Igbokwe, 1994). The enzyme, when released into the general circulation is capable of damaging erythrocytes and vascular endothelium by cleaving sialic acid fractions from the cell membrane in the form of glycopeptides (Cook et al., 1966). It was also reported that aromatic amino acids could be metabolized by trypanosome to produce toxic by-products, which acts directly on the erythrocyte cell membrane to cause osmotic fragility and lyses (Igbokwe, 1994). Similarly, phenylalanine could be catabolized to phenylpyruvate, which is proteolytic in nature and inhibitory to mitochondrial gluconeogenesis (Igbokwe, 1994). Tryptophan can also be broken down during trypanosomosis to indole-ethanol, which damages erythrocyte cell membranes (Igbokwe, 1994).

8. Lipid peroxidation

The mechanism of aneamia in trypanosomosis is greatly associated with the generation of free radicals and super oxides following lipid peroxidation. These oxidative products generally attack the cellular integrity of erythrocytes during trypanosomosis (Anosa & Kaneko, 1983; Igbokwe, 1994; Umar et al., 2007). They also particularly attack erythrocyte membrane polyunsaturated fatty acids and proteins (Slater, 1984) or red blood cells directly leading to oxidative haemolysis (Ameh, 1984; Igbokwe, et al., 1989; Umar et al., 2007). Sialic acids consist of about four derivatives of nine-carbon sugar neuraminic acids (Varki, 1992; Schauer & Kamerling, 1997). It was therefore concluded that anaemia in trypanosomosis might occur due to erythrophagocytosis (Holmes & Jennings, 1976) and may be associated with the formation of antigen-antibody complexes with sialic acids (Audu et al., 1999). Esievo et al. (1982) pointed out that trypanosomosis may cause a deficit in the systematic antioxidant capacity of the infected host. This has been demonstrated in acute T. b. gambiense infection in rats (Ameh, 1984), T. evansi (Wolkmer et al., 2009) and in T. brucei infected mice (Igbokwe et al., 1989), where erythrocytes were susceptible to free radical-damage following hydrogen peroxidation. This process in mice led to enhanced oxidative haemolysis. Peroxidation caused the erythrocytes to produce large quantities of lipid peroxidation by-products. This is suggestive therefore that erythrocytes of the infected animals possessed decreased antioxidant ability, leading to its inability to withstand oxidative stress (Igbokwe, 1994). Trypanosoma vivax produced neuraminidase enzyme, which had a direct relationship with parasitaemia. It was therefore concluded that neuraminidase produced by trypanosomes in-vivo, cleaved off erythrocyte surface sialic acid, making the red cells prone to phagocytosis. Similarly, Nok and Balogun (2003) showed a progressive increase in the level of serum sialic acid corresponding with anaemia and parasitaemia in T. congolense infected mice. Trypanosoma vivax was observed to be highly erythrogenic in mice, which was probably associated with depressed erythropoietin activity following the cleaving of sialic acid fragments (Igbokwe et al., 1989). It has also been reported that glycolysis in trypanosomosis leads to the accumulation of pyruvate in-vivo as parasitaemia increases (Grant & Fulton, 1957; Coleman et al., 1957).

A ten-fold increase of pyruvate has been observed in T. brucei infected rabbits (Goodwin & Guy, 1973). In as much as the influence of pyruvate is debatable, it may not reach toxic levels in the blood during trypanosomosis (Igbokwe, 1994) however, Newton (1978) suggested that pyruvate might lead to acidosis and a lowered affinity of haemoglobulin for oxygen. It also inhibited the tricarboxylic acid cycle (TCA) in human mitochondria during T. b. gambiense infection (Seed & Hall, 1985). After death and autolysis, trypanosomosis releases large quantities of phospholipase A1 and lysophospholipase A1 (Tizard et al., 1978c). These chemical substances can cause erythrocyte degradation, damage to vascular endothelial cells and haemolysis (Colley et al., 1973). Phospholipase A1 was demonstrated in extreme proportions *in-vitro* in tissue fluids and less in plasma of rabbits infected with *T. brucei* (Hambrey et al., 1980). Tizard et al. (1978a, c) observed that phospholipase released free fatty acids (FFA) from phosphatidylcholine *in-vivo*. Most common of them were palmitic, stearic and linoleic acids (Tizard & Holmes, 1977).

Tizard et al. (1978b) reported that linoleic acid possessed a detergent - like activity, which produced severe haemolysis and cytotoxicity *in-vitro*. It was however believed that free fatty acids are easily bound by albumin and may not cause haemolysis *in-vivo*. The author however pointed out that during high parasitaemia in *T. congolense* infection, the FFA released exceeded the binding capacity of albumin and thereby leading to cytotoxicity and haemolysis. Similarly, it was reported that even the albumin bound FFA may cause haemolysis due to the activities of its oxidized products. Nok et al. (1992a, b) reported that trypanosomes could cause certain alterations that invariably affected erythrocyte membrane fluidity hence a decrease in erythrocyte membrane-bound enzymes (NoK-ATpase and CaMg-ATpase). Lipid peroxidation of membranes has been associated with decrease in membranes fluidity and in the activities of membrane-bound enzyme (McCay & King, 1980; Slater, 1984; Igbokwe, 1994). It was however suggested that a comprehensive study in ruminants is needed to highlight the extent of anti-oxidant deficiency and the degree of susceptibility of red cells to oxidative damage during trypanosomosis (Igbokwe, 1994).

9. Idiopathic serum factors

In trypanosomosis, an unknown (idiopathic) serum factor, not of a trypanosome origin but a heat stable-protein has been demonstrated to inhibit activities of erythropoiesis (Kaaya et al., 1979; 1980). It was however reported that serum from cattle infected with *T. congolense* and *T. vivax* did not depress colonies of erythrocytes *in-vitro*. However, an unknown serum factor entirely different from those reported by Kaaya et al. (1979; 1980) had effect on an erythroid colony (Igbokwe et al., 1989).

10. Immune complexes

Immunological mechanisms in trypanosomosis have been advanced as a major reason for the removal of erythro autolologous immunoglobulin (IgM and IgG) antibodies and complement (C3) on the surface of red cells (Kobayashi et al., 1976; Facer et al., 1982; Assoku & Gardiner, 1992; Naessens et al., 2005). The mechanism suggested that autoantibodies appeared after the first peak of parasitaemia that correlated with the decline in packed cell volume (PCV). Red cell surfaces may bind auto or poly reactive antibodies, or may be sensitized by absorption of immune complexes (Naessens et al., 2005). Alternatively, erythrocytes may passively absorb trypanosome molecules followed by binding of antitrypanosome antibodies with subsequent removal from the system (Rifkin & Lansberger, 1990; Naessens et al., 2005). Although Naessen et al. (2005) reported that immunological competence is not essential for the development of anaemia, irradiated rats still became anaemic after *T. brucei* infection (Murray & Dexter, 1988) and when cattle were depleted of T-cells. The authors also reported that specific, non-specific antibody production was drastically reduced, delayed, and at the same time, anaemia was consistent. Several authors (Ikede & Losos, 1972; Mackenzie & Cruickshank, 1973; Mackenzie et al., 1978; Anosa & Isoun, 1983; Igbokwe, 1994) reported an overwhelming proliferation of tissue macrophages during trypanosomosis.

The activation of macrophages was through lymphokines, antigen-antibody complexes and C3b complement fragments (Woo & Kobayashi, 1975; Allison, 1978). It was suggested therefore, that cytokines mediated loss of erythrocytes in trypanosomosis (Naessens et al., 2005). Similarly, strong evidence suggested that anaemia in trypanosomosis was mediated by TNF-a, IFN gamma and other inflammatory cytokines (Jelkmann, 1998). However, in more recent studies (Nemeth et al., 2004) suggested that anaemia in trypanosomosis involving hypofferaemia was caused by IL-6 and hepeidin. Although Naessens et al. (2005) concluded that this is unlikely to cause anaemia in trypanosomosis, some weak evidence of the role of THF-a-in the severity of anaemia in trypanosome-infected cattle (Silegham et al., 1994), mice infected with *T. brucei* (Magez et al., 1999) and in *T. brucei gambiense* infected mice (Naesens et al., 2005) was documented.

11. Malnutrition

Trypanosomosis may cause a drop in feed intake hence there is energy deficit and loss of tissue associated with catabolism of body fat, deficiencies of vitamin C, B and essential amino acids (Igbokwe, 1994). Inadequate energy supply to erythrocytes may alter the erythrocyte membrane surface therefore leading to weakening of the cell membrane, increased osmotic fragility and haemolysis (Jennings, 1976).

12. Tumor necrosis factor/Bone marrow nitric oxide (NO)

It has been reported that tumor necrosis factor (TNF) production by monocytes from cattle infected with *Trypanosoma (Duttonella) vivax* and *T. (Nannomonas) congolense*, was found to play in concert in the severity of anaemia associated with trypanosomosis (Sileghem et al., 1994). Bone marrow cell population from *T. brucei* infected mice exhibited levels of bone marrow nitric oxide production. This was found to coincide with suppressed bone marrow T-cell proliferation in response to stimulation with mitogen concanavalin *in-vivo* and *in-vitro*. It was therefore concluded that nitric oxide might inhibit proliferation of haemopoitic precursors leading to anaemia in trypanosomosis (Mabbot & Sternberg, 1995; Liew & Turner, 1999). A similar synthesis of nitric oxide and cytokines leading to anaemia in human trypanosomosis has been reported (MacLean et al., 2001).

13. Conclusion

The mechanism of anaemia in trypanosomosis was caused mainly by extra vascular haemolysis in the expanded active mononuclear phagocytic system of the host. This was followed by a drastic reduction of all red blood cell indices during successive waves of parasitaemia. The pattern of anaemia varied, depending on whether the specie of trypanosome was "humoral" or "haemic". Although the mechanism of anaemia is complex and multifactorial, it primarily compromised the cellular integrity of erythrocytes leading to either haemolytic anaemia or enhanced erythrophagocytosis. Injuries sustained by red blood cell (RBC) membranes caused by the flagella and microtubule reinforced body of the organisms greatly enhanced erythrophagocyosis of damaged RBC by the MPS. Similarly, erythrocytes, reticulocytes and platelets that adhered to trypanosomes via sialic acid receptors, caused injuries to erythrocyte membrane at the point of contact. Other factors that promoted haemolytic anaemia in trypanosomosis were trypanosome autolysates, immunochemical reactions, platelet aggregation, undulating pyrexia, oxidative stress, lipid peroxidation, nutritional and hormonal imbalances, disseminated intravascular coagulation, idiopathic and tumor necrosis factors (TNF) and bone marrow nitric oxide (NO) activity.

14. Acknowledgement

The authors highly appreciate the efforts of Professor I.O. Igbokwe in providing some of the literature used in this chapter.

15. References

Abenga. J.N. & Anosa, V.O. (2006). Clinical studies on experimental Gambian trypanosomosis in vervet monkeys, *Veternarski Arhiv* 76(1): (February 2008), 11-18, ISSN 0372-5480

Adamu, S., Maashin Useh, N., Ibrahim, D.N., Nok, A.J. & Esievo, K.A.N. (2009). Erythrocyte surface sialic acid depletion as predisposing factor to erythrocyte destruction in sheep experimental   model of African trypanosomosis: A preliminary Report, *Slovenian Veterinary Research* 46(1): (March 2009), 19-28, ISSN 1580-4003

Allison, A.C. (1978). Mechanisms by which activated macrophages inhibit lymphocyte responses, *Immunology Review* 40: (June 1979), 23-27, ISSN 1550-6606

Ameh, D.A. (1984). Depletion of reduced glutathione and the susceptibility of erythrocytes to   oxidative haemolysis in rats infected with *Trypanosoma brucei gambiense*, *Parasitology and Infectious Disease* 12: (March 2008), 130-139, ISSN 1996-0778

Anosa, V.O. (1977). *Studies on the Mechanism of Anaemia and the Pathology of Experimental Trypanosoma   vivax (Zieman, 1905) Infection in Sheep and Goats.* PhD Thesis, University of Ibadan, Ibadan, Nigeria

Anosa, V.O. (1988). Haematological and biochemical changes in human and animal trypanosomosis, Parts I & II, *Revue d' Elevage et de Medicine Ve'te'rinaire des pays Tropicaux* 41(2): (June 1988), 65-78, ISSN 151-164

Anosa, V.O. & Isoun, T.T. (1980). Haematological studies on *Trypanosoma vivax* infection of goats and splenectomized sheep, *Journal of Comparative Pathology* 90 (4): (November 1980), 153-168, ISSN 1695-7504

Anosa, V.O. & Isoun, T.T. (1983). Pathology of experimental *Trypanosoma vivax* infection in sheep and goats, *Zentraiblatt fur veterinarmedizin* 30 (1): (November 1983), 685-700, ISSN 0721-1856

Anosa, V.O. & Kaneko, J.J. (1983). Pathogenesis of *Trypanosoma brucei* infection in deer mice (*Peromyscus maniculatus*), Light and electron microscopic studies on erythrocyte pathologic changes and phagocytosis, *American Journal of Veterinary Research* 44 (4): (August 1983) 645-651, ISSN 0002- 9645

Assoku, R.K.G. & Gardiner, P.R. (1992). Detection of antibodies to platelets and erythrocytes during   haemorrhagic *Trypanosoma vivax* infection of Ayrshire cattle, *Veterinary Parasitology* 31(2): (April 2009) 199-216, ISSN 1932-6203

Audu, P.A., Esievo, K.A.N., Mohammed, G. & Ajanusi, O.J. (1999). Studies of infectivity and pathogenicity of an isolate of *Trypanosoma evansi* in Yankasa sheep, *Veterinary Parasitology* 86 (4): (October 1999) 185-190, ISSN 0304-4017

Banks, K.L. (1980). Injury induced by *Trypanosoma congolense* adhesions to cell membranes, *Journal of Parasitology* 6(1): (October 1980) 34-37, ISSN 0002-9645

Barret-Connor, E., Ugoretz, J.R. & Braude, A.I. (1973). Disseminated intravascular coagulation in trypanosomiasis, *Archives of Internal Medicine* 131(4): (April 1973) 574-577, ISSN 0003-9926

Bungener, W. & Muller, G. (1976). Adharenz phanomene bei *Trypanosoma congolense* [Adgerence phenomena in *Trypanosoma congolense*], *Tropenmedizin und parasitologie* 27 (2): (September 1976) 370-371, ISSN 0303-4208

Coleman, R.M., Brand, T. & von (1957). Blood pyruvate levels of rats during haematophagus infections, *Journal of Parasitology* 43 (1): (June 1957) 263-270, ISSN 0022-3395

Colley, C.M., Zwaal, R.F.A., Roeofsen, B. & Decssen, L.L.M. van (1973). Lytic and non-lytic degradation of phospholipids in mammalian erythrocytes by pure phospholipase, *Biochimica et Biophsica Acta* 307(1): (April 1973) 74-82, ISSN 0006-3002

Cook, G.M.W., Heard, D.H. & Seaman, G.V.F. (1966). A sialomuscopeptide liberated by trypsin from the human erythrocyte, Nature (*London*) 188 (1): (August 1967) 1011-1012, ISSN 1523-1747

Davies, C.E., Robins, R.S., Weller, R.D. & Broude, A.I. (1974). Thrombocytopenia in experimental trypanosomiasis, *Journal of Clinical Investigation* 53(1): (June 1974) 1359-1367, ISSN 1558-8238

Edwards, E.E., Judd, J.M. & Squire, F.A. (1956). Observations on trypanosomiasis in domestic animals in West Africa II, The effect on erythrocyte sedimentation rate, plasma protein, bilirubin, blood sugar, osmotic fragility, body weight and temperature in goats and sheep infected with *Trypanosoma vivax, T. congolense* and *T. brucei, Annals of Tropical Medicine and Parasitology* 50(2): (December 1957) 242-251, ISSN 0003-4983

Esievo, K.A.N. (1979). *In-vitro* production of neuraminidase (sialidase) by *Trypanosoma vivax, Proceedings of the 16th meeting of the International Scientific Council for Trypanosomiasis. Nairobi, Kenya: Organization of African Unity, Scientific, Technical and Research and Control*, pp. 205-210, ISSN 0372-5480, Yaoundé, Cameroon, August 24-29, 1978

Esievo, K.A.N. (1983). *Trypanosoma vivax*, stock V 953: inhibitory effect of type A influenza virus anti HAV8 serum on *in-vitro* neuraminidase (sialidase) activity, *Journal of Parasitology* 69(1): (December 1983) 491-495, ISSN 0022-3395

Esievo, K.A.N., Saror, D.I., Ilemobade, A.A. & Hallaway, M.H. (1982). Variation in erythrocyte surface and free serum sialic acid concentrations during experimental *Trypanosoma vivax* infection in cattle, *Research in Veterinary Science* 32 (2): (January 1982) 1-5, ISSN 0034-5288

Facer, C.A., Crosskey, J.M., Clarkson, M.J. & Jenkins, G.C. (1982). Immune haemolytic anaemia in bovine trypanosomiasis, *Journal of Comparative Pathology* 92(1): (October 1973) 293-401, ISSN 0721-1856

Goodwin, L.G. & Guy, M.W. (1973). Tissue fluids in rabbits infected with *Trypanosoma* (*Trypanozoon*) *brucei, Parasitology* 66 (1): (September, 1973) 499-513, ISSN 0031-1820

Grant, P.T. & Fulton, J.D. (1957). The catabolism of glucose by strains of *Trypanosoma rhodesiense, Biochemical Journal* 66 (2): (October 1957) 242-243, ISSN 0264-6021

Hambry, P.N., Tizard, I.R. & Mellors, A. (1980). Accumulation of phospholipase A1 in tissue fluid of rabbits infected with *Trypanosoma brucei, Tropen medizin und parasitologie* 31(1): (December 1980) 439-443, ISSN 0303-4208

Holmes, P.H. & Jennings, F.W. (1976). *Pathogenicity of parasitic infections*, Academic Press New York, ISBN 0372-5480, New York, USA

Igbokwe, I.O., Obagaiye, I.K., Esievo, K.A.N. & Saror, D.I. (1989). Dyserythropoesis in animal trypanosomiasis, *Revue d'Elavage et de Medicine veterinaire des pays Tropicaux* 42(4): (November 1990) 423-429, ISSN 0035-1865

Igbokwe, I.O. (1994). Mechanisms of cellular injury in African trypanosomiasis, *Veterinary Bulletin* 64(7): (March 1994), 611-620, ISSN 1684-5315

Ikede, B.O. & Losos, G.K. (1972). Pathology of the disease in sheep produced experimentally by *Trypanosoma brucei*, *Veterinary Pathology* 9(2): (July 1972) 278-289, ISSN 0300-9858

Isoun, T.T. & Esuruoso, G.O. (1972). Pathology of natural infection of *Trypanosoma vivax* in cattle, *Nigerian Veterinary Journal* 1(2): (September 1972), 42-45, ISSN 0721-1856

Jelkmann, W. (1998). Proinflamatory cytokines lowering erythropoietin production, *Journal of Interferon Cytokine Research* 18(2): (March 1998), 555-559, ISSN 0022-3751

Jennings, F.W. (1976). The anaemia of parasitic infections, *Proceedings of the 7th International Conference of the World Association for the Advancement of Veterinary Parasitology*, pp. 41-67, ISBN 0-12655 365- 3, Thessalonica, Greece, October 15-19, 1975

Kaaya, G.P., Valli, V.F., Maxie, M.G. & Losos, G.J. (1979). Inhibition of bovine granulocyte/macrophage colony formation *in-vitro* by serum collected from cattle infected with *Trypanosoma vivax* or *T. congolense*, *Tropen medizin und parasitologie* 30(2): (June 1979), 230- 235, ISSN 0303-4208

Kaaya, G.P., Tizard, I.R., Maxie, M.G. & Vall, V.O. (1980). Inhibition of leucopoiesis by sera from *Trypanosoma congolense* infected calves, partial characterization of the inhibitory factor, *Tropen medizin und parasitologie* 30(1): (June 1980), 230-235, ISSN 0303-4208

Karle, H. (1974). The pathogenesis of the anaemia of chronic disorders and the role of fever in erythrogenesis, *Scandinavian Journal of Haematology*, 13 (1): (October 1974), 81-86, ISSN 0036- 5534

Kobayashi, A., Tizard, I.R. & Woo, P.T.K. (1976). Studies on the anaemia in experimental African trypanosomiasis II. The pathogenesis of the anaemia in calves infected with *Trypanosoma congolense*, *American Journal of Tropical Medicine and Hygiene* 25(1): (May 1976), 401-406, ISSN 0002-9637

Liew, F.Y. & Turner, C.M.R. (1999). T. cell responses during *Trypanosoma brucei* infections in mice deficient in inducible nitric oxide synthase, *Infection and Immunology* 67(1): (May 1999), 3334- 3338, ISSN 0022-1767

Lonsdale-Eccles, J.D. & Grab, D.J. (1986). Proteases in African trypanosomes. In: Cytokine proteinases and their inhibitors, V.J. Turk, (Ed.), 189-197, Walter de Grayter, Berlin, Germany

MacLean, L., Odiit, M., & Sternberg, J.M. (2001). Nitric oxide and cytokine synthesis in human African trypanosomiasis, *The Journal of Infectious Disease* 184(4): (July 2001), 1086-1090, ISSN 0022-1899

Mackenzie, P.K.I. & Cruickshank, J.G. (1973). Phagocytosis of erythrocytes and leucocytes in sheep infected with *Trypanosoma congolense* (Broden, 1904), *Research in Veterinary Sciences* 15(1): (February 1973), 256-262, ISSN 0034-5288

Mackenzie, P.K.I., Boyt, W.P., Nesham, V.W. & Pirie, E. (1978). The etiology and significance of the phagocytosis of erythrocytes in sheep infected with *Trypanosoma congolense* (Broden, 1904), *Research in Veterinary Sciences* 24 (1): (April 1978), 4-7, ISSN 0034-5288

Mabbot, N. & Sternberg, J. (1995). Bone marrow nitric oxide production and development of anaemia in *Trypanosoma brucei* infected mice, *Infection and Immunology* 63(4): (June 1995), 1563-1566, ISSN 1098-5522

Magez, S., Radwanaska, M., Beschin, A., Sekikawa, K. & Debaetselier, P. (1999). Tumor necrosis factor alpha is a key mediator in the regulation of experimental *Trypanosoma brucei* infections, *Infection and Immunology* 67(5): (June 1999), 3128-3132, ISSN 1098-5522

Maxie, M.G. & Losos, G.J. (1979). Release of *Trypanosoma vivax* from the microcirculation of cattle by Berenil®, *Veterinary Parasitology* 3: (June 1979), 277-281, ISSN 0019-9867

McCay, P.B. & King, M.M. (1980). Endogenous sources of free radicals, In: Basic and Clinical Nutrition and development of anaemia in *Trypanosoma brucei* infected mice, L.J. Machlin, (Ed.), 269-303, Marcel Decker Inc, New York, USA

Mbaya, A.W., Nwosu, C.O. & Onyeyili, P.A. (2007). Toxicity and anti-trypanosomal effects of ethanolic extract of *Butyrospermum paradoxum* (*Sapotacea*) stem bark in rats infected with *Trypanosoma brucei* and *T. congolence*, *Journal of Ethnopharmacology* 111: (May 2007), 536-530, ISSN 0378-8741

Mbaya, A.W., Aliyu, M.M., Nwosu, C.O., Taiwo, V.O. & Ibrahim, U.I. (2009a). Effects of melarsamine hydrochloride (Cymelarsan®) and diaminazene aceturate (Berenil®) on the pathology of experimental *Trypanosoma brucei* infection in red fronted gazelles (*Gazella rufifrons*), *Veterinary Parasitology*, 163 (1-2): (July 2009), 140-143, ISSN 0304-4071

Mbaya, A.W., Aliyu, M.M., Nwosu, C.O. & Taiwo, V.O. (2009b). An assessment of the efficacy of DFMO in baboons (*Papio anubis*) infected with *Trypanosoma brucei gambiense*, *Global Journal of Pure and Applied Sciences*, 15 (1): (September 2009), 69-78, ISSN 1118-0579

Mbaya, A.W., Aliyu, M.M., Nwosu, C.O. & Ibrahim, U.I. (2009c). Effect of DL-α-difluoromethylornithine on biochemical changes in baboons (*Papio anubis*) experimentally infected with *Trypanosoma brucei gambiense*, *Nigerian Veterinary Journal*, 30(1): (September 2009), 35-44, ISSN 0331-3026

Mbaya, A.W., Aliyu, M.M. & Ibrahim, U.I. (2009d). Clinico-pathology and mechanisms of trypanosomosis in captive and free-living wild animals: A review, *Veterinary Research Communications*, 33: (April 2009), 793 – 809, ISSN 1573-7446

Mbaya, A.W., Aliyu, M.M., Nwosu, C.O. & Egbe-Nwiyi, T.N.C. (2009e). The relationship between parasitaemia and anaemia in a concurrent *Trypanosoma brucei* and *Haemonchus contortus* infection in red fronted gazelles (*Gazella rufifrons*), *Veterenarski Arhiv*, 79 (5): (September 2009), 451-460, ISSN 03720-5480

Mbaya, A.W., Ibrahim, U.I. & Apagu, S. T. (2010). Trypanosomosis of the dromedary camel (*Camelus dromedarius)* and its vectors in the tsetse-free arid zone of northeastern, Nigeria, *Nigerian Veterinary Journal*, 31(3): (September 2010), 195-200, ISSN 0331-3026

Mbaya, A.W. & U.I. Ibrahim (2011). In-vivo and in-vitro activities of medicinal plants on haemic and humoral trypanosomes: A review, *International Journal of Pharmacology*, 7(1): (January 2011), 1- 11, ISSN 1812-5700

Mbaya, A. W. Nwosu, C. O. & Kumshe, H. A. (2011). Genital lesions in male red fronted gazelles (*Gazella rufifrons*) experimentally infected with *Trypanosoma brucei* and the effect of melarsamine hydrochloride (Cymelarsan®) and diminazene aceturate

(Berenil®) in their treatment. *Theriogenology,* 16: (May 2011) 721-728, ISSN 1879-3231

Morrison, W.I., Max Murray, Sayer, P.D. & Preston, J.M. (1981). The pathogenesis of experimentally induced *Trypanosoma brucei* infection in the dog, Tissue and organ damage, *American Journal of Pathology* 102: (September 1981), 168-181, ISSN 0001-5598

Murray, M. & Dexter, T.M. (1988). Anaemia in bovine African trypanosomiasis: A review, *Acta Tropica* 45: (December 1988), 389-432, ISSN 0001-706X

Murray, M. & Morrison, W.I. (1978). Parasitaemia and host susceptibility in African trypanosomiasis, *Proceedings of a workshop,* pp.71`-81, ISBN 0-088936-214−9, *Nairobi, Kenya,* Nov. 20-23, 1978

Naessens, J., Kitani, H., Yagi, Y., Sekikawa, K., Iraqqi, F. (2005). TNF-a mediates the development of anaemia in a murine *Trypanosoma brucei rhodesiense* infection, but not the anaemia associated with a murine *T. congolense* infection, Clinical and Experimental Immunology 139(3): (March 2005), 403-410, PMID: PMC 180 9320

Nazrul-Islam, A.K.M. & Woo, P.T.K. (1991). Anaemia and its mechanism in goldfish (*Carassius auratus*) infected with *Trypanosoma danilewsky, Disease of Aquatic Organisms* (11): (November 1991), 37- 43, ISSN 0177-5103

Nemeth, E., Rivera, S., Gabayan, V., Keller, C., Taudorf, S., Pedersen, B.K. & Ganz, T. (2004). IL-6 mediates hypoferremia of inflammation by inducing the synthesis of the iron regulatory hormone hepcidin, *Journal of Clinical Investigation* 113: (May 2005), 1271-1276, ISSN 0021- 9738

Newton, B.A. (1978). The metabolism of African trypanosomiasis in relation to pathogenic mechanisms, In: *Pathogenicity of trypanosomes,* G. Losos, A. Chouinard, (Eds.), pp. 17-22, ISBN 0-88936-214-9 Proceedings of a workshop, Nairobi Kenya, November 20-23, 1977

Nwosu, C.O. & Ikeme, M.M. (1992). Parasitaemia and clinical manifestations in *Trypanosoma brucei* infected dogs, *Revue d'Elavage et de Medicine veterinaire des pays Tropicaux* 45(3-4): (September 1992), 273-277, ISSN 0035-1865

Nok, A.J. & Balogun, E.O. (2003). A blood stream *Trypanosoma congolense* sialidase could be involved in anaemia during experimental trypanosomiasis, *The Journal of Biochemistry* 133(6): (June 2003), 725-730, ISSN 1756-2651

Nok, A.J., Esievo, K.A.N., Ukoha, A.I., Ikediobi, C.O., Baba, J., Tekdek, B. & Ndams, I.S. (1992a). Kidney NaK-ATPase: kinetic study of rats during chronic infection with *Trypanosoma congolense, Journal of Clinical Biochemistry and Nutrition* 13: (September 1992), 73-79, ISSN 0912- 0009

Nok, A.J., Esievo, K.A.N., Ajibike, M.O., Achoba, I.I., Tekdek, K., Gimba, C.E., Kagbu, J.A. & Ndams, I.S. (1992b). Modulation of the calcium pump of the kidney and testes of rats infected with *Trypanosoma congolense, Journal of Comparative Pathology,* 107: (July 1992), 119-123, ISSN 0021- 9975

Ogwu, D., Njoku, C.O. & Ogbogu, V.C. (1992). Adrenal and thyroid dysfunction in experimental *Trypanosoma congolense* infection in cattle, *Veterinary Parasitology* 42: (April 1992), 15-26, ISSN 0304-4017

Rabo, J.S. (1995). Toxicity studies and trypanosuppressive effects of stem bark extract of *Butyrospermum paradoxum* in laboratory animals, PhD Thesis, University of Maiduguri, Maiduguri, Nigeria

Rautenberg, P., Schedler, R., Reinwalde, E. & Risse, H.J. (1982). Study on a proteolytic enzyme from *Trypanosoma congolense*, Purification and some biochemical properties, Molecular and some biochemical properties, *Molecular and Cellular Biochemistry* 47: (September 1982), 151-159, ISSN 0300-8177

Rifkin, M.R. & Landsberger, F.R. (1990). Trypanosome variant surface glycoprotein transfer to target membranes: A model for the pathogenesis of trypanosomiasis, *Proceedings of the National Academy of Science*, pp. 801-806, ISSN 0027-8424, May 23-27 USA, 1990

Saror, D.I. (1982). Aspects of the anaemia of acute bovine trypanosomiasis, *Proceedings of the first National Conference on Tsetse and Trypanosomiasis Research*, pp. 12-14, ISSN 0049-4747, August 10-12, Kaduna, Nigeria, 1981

Schauer, R. & Kamerling, J.P. (1997). Chemistry, biochemistry and biology of sialic acid. In: *Glycoptroteins*, J. Montrevil, J. .F. G. Vigenther & H. Shachter (Eds.) 241-400, Elsevier, ISBN 0- 444-80303-3, Amsterdam, The Netherlands

Seed, J.R. and Hall, J.E. (1985). Pathophysiology of African trypanosomiasis. In: *Immunology and pathogenesis of trypanosomiasis*, I.J. Tizard (Ed.), CRC Press, ISBN 0-8493-5640-7, Boca Raton, Florida, USA

Shehu, S.A., Ibrahim, N.D.G., Esievo, K.A.N. & Mohammed, G. (2006). Role of erythrocyte surface sialic acid inducing anaemia in Savannah Brown bucks experimentally infected with *Trypanosoma evansi, Veterenarski Arhiv* 26(6): (October 2006), 521-530, ISSN 0372-5480

Sileghem, M., Flynn, J.N., Logan-Henfrey, L. & Ellis, J. (1994). Tumour necrosis factor production by monocytes from cattle infected with *Trypanosoma (Dutonella) vivax* and *T. (nannomonas) congolense*, Possible association with severity of anaemia associated with the disease, *Parasite Immunoassay*, 16(1): (January, 1994), 51-54, ISSN 0141-9838

Slater, T.F. (1984). Free radical mechanism in tissue injury, *Biochemistry Journal* 222: (August 1984), 1-15, ISSN 0264-6021

Solano, P., Dela Roqoes, S. & Duvalet, G. (2003). Biodiversity of trypanosomes pathogenic for cattle and their epidemiological importance, *Annals of Society* 68: 169 – 171.

Soulsby, E.J.L. (1982). *Helminthes, Arthropods and Protozoa parasites of domesticated Animals*, Bailere Tindal, ISBN 0702008206 9780702008207, London

Swallow, B.M. (2000): Impacts of trypanosomosis in African agriculture, Programme against African Trypanosomosis Technical and Scientific series, Food Agriculture Organization (F. A. O.) 2: (April 2000), 45 – 46, ISSN 1020-7163

Tizard, I.R. & Holmes, W.L. (1976). The generation of toxic activity from *Trypanosoma congolense*, *Experentia* 32: (May 1977), 1533-1534, 0014-4754

Tizard, I.R. & Holmes, W.L. (1977). The release of suitable vasoactive material from *Trypanosoma congolense* intraperitoneal diffusion chambers, *Transactions of the Royal Society of Tropical Medicine and Hygiene*, 71: (June 1977), 52-55, ISSN 0035-9203

Tizard, I.R., Holmes, W.L., Yorke, D.A. & Mellors, A. (1977). The generation and identification of haemolysin of *Trypanosoma congolense, Experintia* 33: (July, 1977), 901-902, ISSN 0014-4754

Tizard, I.R., Holmes, W.L. & Nielsen, K. H. (1978a). Mechanisms of anaemia in trypanosomiasis: Studies on the role of haemolytic fatty acids derived from

Trypanosoma congolense, Tropen medizin und parasitologie 29: (March, 1978), 108-114, ISSN 0303-4208

Tizard, I.R., Nielsen, K. H., Mellors, A. & Assoku, R.K.G. (1978b). Biologically active lipids generated by autolysis of *Trypanosoma congolense*. In: *Pathogenecity of Trypanosomes. Proceedings of a workshop*, pp. 103-110, ISBN 0-88936-214-9, Nairobi, Kenya, November 20-23, 1978

Tizard, I.R., Sheppard, J. & Nielsen, K. (1978c). The characterization of a second class of haemolysin from *Trypanosoma brucei, Transactions of the Royal Society of Tropical Mediciene and Hygiene* 72: (July 1978), 198-2000, ISSSN 0035-9203

Umar, I.A., Ogenyi, E., Okodaso, D., Kimeng, E., Stanecheva, G.I., Omage, J.J., Isah, S. & Ibrahim, M.A. (2007). Amelioration of anaemia and organ damage by combined intraperitoneal administration of vitamin A and C to *Trypanosoma brucei brucei* infected rats, *African Journal of Biotechnology* 6(18): (July 2007), 2083-2086, ISSN 0035-9203

Van den Ingh. T.S.G.A.M., Zwart, D., Schotman, A.J.H., Van miert, A.S.J.P.A.M. & Veenaidal, G.H. (1976). The pathology and pathogenesis of *Trypanosoma vivax* infection in the goat, *Research in Veterinary Science* 21: (June 1977), 264-270, ISSN 0034-5288

Varki, A. (1992). Diversity in the sialic acids, *Glycobiology* 2: (February 1992), 25-40, ISSN 0959-6658

Verma, B.B. & Gautam, O.P. (1978). Studies on experimental surra (*T. evansi* infection) in Buffalo and cow calves, *Indian Veterinary Journal* 55: (August 1978), 648-653, ISSN 0019-6479

Vickerman, K. & Tetley, L. (1978). Biology and ultra structure of trypanosomes in relation to pathogenesis. In: *Pathogenecity of trypanosomes*, Proceedings of a workshop, pp. 231-31, ISBN 0- 88936-214-9, Nairobi, Kenya, November 20-23, 1978

Woodruff, A.W., Topley, E., Knight, R. & Downie, C.G.B. (1972). The anaemias of Kalaazar. *British Journal of Haematology* 22: (March 1973), 319-329, ISSN 0007-1048

Wolkmer, P., Shafer da Silva, A., Treasel, C.K., Paim, F.C., Cargncutti., J.F., Pagononcelli, M., Picada,   M.E., Monterro, S.G. & Anjus Lopes, S.T. (2009). Lipid peroxidation associated with anaemia in rats experimentally infected with *Trypanosoma evansi, Veterinary Parasitology* 165: (1-2): (October 2009), 41-46, ISSN 1873-2550

Woo P.T.K. & Kobayashi, A. (1975). Studies on the anaemia in experimental African trypanosomiasis, Preliminary communication on the mechanism of the anaemia. *Annals Society Belge Medicine Tropicale* 53(1): (October 1973), 37-45, ISSN 0772-4128

Zwart, D. & Veenendal, G.H. (1978). Pharmacologically active substances in *Trypanosoma vivax* infections. In: *Pathogenecity of trypanosomes*. Proceedings of a workshop, pp. 111-113, ISBN 0-88936-214-9, Nairobi, Kenya, November 20-23, 1978

6

Molecular Basis of Thalassemia

Michela Grosso, Raffaele Sessa, Stella Puzone,
Maria Rosaria Storino and Paola Izzo
Dipartimento di Biochimica e Biotecnologie Mediche,
University of Naples Federico II
Italy

1. Introduction

Hemoglobinopathies are a heterogeneous group of monogenic disorders widespread overall. They are commonly subdivided into three partially overlapping subgroups: structural variants which comprise the sickle cell anemia syndrome; thalassemias, characterized by a reduced rate of synthesis of one or more globin chains of hemoglobin; conditions of high persistence of fetal hemoglobin in adulthood (HPFH) (Weatherall & Clegg, 2001).

As a group, they are the commonest monogenic disorders in the world population. It is thought that the high prevalence of these defects could be due to selective advantage of the carrier state to malaria infection. However, in spite of epidemiological evidences supporting this hypothesis as well as of extensive hematological studies, the mechanisms underlying this protection still remain unknown. It is, however, evident that as a consequence of this positive selection, these diseases are mostly common in geographic areas extending from the Mediterranean region through tropical countries including Sub-Saharian Africa, the Middle East, India, Southeast Asia and Indonesia, where malaria was or still is endemic (Weatherall & Clegg, 2001). In many of these areas the estimated frequencies of these disorders range from 3 to 10 percent, even though in some specific areas the carrier frequencies may be higher, reaching 80-90% in some tribal populations in India (Harteveld & Higgs, 2010). Because of their high frequencies, different hemoglobin defects may be co-inherited, giving rise to an extremely complex series of genotypes and clinical phenotypes. In fact, in many regions thalassemic defects coexist with structural Hb variants; it is also quite common for individuals from areas at high frequency of thalassemic defects to inherit genes for more than one type of thalassemia. Furthermore, some Hb variants are synthesized at reduced rate or are highly instable, leading both to functional and structural deficiency of the affected globin chain, thus resulting in a thalassemic condition, generally showing dominant inheritance. These complex interactions contribute to generate a wide range of clinical disorders that, taken together, constitute the thalassemic syndromes (Weatherall, 2001).

The complex and heterogeneous spectrum of molecular defects underlying these inherited conditions is regionally specific and in most cases the geographic and ethnic distributions have been determined, providing support for prevention programs based on screening, genetic counselling and prenatal diagnosis in couples at risk.

On the other hand, as the result of mass migration of populations from areas at high risk, hemoglobinopathies are being seen with increasing frequency even in regions where they were rather uncommon.

In Italy eight point mutations represent about 90% of β-thalassemia defects (Rosatelli et al., 1992) with the remaining 10% being represented by a wide array of molecular defects, some of which very rare. Furthermore, recent intensive immigration flows moving from countries with high incidence of hemoglobinopathies (Middle East, Southeast Asia and Northern Africa) with their own specific pattern of mutations as well, has rapidly increased the molecular heterogeneity of hemoglobinopathies in our region. This condition requires additional efforts to allow rapid and feasible carrier and prenatal screening programs.

2. Organization and structure of human globin genes

Hemoglobin tetramer is composed by two α-like and two β-like globin chains which are encoded by genes localized in two clusters where they are arranged in a sequential mode in the $5'{\rightarrow}3'$ direction, according to their order of activation and expression during ontogenesis (Weatherall & Clegg, 2001). The α-like gene cluster is located in a region of about 30 kb in the telomeric region on the short arm of chromosome 16 (Fig. 1). It includes in the $5'{\rightarrow}3'$ order an embryonal gene (ζ2), three pseudogenes, (Ψζ1, Ψα2, Ψα1), the α2 and α1 genes and the pseudogene θ. The β-like gene cluster is located in a region of DNA of about 60 kb on the short arm of chromosome 11 (Fig. 2). It includes in the $5'{\rightarrow}3'$ order the genes ε, $^Gγ$, $^Aγ$, the pseudogene Ψβ followed by the δ and β genes (Weatherall & Clegg, 2001). All globin genes share a similar structure which includes three coding exons separated by two introns. Conserved sequences critical for gene expression are found in the proximal promoter regions, at the exon-intron boundaries and in the 5' and 3' untranslated (UTR) regions. The fetal globin chains are encoded by two genes, $^Gγ$ and $^Aγ$ which share the same sequence, except in the proximal promoter region and at codon 136, where a glicine residue ($^Gγ$) is replaced by alanine ($^Aγ$). Besides typical promoter and enhancer elements, each globin gene cluster has an upstream regulatory region which plays a crucial role to promote erythroid-specific gene expression and to coordinate the developmental regulation of each gene. In the β-gene cluster this region is known as Locus Control Region (LCR), a relatively large element, encompassing ~20 Kb. It is located approximately 25 Kb upstream of the most proximal ε-globin gene and contains five DNase I hypersensitive (HS) erythroid specific sites (HS-1 HS-2 HS-3 HS-4 HS-5). These sites define sub-regions of open chromatin that are bound by multi-protein complexes (Fig. 2). Similarly a regulatory region, known as HS-40, is located in the α-gene cluster, upstream of the embryonal α-like globin gene (Fig. 1) (Cao & Moi, 2002; Ho & Thein, 2000; Weatherall & Clegg, 2001).

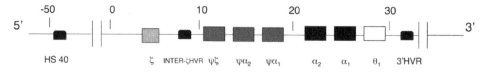

Fig. 1. **Structure of the α-gene cluster on chromosome 16.** The genes are arranged spatially in the order of their expression during ontogeny.

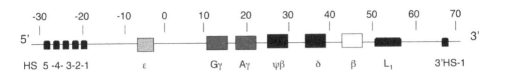

Fig. 2. **Structure of the β-gene cluster on chromosome 11.** The genes are arranged spatially in the order of their expression during ontogeny.

3. Regulation of globin gene expression

The expression of human globin genes is regulated throughout ontogeny by fine and complex mechanisms involving transcriptional, post-transcriptional and post-translational processes. The function of such a tight control is to assure that, at any stage of development, the production of α-like globin chains equals that of β-like globin chains (α/non-α ratio = 1) for the correct hemoglobin assembling (Cao & Moi, 2000). However, this mechanism of control is not able to detect whether a gene which is to be activated is functional or not. Therefore if a mutation that impairs gene expression occurs in any globin gene, it will give rise to an imbalanced globin chain production. When synthesis of α-globin genes is defective, β-like globin chains will be in excess, thus leading to α-thalassemia, whereas impaired β-globin chain output will lead to excess of α-globin chains and β-thalassemia conditions.

Transcriptional control of each globin gene expression requires distant upstream regulatory regions as well as proximal promoter regions. All proximal regulatory elements are located within the first 500 base pairs (bp), 5' to the transcriptional start (Cap) site. The promoters of all the globin genes share high homology but they also show unique sequences that may be responsible for their developmental stage-specific regulation. Three major regulatory elements with minor sequence variations are common to all globin promoter regions: the TATA, CCAAT and CACCC boxes. In the β-globin gene promoter the TATA box is located at positions -28 to -31, the CCAAT box at positions -72 to -76 and the duplicated CACCC sequences at positions -86 to -90 (proximal element) and at position -101 to -105 (distal element), respectively. It is noteworthy that, with respect to the β-globin gene promoter, the γ-globin gene shows a single CACCC element and a duplication of the CAAT box, which may have implications in the different developmental regulation of these genes. All promoter regions also contain binding sites for specific erythroid transacting factors (Cao & Moi, 2002; Ho & Thein, 2000).

All these elements, through direct interactions with the LCR and transcriptional factors, act as positive regulators and are required for optimal transcription. In fact, mutations in these sequences lead to impaired globin gene expression levels.

Several other positive regulatory elements known as enhancers have been identified within gene sequences or in intergenic regions which increase transcriptional activity of certain promoters. In the β-globin gene, enhancers are found in intron 2 and 3' to the gene, 600 to 900 bp downstream of the polyadenylation site. Silencer elements which repress gene expression play a role in the developmental control of globin gene expression, in the switch from embryonal to fetal to adult hemoglobin production. Indeed, these elements are found in the distal promoter region of the ε-globin gene and in the γ-globin genes (Oneal et al., 2006).

The primary role of the LCR in the β-globin cluster is to confer a tissue specific state of open chromatin at the globin gene loci and also to allow interaction of transacting factors with specific globin gene promoters in a developmental stage-specific manner. Specific binding site for EKLF, GATA-1 and NF-E2, three erythroid-specific transcriptional factors that play critical roles in activation of the β-globin genes, have been described both in the LCR and in the promoters of the globin genes, thus allowing speculations on the complex function of the LCR on globin gene expression. Therefore, the stage-specific expression of globin genes could depend on the location of the genes in the cluster as well as on the availability of stage-specific transcription factors (Cao & Moi, 2002; Ho & Thein, 2000).

4. Switching of globin gene expression

During ontogenesis, physiological changes in oxygen requirements are accompanied by the switching of globin gene expression (Stamatoyannopoulos G. & Gronsveld F., 2001). This process represents one of the most intriguing and studied regulatory mechanisms of gene expression which leads to progressive and sequential changes in the expression of embryonic, fetal and adult globin genes and thus allows to synthesize different types of hemoglobin tetramers. However, the detailed mechanisms that control this process are still not fully understood (Pi et al., 2010; Ross et al., 2009).

Human hemoglobin synthesis requires two switches: from embryonic to fetal hemoglobin at 6 week of gestation and from fetal to adult production at birth (Fig. 3). The first genes to be expressed are those of the ζ-chain (α-like) and ε-chain (β-like), synthesized in the embryonic yolk sac until 4-5 weeks of gestation, which lead to the formation of Hb Gowers I (ζ2ε2). Then, with the change of the liver as the main erythropoietic compartment, synthesis of α and γ chains is activated. At this stage the embryonic Hb Gowers II (α2ε2) and Hb Portland (ζ2γ2) are progressively and completely substituted by the fetal hemoglobin Hb F (α2γ2). Around birth, when the bone marrow becomes the main erythropoietic site, β-globin gene expression is activated to synthesize the adult Hb A (α2β2), which at birth is about 20% of total hemoglobin. The switch from fetal to adult hemoglobin is completed within the first two years of life and leads to the pattern in which adult globin expression HbA (α2β2) comprises about 97%, HbA2 (α2δ2) 2-3% and HbF (α2γ2) less than 1% of total hemoglobin, respectively (Stamatoyannopoulos G. & Gronsveld F., 2001).

The control of tissue and developmental expression of specific globin genes is exerted by physical interactions between the different globin gene promoters and the LCR through binding of both ubiquitous and erythroid-specific transacting factors. The sequential expression of different globin genes requires coordinated mechanisms of gene silencing and gene competition for the LCR sequences, as well as chromatin remodelling and complex chromosomal looping and tracking processes (Pi et al., 2010; Ross et al., 2009).

The switching of the expression of β-globin genes is not only a fascinating and complex model used for studying regulation mechanisms of gene expression in space and time, but its full understanding could also have important therapeutic implications in the treatment of sickle cell anemia and β-thalassemia. Indeed, the clinical picture of these conditions can improve in the presence of sufficiently high levels of HbF: in β-thalassemia syndromes, in fact, hereditary persistence or drug-mediated reactivation of γ-globin chain output may result in a reduction of the α/non α globin chain imbalance which represents the main pathogenetic factor influencing the severity of these conditions, whereas in sickle cell anemia an increase in HbF contributes to ameliorate the severity of disease by inhibiting the polymerization of sickle hemoglobin and its related pathophysiological effects (Fathallah & Atweh, 2006).

Persistent expression of fetal hemoglobin may be associated with specific genotypes (as described below in detail) or induced by appropriate drug treatments. In fact, fetal globin genes can be reactivated by demethylation of regulatory sequences generated by hydroxyurea or 5-azacytidine or by histone deacetylation induced by treatment with short-chain fatty acids (Fathallah & Atweh, 2006). However, besides toxic side effects of these drugs, response to treatment is transient and highly variable. Thus, a better understanding of the switching processes and regulatory mechanisms of fetal globin genes may indicate new therapeutic approaches in the treatment of thalassemia and sickle cell anemia by means of a permanent reactivation of the γ-globin genes.

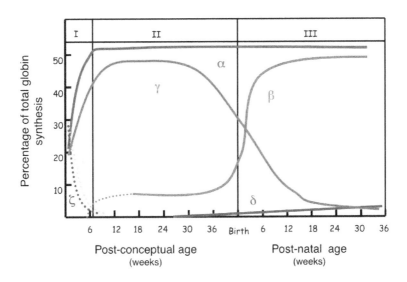

Fig. 3. **Changes in globin gene expression profile during ontogeny.** The x-axis represents the age of the fetus in weeks. The y-axis corresponds to the expression of each globin gene as a percentage of total globin gene expression. Time of birth is denoted with a vertical line. The embryonic genes are expressed during the first six weeks of gestation. The first switch from ε- to γ-globin occurs within 6 weeks after conception, and the second switch from γ- to β-globin occurs shortly after birth.

5. Molecular basis of hemoglobinopathies

With few exceptions, molecular defects affecting the globin genes are transmitted in an autosomal recessive manner and can result in:

1. Structural variants, characterized by the production of abnormal globin chains;
2. Thalassemias due to a quantitative defect in the synthesis of one or more globin chains;
3. Hereditary persistence of fetal haemoglobin (HPFH), a heterogeneous group of defects in the switch from fetal to adult globin gene expression which leads to persistent fetal hemoglobin synthesis in adult life. This condition, without any clinical relevance, is of great interest because it represents a useful model for studying the regulation of globin gene switching during development and because of its potential therapeutic role, since high HbF levels can ameliorate the severity of clinical phenotypes associated with some structural hemoglobin variants or thalassemias.

5.1 The structural variants

Over 900 hemoglobin variants have been identified so far (Weatherall & Clegg, 2001). Although their frequencies vary greatly in different ethnic groups, only three of them occur at high frequency in different populations: the Hb S, responsible of the sickle cell anemia which is distributed in the sub-Saharan region, in the Mediterranean area, in Middle East and in some Indian regions; the Hb C which is present in West Africa and certain parts of the Mediterranean area; the Hb E which occurs at very high frequency in Indian and Southern Asian populations.

The majority of human Hb variants result from single amino acid substitutions in one of the globin chains. Some rarer variants are instead characterized by elongated or shortened globin chains. Another type of structural variant is due to unequal crossing-over events with the formation of hybrid or fusion globin chains, as in the case of the Hb Lepore which involves the δ- and β-globin genes. All variants have the $\alpha_2\beta_2$ tetrameric structure, with the exception of the non-functional Hb Bart's and HbH, which are γ_4 and β_4 homotetramers, respectively.

5.2 The thalassemias

The thalassemias are a heterogeneous group of inherited disorders of hemoglobin synthesis, all characterized by the absent or reduced output of one or more globin chains. They are classified into α-, β-, δβ-, γδβ- and εγδβ-thalassemias, according to the particular globin chain(s) which is ineffectively synthesized. However, since the prevalent hemoglobin tetramer in adulthood is composed by α- and β-globin chains ($\alpha_2\beta_2$), the most relevant clinical forms are thus α- and β-thalassemias, respectively. In recent years, the molecular basis of the thalassemia syndromes have been described in detail, revealing the wide range of mutations encountered in each type of thalassemia (Galanello & Ortiga, 2010).

5.2.1 The β-thalassemias

The β-thalassemias are subdivided into the β^0-, β^+ and β^{++} groups, to designate a complete, severe or mild defect in β-globin chain synthesis, respectively (Weatherall & Clegg, 2001). This results in excess of α-globin chains and, consequently, various degrees of imbalanced α/non α chain output, which is the main determinant of the typical hematological phenotypes and the clinical severity of these conditions (Cao & Moi, 2000; Weatherall, 2001).

Molecular basis of β-thalassemia are extremely heterogeneous. So far, more than 200 different β-thalassemic mutations have been described. Most of them are point mutations (single base changes, small deletions or insertions), whereas only a minority are due to large deletions encompassing the β-globin cluster (a comprehensive database of thalassemia and other globin gene defects is available at http://globin.cse.psu.edu/).

These mutations may occur in exon or intron sequences, as well as in the promoter or the 5' and 3' flanking UTR sequences (Fig. 4). As a consequence of the type and the position in which these defects fall, they have been reported to affect expression of the β-globin gene at the following stages:

- transcription efficiency, for mutations occurring in the promoter region, i.e., recognition sequences for proteins involved in transcriptional or post-transcriptional mechanisms such as the conserved TATA, CCAAT and CACCC boxes. Generally, such mutations are of β^+ or β^{++} types, thus resulting in mild forms of β-thalassemia;

- maturation of pre-mRNA, if they fall into splicing or polyadenylation sites. RNA-splicing mutations are fairly common and represent a large portion of all β-thalassemic mutations. These mutations affect the splicing process at variable degree, depending on the position in which the mutation occurs. Mutations that affect either of the invariant dinucleotide at the intron-exon junction (the GT motif at the 5' or donor site and the AG motif at the 3' or acceptor site) completely abolish normal splicing and result in β^0-thalassemia. Mutations occurring in the splicing consensus sequences are instead of β^+ type, resulting in variable degrees of defective splicing and causing milder types of β-thalassemia. Other mutations occurring in exon or intron sequences may activate a cryptic splicing site, thus leading to abnormal mRNA processing. Even in these cases defective splicing occurs at variable degrees, resulting in phenotypes that range from mild to severe;

- RNA stability, if they occur in the 5' UTR, Cap site, 3' UTR or the polyadenylation site. These mutations are generally associated with mild β-thalassemia phenotypes. In particular, mutations occurring in the 5' UTR are so mild that they act as silent β-thalassemic alleles which generally show normal hematological phenotypes in heterozygotes.

- mRNA translation, if they generate premature nonsense codons. Premature termination of globin chain synthesis generally leads to the production of short, nonviable β-chains or to nonsense mediated decay (NMD) of abnormal mRNA. In all these cases mutations are of β^0-type and result in severe thalassemia;

- protein instability, if they give rise to truncated or elongated globin chains which tend to form insoluble tetramers.

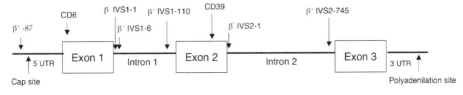

Fig. 4. **Schematic representation of the β-globin gene.** The arrows show the positions of the most frequent β-thalassemic mutations in the Mediterranean area (Rosatelli et al., 1992).

5.2.2 The α-thalassemias

Alpha thalassemias are characterized by absent (α^0-thalassemia) or reduced (α^+-thalassemia) output of α-globin chains, thus resulting in globin chain imbalance. As a consequence, there is a relative excess of γ-and β-globin chains which aggregate to form the homotetramers Hb Bart's and HbH, respectively, and are responsible of a severe hemolytic anemia. The two main groups of α-thalassemia can be further subdivided into deletional and non-deletional forms, according to the specific type of the underlying molecular defect. In fact, the majority of the α-thalassemia defects result from deletions involving one or both α-globin genes on the same chromosome whereas point mutations affecting the functional expression of one of the two α-globin genes (α_2 or α_1 globin gene) are less common (Harteveld & Higgs, 2010; Higgs & Gibbons, 2010). The cause of the increased susceptibility to such deletional defects for the α-globin cluster with respect to the β-globin cluster is due to the presence of highly homologous regions scattered within this cluster which predispose to events of unequal recombination. Normal individuals have four α-globin genes since each chromosome 16 carries two α-globin genes (Fig. 1); therefore, normal genotypes can be written as $\alpha\alpha/\alpha\alpha$. Deletions so far reported result in loss of one (-α) or both (--α) of the duplicated α-globin genes from the same chromosome (Kattamis et al., 1996). The clinical picture of α-thalassemia is determined by the number of the remaining functional genes. The deletional loss of the α_2 or α_1 gene (namely, the $-\alpha^{4.2}$ and $-\alpha^{3.7}$ deletion, respectively) are the most common molecular defects responsible for α-thalassemia. These two mutations have been found, even with different frequencies, in all populations in which thalassemia defects are common. The unequal crossing-over events responsible for their origin give also rise to the corresponding triplicated or quadruplicated α-gene arrangements which are referred to as $\alpha\alpha\alpha^{anti3.7}$ and $\alpha\alpha\alpha^{anti4.2}$ or $\alpha\alpha\alpha\alpha^{anti3.7}$ and $\alpha\alpha\alpha\alpha^{anti4.2}$, respectively. In α^0-thalassemias large deletions almost entirely remove the α-globin cluster region. The two most common α^0-thalassemias, the $--^{SEA}$ and $-^{MED}$ occur in Southeast Asia and Mediterranean area, respectively (Sessa et al., 2010; Harteveld & Higgs, 2010; Kattamis et al., 1996; Mesbah-Amroun et al., 2008) (Fig. 5).

Non-deletional α-thalassemias (indicated at the heterozygous state as $\alpha\alpha^T/\alpha\alpha$) are due to point mutations that, similarly to the mutations responsible for β-thalassemia, occur in genomic regions critical for normal expression of the α-genes. Furthermore, as for the β-thalassemia defects, they may be classified according to the level of gene expression that is affected and also their distribution is population-specific. However, point mutations affecting the α_2 gene are able to impair more greatly α-globin gene expression since in normal conditions the α_2 globin gene expression is about three times greater than that of the α_1 gene. Therefore, such mutations have more relevant effects on phenotype and it is expected that they could provide a greater selective advantage with respect to malaria infection. It is thus evident that they are more common than those occurring in the α_1 gene. On the other hand, non deletional α-thalassemia mutations have also a greater effect on phenotype than –α deletions. In fact, the $-\alpha^{4.2}$ deletional form of α-thalassemia which involves the α_2-globin gene results in a compensatory increase in the remaining intact α_1 gene, whereas no increased expression in the remaining functional gene is detected when the α_2 globin gene is inactivated by a point mutation.

Alpha thalassemia point mutations so far detected may have effects either on RNA processing, as in the case of α^{Hph} mutation, or on RNA translation, as for the α^{Nco} defect, or on protein instability, as for the Hb Suan Dok or the Hb Evanston. Some point mutations affecting the termination codon give rise to elongated α-globin chains, as in the case of Hb Constant Spring which is found with relatively high frequency in Southeast Asia (Harteveld & Higgs, 2010; Weatherall, 2001).

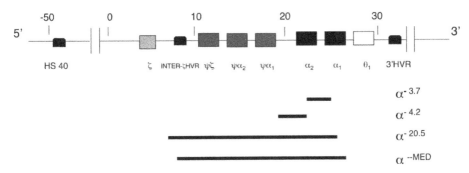

Fig. 5. Schematic representation of the α-globin cluster showing the regions removed by the most frequent α-thalassemic deletions in the Mediterranean area (Harteveld & Higgs, 2010).

5.3 High persistence of fetal hemoglobin (HPFH)

Generally, fetal hemoglobin production declines rapidly within few months after birth and in adult life it is detected only in traces (<1% of total hemogobin). This production is normally confined to a particular small subpopulation of red cells, called F cells (fetal cells), in which the fetal profile of globin gene expression is still active. Persistent expression of fetal hemoglobin in adulthood represents a group of conditions which are referred to as HPFH (high persistence of fetal hemoglobin). The mechanisms and the molecular basis underlying these conditions are very heterogeneous. In conditions of hematopoietic stress, such as β-thalassemia, an increased number of F cells may be detected along with higher HbF levels. In these cases the γ-chains have an ameliorative effect on the thalassemic phenotype, since they reduce the excess of α-globin chains. Consequently, the erythroid precursors which produce high γ-chain levels undergo positive selection, thus increasing the number of circulating F cells.

However, because the number of F cells is largely under genetic control, the HbF levels vary considerably in these patients and this contributes to the remarkable diversity in the severity of these diseases (see also the 6.1 paragraph, for further discussion). HbF levels vary considerably not only in thalassemic patients but also in healthy adults, where it represents a benign and clinically silent condition (Thein et al., 2009; Weatherall, 2001).

Besides epigenetic factors such as gender and age (Chang et al., 1995), the molecular basis of this variation largely depends on genetic determinants which may be linked or unlinked to the β-globin cluster. Forms of HPFH may be caused by large deletions within the β-globin cluster or point mutations in the proximal or distant promoter regions of the fetal globin genes (Cao & Moi, 2000). These rare forms, in which all red blood cells show increased levels of HbF, are referred to as pancellular HPFH and are transmitted in a simple Mendelian manner. Large deletions involving intergenic γ-δ sequences, the structural δ- and β-globin genes as well as regulatory regions at the 3' end of the β-globin cluster (Thein et al., 2009) are associated with reactivation of fetal globin gene expression. These types of rearrangements may indeed cause a loss of regulatory regions involved in globin gene switching or may result in enhancer regions brought in apposition to the γ genes as well. Examples of HPFH deletions in the β-globin cluster are the Sicilian δβ⁰ deletion (Esposito G. et al., 1994) and the Corfù deletion (Bank A. et al., 2005). A similar but less marked effect on HbF increase is found in the Hb Lepore, a δβ hybrid hemoglobin variant caused by a deletion originated from a mechanism of non homologous recombination between the δ- and β-globin genes. It is thought that this deletion also removes putative elements involved in globin gene switching located between these two genes, thus leading to persistent expression of fetal hemoglobin (Weaterall & Clegg, 2001).

Point mutations responsible for this form of HPFH are thought to modify the binding of transacting factors involved either in the mechanisms of globin gene switching or in γ-globin gene silencing. Among these defects, the most common mutations are those occurring in the proximal promoter region of the $^Gγ$ gene at position -202 (C→G) and –175 (T→C) or in the proximal promoter of the $^Aγ$ gene at position -196 (C→T), -175 (T→C) and -117 (G→A) (Olave et al., 2007). A relatively common C→T polymorphism at position -158 in the $^Gγ$-globin gene, altering a Xmn I recognition site, is associated with increased HbF levels in conditions of hematopoietic stress whereas it has no or little effects in normal individuals. Its presence has also been associated with a delayed decline of γ-globin gene expression in infant age (Grosso et al., 2007).

In heterocellular HPFH, a more common set of conditions, the HbF is distributed in an uneven fashion among F cells. Heterocellular HPFH forms are generally characterized by a structurally intact β-globin cluster and are inherited as a quantitative genetic trait (Thein et al., 2009). Extensive linkage studies have so far identified three major quantitative trait loci (QTLs) involved in the heterocellular HPFH phenotype: the Xmn I-158 $^Gγ$ polymorphism, the HBS1L-MYB intergenic region on chromosome 6q23 and the BCL11A on chromosome 2p16 (Craig et al., 1996; Manzel et al., 2007). The role for one of these QTLs has been recently described. It had been found that the BCL11A locus codifies for a transfactor acting as repressor of fetal globin genes (Xu et al., 2011). Recently, another repressor of fetal globin genes, the Cold Shock Domain Protein A or CSDA, has been identified and characterized (Petruzzelli et al., 2010). Therefore, both these two factors may be directly involved in the switching of globin gene expression through silencing of the transcriptional activity of γ-globin genes in adult life, although additional studies are required in order to define better their role in the regulation of this complex mechanism of gene expression.

6. Clinical phenotypes

6.1 β-thalassemias

The hallmark of β-thalassemias is the quantitative defect in the production of β-globin chains which leads to imbalanced α-/non α-globin chain ratio and an excess of α-chains. This condition is the main determinant in the pathophysiology of β-thalassemia. Alpha-globin chains in excess precipitate in red-cell precursors, causing oxidative membrane damage, abnormal cell maturation and erythroid premature destruction in the bone marrow with consequent ineffective erythropoiesis. These abnormalities are responsible for the subsequent erythroid marrow expansion and characteristic skeletal deformities. Marrow expansion leads ultimately to increased iron absorption and progressive deposition of iron in tissues (Weatherall & Clegg, 2001). Severity of clinical conditions is thus clearly related to the degree of globin chain imbalance which gives rise to a wide array of extremely diverse hematological phenotypes. The most severe forms are represented by β-thalassemia major, a set of conditions characterized by severe anemia requiring regular blood transfusion treatments for survival since early childhood. These forms most often result from homozygosity or compound heterozygosity for β-globin gene mutations and, in rarer cases, from heterozygosity for dominant mutations. In some cases, however, the same genotypes may lead to milder conditions, referred to as thalassemia intermedia. These intermediate forms show very heterogeneous clinical pictures that range in severity from the asymptomatic condition to transfusion-dependent anemia, generally only slightly less severe than thalassemia major. Since, as above discussed, severity of disease is related to the degree of globin chain imbalance, the milder clinical phenotype of these conditions can be explained by coinheritance of genetic factors that are able to reduce the excess of α-globin chains, such as α-thalassemia that reduce the α-globin chain production, or genetic determinants that lead to persistent expression of γ-globin chains in adulthood, thus increasing the β-like globin chain production. Alternatively, these attenuated phenotypes may also be due to homozygosity for mild mutations or compound heterozygosity for a mild or silent mutation and a more severe defect in the β-globin genes. On the other hand, triplication or quadruplication rearrangements of α-globin genes may produce a more marked imbalance in globin chain production thus leading to a clinical picture of thalassemia intermedia even in simple heterozygotes for β-thalassemia, who are otherwise generally clinically silent (Cao & Moi, 2002; Thein, 2005; Weatherall, 2001; Wong et al., 2004). This latter condition, also referred to as β-thalassemia minor, is characterized by mild anemia and morphological changes of the red blood cells, which are tipically hypochromic and microcitic. Other typical features are represented by increased HbA$_2$ levels and slight increase of HbF (Steinberg & Adams J.G. III, Weatherall & Clegg, 2001). Finally, a rarer form of β-thalassemia trait is characterized by normal HbA$_2$ and thalassemia-like red cell indices (Moi et al., 1988). This condition may represent co-inheritance of mutations, associated or not on the same chromosome and decreasing both β- and δ-globin gene function. Increased HbF levels are usually detected in δβ-thalassemia characterized by deletions involving both δ- and β-globin genes.

6.2 α-thalassemias
The clinical phenotypes of α-thalassemia are classified in four types that range from mild to severe conditions, depending on the degree of defective α-globin gene output. The wide heterogeneity in clinical and hematological pictures is largely related on the wide spectrum of molecular defects which may lead to a great variety of genotypes characterized by loss of one, two, three or all four α-globin genes. In general, the loss of only one α-gene leads to very mild clinical conditions, with the -α$^{3.7}$ producing milder phenotypes respect to the –α$^{4.2}$. Non deletional mutants involving the α$_2$ gene are responsible of a more pronounced phenotype, as already discussed, whereas deletional loss of both α genes leads to more severe conditions (Higgs & Gibbons, 2010; Weatherall, 2010).
Deletion of one α gene (-α/αα) is associated to the milder clinical forms of α-thalassemia, referred to as silent carrier state, which are characterized by slight imbalanced α/non-α globin chain production, normal values of HbA$_2$ and mild microcytosis, with or without anemia. The α-thalassemia trait is instead characterized by mild or moderate microcytic and

hypochromic anemia, which is clinically asymptomatic and is generally diagnosed during regular health checks or prenatal screening. This condition is commonly generated by loss of two α genes (-α/-α or --/αα genotypes). On the other hand, the homozygous condition of the non deletional form of α-thalassemia responsible for the synthesis of Hb Constant Spring ($\alpha\alpha^{CS}/\alpha\alpha^{CS}$) causes a more severe phenotype respect to the α-thalassemia trait. This condition is characterized by severe anemia, typical thalassemic changes in hematological indices, moderate jaundice and a variable degree of hepatosplenomegaly, a clinical picture more similar to the HbH disease than to the mild thalassemic trait. The HbH disease is most frequently the result of compound heterozygosity for α^+ and α^0 mutations (--/-α) and is therefore predominantly found in Southeast Asia and in the Mediterranean region, where these defects are more common. HbH disease forms produced by non deletional defects are more severe than those caused by the more common deletional α-thalassemic types. The clinical conditions resemble those of β-thalassemia intermedia. Similarly to these intermediate conditions, the HbH disease is characterized by considerable variation in the severity of hematological conditions. The predominant features are variable degrees of anemia, with hemoglobin levels ranging from 2.6 to 12.4 g/dl, and amounts of HbH from 2 to 40% of total hemoglobin. Hb Bart's is occasionally detected in the peripheral blood. HbH patients usually have hepatosplenomegaly, jaundice in variable degrees, gall stones and acute hemolytic episodes induced by infections or drug treatments. In fact, with respect to the β-thalassemia conditions characterized by ineffective erythropoiesis, in α-thalassemia the main mechanism of anemia is due to hemolysis. The most severe deficiencies in α-globin chain production lead to Hb Bart's hydrops fetalis syndrome, which is commonly the result of inheritance of two α^0 determinants, although it may also result from compound heterozygosity for a severe non deletional determinant with a deletional α^0 mutant allele. In this syndrome most of the circulating hemoglobin is constituted by the non functional homotetramers γ4 and β4, with also variable amounts of the embryonic Hb Portland, the only functional type of hemoglobin in these patients. The severity of anemia conditions and cardiac failure, along with the other prominent features of this syndrome, often leads to death *in utero* (23-38 weeks of pregnancy) or soon after birth (Weatherall & Clegg, 2001).

7. Unusual forms of thalassemia

Over the last two decades, our group has been involved in a prevention program for hemoglobinopathies based on screening and molecular characterization of carriers and on prenatal diagnosis in couples at-risk. In the course of this activity we have defined the molecular basis of several atypical thalassemic phenotypes which have been found to be associated with complex and unusual interactions of mutations affecting the expression of one or more globin genes. Our study provides further indications on the complexity and heterogeneity of molecular basis of thalassemia in our region. Our experience also highlights the potential pitfalls in genetic counselling in areas where globin gene disorders are most common. Some of the most intriguing cases are now being discussed in detail.

7.1 A δβ-thalassemia phenotype associated with a complex interaction of mutations in the γ-, δ- and β-globin genes

In this case the propositus was a 2 year-old girl of Italian descent showing a mild hypochromic microcytic anemia (Fig. 6) (Grosso M al., 2007). The peripheral blood film showed anisopoikilocytosis and marked microcytosis; she had normal serum iron values and increased osmotic fragility; the hemoglobin analysis, carried out by cation exchange HPLC, revealed normal Hb A$_2$ (2.5%) and increased Hb F (6.4%) levels. This condition was consistent with a δβ-thalassemia trait. To confirm this hypothesis, hematological studies were extended to all family members. Unexpectedly, the father was found to be a typical β-thalassemia carrier with a mild increase of Hb A$_2$ (3.5%) and no Hb F, while the mother showed normal red blood cell indices and iron balance with a low Hb A$_2$ level (1.5%) and no HbF. Her two siblings, a 4 year old brother and a 13 month old sister, had both normal red blood cell indices and iron balance with HbA$_2$=2.1% , HbF=1% and HbA$_2$ 0.8%, HbF 6%, respectively.

Molecular analysis was performed for all family members on genomic DNA. The propositus and her father were heterozygotes for the β$^+$IVS I-6 (C→T) mutation. The propositus, her mother and the younger sister were all carriers of the δ+27 (G→T), the Mediterranean most common δ-thalassemia defect (Pirastu et al., 1983) and the –158 ^{G}γ gene polymorphism (C→T) (Fig. 6). The molecular study thus showed that in the propositus co-inheritance of the β$^+$IVS I-6 with the δ+27 mutation was responsible for the normalization of the HbA$_2$ level, whereas the HbF increase was associated with the –158 ^{G}γ-globin gene polymorphism. The δ- and γ-globin gene defects had been co-inherited *in cis* on the maternal chromosome. However, the mother had normal HbF values. In fact, carriers for the –158 ^{G}γ- gene polymorphism have increased HbF levels only in conditions of erythropoietic stress, which may be caused by a β-thalassemic trait, as found in the propositus and not in her mother. This case also allowed us to detect a novel *in cis* association of the –158 ^{G}γ polymorphism with a δ-thalassemic defect, thus providing further evidence of the complex effects on the hematological phenotype when different thalassemic defects are co-inherited.

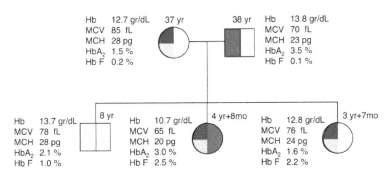

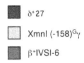

Fig. 6. **Complex interaction of mutations in the γ-, δ- and β-globin genes.** Pedigree with hematological data of the propositus and her family. The propositus had inherited the β-thalassemic defect from her father and the maternal chromosome bearing both the δ+27 mutation, which is responsible for the normalization of the HbA$_2$ level, and the –158 (C→T) ^{G}γ-globin gene polymorphism associated with increased HbF levels.

7.2 An unusual δβ-thalassemia phenotype associated with a complex interaction of mutations in the δ- and β-globin genes

We investigated the molecular basis of a mild hypochromic microcytic anemia in a 5-year-old boy from Naples, Italy (Grosso et al., 2001). The patient had normal HbA$_2$ (2.5%) and no HbF. Osmotic resistance, serum iron and transferrin concentrations were within normal values. His father had normal red blood indices and iron balance, low HbA$_2$ (1.5%) and normal HbF (0.3%) levels. His mother had mildly hypochromic microcytic red blood indices, normal HbA$_2$ (2.7%) and HbF (0.6%). This phenotype could have been explained by either double heterozygosity for δ- and β-thalassemia or heterozygosity for α-thalassemia. Globin chain synthesis analysis allowed to exclude the α-thalassemia carrier status since the α/non-α globin chain ratio was 2.27 for the patient, and 1.66 and 0.96 for his mother and father, respectively. Reverse phase HPLC performed in the course of globin chain synthesis analysis revealed in the patient and his mother an anomalous β-globin peak that showed features comparable to those of Hb Neapolis (beta 126 (H4) Val→Gly). Hb Neapolis is a rare unstable hemoglobin variant undetectable by conventional hematological HPLC screening methods and showing mild thalassemic features. Subjects heterozygous for this variant are characterized by mild microcytosis and slightly increased Hb A$_2$ levels (Pagano et al., 1991; Pagano et al., 1997). DNA sequence analysis confirmed the presence of the mutation causing the synthesis of Hb Neapolis in the propositus and his mother.

Our study also revealed the δ+27 (G→T) mutation in the heterozygote state, in the patient and his father.

These results indicated that the atypical δβ-thalassemia phenotype was determined in this patient by coinheritance *in trans* of δ+27 (G→T) and β-globin codon 126 (T→G) mutations. The δ-thalassemic trait completely normalized HbA$_2$ concentration, thus almost completely silencing the mild β-thalassemic phenotype produced by Hb Neapolis (Fig. 7).

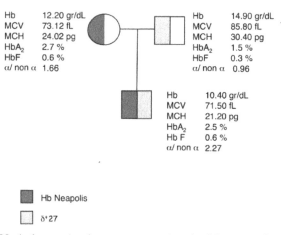

Fig. 7. **An unusual δβ-thalassemia phenotype associated with a complex interaction of mutations in the δ- and β-globin genes.** Pedigree with hematological data of the propositus and his family. The propositus was found to be a compound heterozygous for two rare mutations: a rare hemoglobin variant, the Hb Neapolis, associated with a mild thalassemic phenotype, inherited from his mother, and a δ-thalassemic defect (δ+27) of paternal origin, which was responsible for the normalization of the HbA2 level (2.5%).

It is noteworthy that the HbA$_2$ level detected in the mother is lower comparable to that expected for carriers of the Hb Neapolis variant. In this case the slightly increased HbA$_2$ level reported for this mutation was reduced to normal values by coexistence of iron deficiency (Moi et al., 1988). This condition might have masked the underlying mild β-thalassemia carrier status, thus strengthening the importance of accurate evaluation of hematological features in families at-risk for hemoglobinopathies.

7.3 Interaction of α- and β-globin gene mutations in a couple at risk for thalassemia

A couple at risk for hemoglobinophaties, originated from Nigeria, was referred to our Prenatal Centre for genetic counselling. The woman showed slight microcytic indices with normal iron and ferritin serum values. Cation exchange HPLC analysis of hemoglobin showed mild increase of Hb F and normal HbA2 level, along with an abnormal peak consistent with the presence of the HbS variant at the heterozygous state. The Hb S is characterized by the replacement of the glutamic acid residue at position 6 with a valine residue in the β-globin chain. At the DNA level a point mutation (A→T) at codon 6 modifies the codon GAG (glutamic acid) into GTG (valine) (Weatherall & Clegg, 2001). Molecular analysis confirmed the presence of this mutation and excluded other β-globin gene defects.

Her partner showed a slight microcytic anemia, normal HbA2 values (2.9%) with both serum iron and ferritin low levels (Fig. 8).

We hypothesized that the hematological phenotype in both cases could be explained by the presence of α-thalassemia defects. Indeed, both partners were found to be heterozygous for the -α$^{3.7}$ deletion, one of the most common *thalassemic* defects in their country of origin along with the hemoglobin variant HbS (Galanello & Origa, 2010). Transmission of both these defects does not represent a factor of risk for hemoglobinopathy since when combined with α-thalassemic determinants, the HbS defect remains in a carrier state (Cao & Moi, 2000).

However, it is known that iron deficiency contributes to slightly reduce HbA2 levels. Therefore, we could not exclude that the normal HbA2 value detected in the male could have been the result of a complex combination of both genetic and epigenetic factors. We thus performed extensive β-globin gene sequence analysis also in this subject, in order to verify the hypothesis that the α-thalassemic defect associated with iron deficiency could have masked a mild β-thalassemic trait. Indeed, if this was the case, co-inheritance of the paternal β-thalassemic allele with the maternal HbS defect, which also occurs within the β-globin gene, would affect the production of functional hemoglobin with varying degree of severity and cause a disease known as HbS-β thalassemia (Weatherhall & Clegg, 2001).

This analysis showed the presence at the heterozygous state of a single nucleotide substitution at the position 108 in the first intron of the β-globin gene (IVS1-108), a defect reported to be associated with a mild β-thalassemic trait phenotype in a Cuban patient of European origin (Muñiz et al., 2000). It has been hypothesized that this point mutation may activate an intronic cryptic branch site, resulting in defective β-globin gene splicing efficiency.

Our study thus allowed us to define the risk of this couple having a child with HbS-β thalassemia disease which, on the basis of the mild β-thalassemic defect, we might expect would present with mild or moderate symptoms.

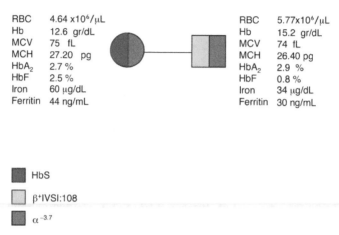

RBC	$4.64 \times 10^6/\mu L$		RBC	$5.77 \times 10^6/\mu L$
Hb	12.6 gr/dL		Hb	15.2 gr/dL
MCV	75 fL		MCV	74 fL
MCH	27.20 pg		MCH	26.40 pg
HbA_2	2.7 %		HbA_2	2.9 %
HbF	2.5 %		HbF	0.8 %
Iron	60 $\mu g/dL$		Iron	34 $\mu g/dL$
Ferritin	44 ng/mL		Ferritin	30 ng/mL

■ HbS

□ β^+IVSI:108

■ $\alpha^{-3.7}$

Fig. 8. Interaction of α- and β-globin gene mutations in a couple at risk for thalassemia.
Genotypes and hematological phenotypes of the couple at-risk for hemoglobinopathy.
Serum iron and ferritin values are also reported, showing a mild hyposideremic condition in
the male partner.

7.4 Rare α-thalassemic genotypes detected in a family at-risk for thalassemia.

A couple of Italian descend at risk for thalassemia was referred to our Prenatal Centre for
genetic counselling and further investigations. The woman who was at the 8th week of
pregnancy showed slight microcythemia (MCV=78.40 fl) with normal values of HbA_2 and Hb
F. This phenotype was consistent with a typical α-thalassemia carrier state. However, the
proband was found negative for the most common deletional forms of α-thalassemia. Since
her partner was a typical carrier of β-thalassemic trait, extensive molecular studies were
performed in the woman to exclude the presence of any silent or mild β-thalassemia defect.
Furthermore, to investigate the molecular basis of this very mild phenotype, we extended
our study to her parents.
We found that whereas her mother had normal hematological indices, her father showed a
more relevant reduction of both MCV and HbA_2 values with respect to her daughter (Fig. 9).
In this subject, analysis of α-thalassemic deletions revealed the heterozygous condition for
the thalassemic $-\alpha^{-3.7}$ defect. Sequencing analysis performed on the α-globin genes revealed
in both the propositus and her father the heterozygous state for a deletion of five
nucleotides in the 5' donor site of the first intron (-TGAGG) of the α2-globin gene that
abolishes a restriction site for the Hph I restriction enzyme. This mutation, like other non
deletional α-thalassemic determinants, has a more severe effect on the hematological
phenotype with respect to deletions of single α-globin genes. Our study thus allowed us to
define the complex α-globin gene genotypes in this family: the propositus was a carrier of a
non deletional defect ($\alpha\alpha^T/\alpha\alpha$) whereas her father had a more complex genotype ($\alpha\alpha^T/-\alpha$),
consistent with his more prominent α-thalassemic phenotype.
These investigations also allowed us to exclude the risk for thalassemia and the requirement
for prenatal diagnosis in this couple since, as already discussed, co-inheritance of α-
thalassemia trait has ameliorative effects on the β-thalassemic phenotype.

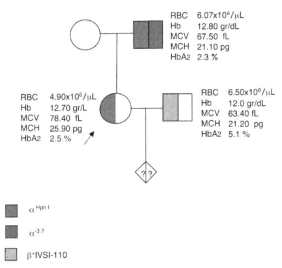

RBC 6.07x10⁶/μL
Hb 12.80 gr/dL
MCV 67.50 fL
MCH 21.10 pg
HbA2 2.3 %

RBC 4.90x10⁶/μL
Hb 12.70 gr/L
MCV 78.40 fL
MCH 25.90 pg
HbA2 2.5 %

RBC 6.50x10⁶/μL
Hb 12.0 gr/dL
MCV 63.40 fL
MCH 21.20 pg
HbA2 5.1 %

α^Hph I

α^-3.7

β⁺-IVSI-110

Fig. 9. **Rare α-thalassemic genotypes detected in a family at-risk for thalassemia.** Pedigree with hematological data of the propositus and her family. The arrow shows the proband who was found to be a carrier of a rare point mutation in the α-globin gene (α^Hph I), inherited from her father who instead is a compound heterozygous for a common deletional defect (-α^-3.7) and the rarer non deletional α^Hph I mutation.

8. Conclusions

The thalassemias, together with sickle cell anemia, are the most common group of inherited monogenic disorders in the world. Their high incidence is related to selective advantage of the carrier state to malaria infection. As a result, these diseases are mostly common in geographic areas extending from the Mediterranean region through tropical countries including Sub-Saharian Africa, the Middle East, India, Southeast Asia and Indonesia, where malaria was or still is endemic. Their clinical severity varies greatly, from asymptomatic hypochromia and microcytosis conditions to life-threatening ineffective erythropoiesis and hemolytic anemia. The more severe conditions require intensive medical treatments throughout life, even though, as a result of advances in transfusion, iron chelation and bone marrow transplantation therapies, expectancy as well as quality of life have increased very considerably in the last years.

Among the first diseases to be studied at the molecular level, the thalassemias still remain a paradigm for understanding the pathogenetic basis of inherited disorders, as well as the molecular mechanisms involved in the regulation of gene expression. In fact, since late 70's when DNA recombinant technologies emerged as a powerful tool for the identification of the molecular defects of the human inherited diseases, the experimental strategies and the methods firstly developed to study hemoglobinopathies were subsequently applied to define the molecular basis of other genetic diseases. These studies have also contributed to define the complex pathophysiological mechanisms underlying these syndromes and have made possible prevention programs based on large-scale screening and prenatal diagnosis in populations at high risk for hemoglobinopathies.

Molecular and clinical investigations have also provided powerful insights into the relationships between the molecular basis of thalassemias and their clinical diversity and have contributed to clarify the effects of the interactions among different genetic determinants on the thalassemic phenotypes, providing in the meantime the basis for accurate genetic counselling and preventive medicine services.

More recently, many efforts have been made toward the definition of the molecular basis of globin gene switching which represents a fascinating and unique model to study the mechanisms of gene expression regulation in space and time. Furthermore, these studies are also expected to provide novel therapeutic targets in the treatment of sickle cell anemia and β-thalassemia, as conditions of high persistence of fetal hemoglobin (HPFH) or drug-mediated reactivation of fetal globin gene expression have considerable ameliorating effects on the severity of these conditions.

A vast body of knowledge has been gained so far and great progress has been made in the understanding of these mechanisms. It is expected that these advances will rapidly lead to novel molecular approaches to the treatment of hemoglobinopathies, before definitive gene therapy strategies will enter clinical practice.

9. References

Bank A., O'Neill D., Lopez L., Pulte D., Ward M., Mantha S. & Richardson C. (2005). Role of intergenic human γ-δ globin sequences in human hemoglobin switching and reactivation of fetal hemoglobin in adult erythroid cells. *Annals of the New York Academy of Science*, 1054, pp. 48-54

Cao A. & Moi P. (2000). Genetic modifying factors in beta-thalassemia. *Clinical Chemistry and Laboratory Medicine*, 38, pp. 123-132

Cao A. & Moi P. (2002). Regulation of the globin genes. *Pediatric Research*, 51, 4, pp. 415-421

Chang Y.C., Smith K.D., Moore R.D., Serjeant G.R. & Dover G.J. (1995). An analysis of fetal hemoglobin variation in sickle cell disease: the relative contribution of the X-linked factor, β-globin haplotypes, α-globin gene number, gender and age. *Blood*, 8, pp.1111-1117

Craig J.E., Rochette J., Fisher C.A., Weatherall D.J., Marc S., Lathrop G.M., Demenais F. & Thein S.L. (1996). Dissecting the loci controlling fetal haemoglobin production on chromosomes 11p and 6p by the regressive approach. *Nature Genetics*, 12, pp. 58-64.

Esposito G., Grosso M., Gottardi E., Izzo P., Camaschella C. & Salvatore F. (1994). A unique origin for the Sicilian (δβ)°-thalassemia in 33 unrelated families and its rapid diagnostic characterization by PCR analysis. *Human Genetics*, 93, pp. 691-693.

Fathallah H. & Atweh G.F. (2006). Induction of fetal hemoglobin in the treatment of Sickle Cell Disease. *Hematology American Society of Hematological Education Program*, pp. 58-62

Galanello R. & Origa R. (2010). β-thalassemia. *Orphanet Journal of Rare Diseases*, 5: 11

Grosso M., Rescigno G., Zevino C., Matarazzo M., Poggi V. & Izzo P. (2001). A rare case of compound heterozygosity for δ+27 and Hb Neapolis (Dhonburi) associated to an atypical β-thalassemia phenotype. *Haematologica*, 86, pp. 985-986

Grosso M., Amendolara M., Rescigno G., Danise P., Todisco N., Izzo P. & Amendola G. (2008). Delayed decline of γ-globin expression in infant age associated with the presence of $^G\gamma$-158 (C→T) polymorphism. *International Journal of Laboratory Hematology,* 31, pp. 359-363.

Harteveld C.L. & Higgs D.R. (2010). α-thalassaemia. *Orphanet Journal of Rare Diseases,* 5: 13

Higgs D.R. & Gibbons R.J. (2010). The molecular basis of α-thalassaemia: a model for understanding human molecular genetics. *Hematology/Oncology Clinics of North America,* 24, 6, pp. 1033-1054

Ho P.J. & Thein S.L. (2000). Gene regulation and deregulation: a β globin perspective. *Blood reviews,* 14, pp. 78-93

Kattamis A.C., Camaschella C., Sivera P., Surrey S. & Fortina P. (1996). Human α-thalassemia syndromes: Detection of molecular defects. *American Journal of Hematology,* 53, pp. 81-91

Mesbah-Amroun H., Rouabhi F., Ducrocq R. & Elion J. (2008). Molecular basis of alpha-thalassemia in Algeria. *Hemoglobin,* 32, 3, pp. 273-278

Menzel S., Garner C., Gut I., Matsuda F., Yamaguchi M., Health S., Foglio M., Zelenika D., Boland A., Rooks H., Best S., Spector T.D., Farrall M., Lathrop M. & Thein S.L. (2007). A QTL influencing F cell production maps to a gene encoding a zinc-finger protein on chromosome 2p15. *Nature Genetics,* 39, 10, pp. 1197-1199

Moi P., Paglietti E., Sanna A., Brancati C., Tagarelli A., Galanello R., Cao A. & Pirastu M. (1988). Delineation of the molecular basis of delta- and normal HbA$_2$ β-thalassemia. *Blood,* 72, pp. 530-533

Muñiz A., Martinez G., Lavinha J. & Pacheco P. (2000).Beta-thassaemia in Cubans: novel allele increases the genetic diversity at the HBB locus in the Caribbean. *American Journal of Hematology,* 64, 1, pp. 7-14

Olave I.A., Doneanu C., Fang X., Stamatoyannopoulos G. & Li Q. (2007). Purification and identification of proteins that bind the Hereditary Persistence of fetal Hemoglobin - 198 mutation in the γ-globin gene promoter. *The Journal of Biological Chemistry,* 282, 2, pp. 853-862

Oneal P., Gantt N.M., Schwartz J.D., Bhanu N.V., Lee Y.T., Moroney J.W., Reed C.H., Schechter A., Ludan N.L. & Miller J.L. (2006). Fetal hemoglobin silencing in human. *Blood,* 108, pp. 2081-2086

Pagano L., Lacerra G., Camardella L., De Angioletti M., Fioretti G., Maglione G., de Bonis C., Guarino E., Viola A. & Cutolo R. (1991). Hemoglobin Neapolis, beta 126 (H4) Val → Gly: a novel beta-chain variant associated with a mild beta-thalassemia phenotype and displaying anomalous stability features. *Blood,* 78, pp. 3070-3075

Pagano L., Carbone V., Fioretti G., Viola A., Buffardi S., Rametta V., Desicato S., Pucci P. & De Rosa C. (1997). Compound heterozygosity for Hb Lepore-Boston and Hb Neapolis (Dhonburi) (beta 126 (H4) Val→Gly) in a patient from Naples, Italy. *Hemoglobin,* 21, pp. 1-15

Petruzzelli R., Gaudino S., Amendola G., Sessa R., Puzone S., Di Concilio R., d'Urzo G., Amendolara M., Izzo P. & Grosso M. (2010). Role of the Cold Shock Domain Protein A in the transcriptional regulation of HBG expression. *British Journal of Haematology,* 150, 6, pp. 689-699

Pi W., Zhu X., Wu M., Sessa R., Whang Y., Fulzele S., Eroglu A., Ling J. & Tuan D. (2010). Long-range function of the intergenic retrotransposon. *Proceedings of the National Academy of Sciences, USA,* 150, 6, pp. 689-699

Pirastu M., Galanello R., Melis M.A., Brancati C., Tagarelli A., Cao A. & Kan Y.W. (1983). Delta (+)-thalassemia in Sardinia. *Blood*, 62, pp. 341-345

Rosatelli M.C., Tuveri T., Scalas M.T., Leono G.B., Sardu R., Faà V., Meloni A., Pischedda M.A. & Monni G. (1992). Molecular screening and fetal diagnosis of β-thalassemia in the Italian population. *Human Genetics*, 89, pp. 585-589

Ross J., Bottardi S., Bourgoin V., Wollenschlaeger A., Drobetsky E., Trudel M. & Milot E. (2009). Differential requirement of distal regulatory region for pre-initiation complex formation at globin gene promoters. *Nucleic Acids Research*, 37, 16, pp. 5295-5308

Sessa R., Puzone S., Ammirabile M., Piscopo C., Pagano L., Colucci S., Izzo P. & Grosso M. (2010). Identification and molecular characterization of the --CAMPANIA deletion, a novel alpha (0)-thalassemic defect, in two unrelated Italian families. *American Journal of Hematology*, 85, pp.143-144

Stamatoyannopoulos G. & Gronsveld F. (2001). Hemoglobin switching, In: *The Molecular Basis of Blood Diseases*, G. Stamatoyannopoulos G., Majerus P.W., Perlmutter R.M. & Varmus H. Eds., pp. 135-182, Saunders, ISBN-10: 0721676715, Philadelphia, PA, USA

Steinberg M.H. and Adams J.G. III (1991). Hemoglobin A$_2$: origin, evolution and aftermath. *Blood*, 78, pp. 2165-2177

Thein S.L. (2005). Genetic modifiers of beta-thalassemia. *Human Molecular Genetics*, 18, 90, 5, pp. 649-660

Thein S.L., Menzel S., Lathrop M. & Garner C. (2009). Control of fetal hemoglobin: new insights emerging from genomics and clinical implications. *Human Molecular Genetics*, 18, pp. 216-223

Weatherall D.J. (2001). Phenotype-genotype relationships in monogenic disease: lessons from the thalassaemias. *Nature Reviews*, 2, pp. 245-255

Weatherall D.J. & Clegg J.B. (2001). *The thalassaemia syndrome* (Fourth edition), *Blackwell Science, ISBN*-10: 0865426643, *Oxford, UK*

Wong W.S., Chan A.Y., Yip S.F., Ma E.S. (2004). Thalassemia intermedia due to co-inheritance of beta0/beta(+)-thalassemia and (--SEA) alpha-thalassemia/Hb Westmead [alpha122 (H5) His→Gln (alpha2)] in a Chinese family. *Hemoglobin*, 28, 2, pp. 151-156

Xu J., Sankaran V.G., Ni M., Menne T.F., Puram R.V., Kim W. & Orkin S.H. (2011). Transcriptional silencing of γ-globin by BCL11A involves long-range interactions and cooperation with SOX6. *Genes & Development*, 24, pp. 783-798

7

Paroxysmal Nocturnal Hemoglobinuria

Antonio M. Risitano
Head of Bone Marrow Transplant Clinical Unit
Department of Biochemistry and Medical Biotechnologies
Federico II University of Naples, Naples
Italy

1. Introduction

Paroxysmal nocturnal hemoglobinuria (PNH) is a complex hematological disorder resulting in a quite unique clinical syndrome. In fact, the typical clinical presentation encompasses three distinct hematological manifestations, i.e., hemolytic anemia, bone marrow failure and thrombophilia (Dunn et al 2000; Parker & Ware 2003; Notaro & Luzzatto 2003). Thus, the term PNH covers only one feature of the disease – the one that is the most evident to patients, even if it does not reveal the actual clinical and pathophysiological complexity of the disease. The first extensive description of PNH was made by Dr. Strübing in 1882, although some cases could be identified even in older reports (maybe the first one dates back to 1678 by Dr. Schmidt from Gdanks). Remarkably, Dr. Strübing recognized the uniqueness of the clinical syndrome (hemolytic anemia with possible thrombosis), anticipating some of the pathophysiological implications that were unraveled decades later. In fact, he hypothesized that hemoglobinuria was due to *"red blood cells which dissolve into the vessels"* (corresponding to intravascular hemolysis in current terminology), possibly secondary to a *"disordered blood production"* of erythrocytes which are *"abnormally sensitive"* to acidification (namely, the production of blood cells with the aberrant PNH phenotype, that makes them susceptible to complement-mediated lysis) (Crosby 1951). However, it was with Marchiafava and Nazari (Marchiafava & Nazari 1911) in 1911 that the disease was recognized as a distinct medical entity, characterized by *"chronic hemolytic anemia with perpetual hemosiderinuria"*, subsequently known as the *Marchiafava-Micheli syndrome* (Micheli 1928); the current name *"paroxysmal nocturnal hemoglobinuria"* was eventually coined by Dr. Enneking in 1928 (Enneking 1928). In the last century, a number of reports on PNH were subsequently published because the puzzling nature of the disease has intrigued generations of investigators; however, PNH remained a mystery until the 1980s, when most of its pathophysiology was progressively elucidated, first with the description of the molecular defect of PNH cells, and then with the identification of the underlying genetic defect. By that time it was already known that PNH erythrocytes are exquisitely sensitive to lysis upon complement activation, both *in vivo* and *in vitro*. Thus, the observation that PNH cells lack from their surface some complement regulators, all included in a specific class of membrane-bound proteins (the so-called glycosyl phosphatidyl-inositol (GPI)-anchored proteins [GPI-APs]), clearly explained the reason for such sensitivity. Thereafter, the biochemical pathway accounting for GPI-AP surface expression was described, as well as its impairment in PNH cells. Finally, the genetic lesion leading to the aberrant phenotype was identified in distinct mutations in the *phosphatidyl-inositol glycan class A (PIG-A)* gene. This formally demonstrated that PNH is a clonal hematological disorder characterized by the expansion of abnormal (GPI-AP deficient, *PIG-A* mutated) hematopoietic stem cells (HSCs) carrying an intrinsic defect, that accounts for the clinical phenoptype of the disease. Nowadays most pathophysiological events occurring in PNH patients have been extensively described, even if definitive explanations for some disease manifestations (i.e., thromboembolic events) are still elusive. In the last few years, insights into the field pertain to the new treatment strategies that have drastically changed the management and clinical outcome of PNH patients. In fact, the availability of an inhibitor of the complement cascade – the actual effector mechanism of hemolysis in PNH – has led to the first etiological treatment for PNH, which seems to have a superb impact on the natural history of the disease.

2. Epidemiology

PNH is a rare acquired disease, with a worldwide prevalence estimated in the range of 1-5 cases per million (Rosse 1996; Orphanet 2004) regardless of the ethnicity; however, given the rarity of the disease and possible reporting biases, its incidence and prevalence remain largely unknown. Indeed, most reports deal with retrospective data, but formal epidemiological studies are lacking. A recent analysis from a well-defined geographical area (Hill et al 2006c) suggests that the actual incidence could be higher than previously reported, in the range of about 1.3/1,000,000/year, leading to a prevalence of about 15 cases per million in a 15 year observation period; however, these data may suffer from biases due to referral center, as well as to inclusion criteria (Parker et al 2005; De Latour et al 2008) In fact, a higher incidence might reflect the inclusion of patients with subclinical PNH, who have not been included in previous studies. In additional, geographical variations in PNH incidence should be considered; for instance, an increased prevalence is reported in some regions which also harbor higher incidence of aplastic anemia (e.g., Thailand and some other Asian countries) (Pramoonjago et al 1999). A multi-national prospective PNH registry is currently ongoing, and possibly will provide more definitive data on the actual incidence and prevalence of PNH in different geographical areas (Muus et al 2010). The incidence of PNH is similar in both genders, and most patients are diagnosed in their middle age (third or fourth decades), although cases have been reported in adolescents, children and even the elderly (De Latour et al 2008; Ware et al 1991).

3. Genetic basis

3.1 The GPI anchor and the *PIG-A* gene
The hallmark of PNH is hemolytic anemia secondary to the intrinsic susceptibility of affected red cells to complement activation (Ham & Dingle 1939; Rosse & Dacie 1966); thus, the presence of intrinsically abnormal blood cells is the cause of the disease phenotype. However, in PNH patients not all blood cells are affected, as they in fact present a mosaicism of normal and abnormal blood cells; therefore, a putative genetic cause was unlikely to be inherited or transmitted to the progeny. The clonal origin of PNH hematopoiesis was first demonstrated in 1970 by Dr. Luzzatto's group, who showed that, in

patients heterozygous for the glucose-6-phosphate-dehydrogenase (G6PD), affected red blood cells (RBCs) all share the same G6PD allele (which, on the other hand, is not involved in pathophysiology of the disease *per se*) (Oni et al 1970). Subsequently, the biochemical defect of PNH cells was identified in a specific molecular abnormality, consisting in the bizarre lack of several proteins from the cell surface. This peculiar defect was first described in the 1980s (Kunstling & Rosse 1969; Nicholson-Weller et al 1983; Selvaraj et al 1988), and rapidly became the hallmark of PNH, although its relationship with the pathophysiology of the disease remained obscure at that time. Notably, this abnormal phenotype pertained not only to erythrocytes, rather it included myeloid and megakaryocytic lineages too, suggesting that it derived from either multi-potent hematopoietic progenitors or even hematopoietic stem cells (Kinoshita et al 1985). Focusing on the underlying intrinsic abnormality rather than on the consequences of individual protein deficiency (which accounts for the susceptibility to hemolysis, as discussed later on), it became clear that all the proteins missing from the PNH cell surface shared a common mechanism responsible for their attachment to the cell membrane (Medof et al 1987). This is a specific glycolipid structure named glycosyl-phosphatidyl inositol (GPI) anchor (Mahoney et al 1992). The functional implications of the GPI-anchoring of proteins are not completely understood; they include ease of assemblage and shedding, lateral mobility, capping, involvement in endo-, exo-, and potocytosis (a clathrin-independent form of endocytosis and recycling). The strongest evidence that this type of membrane anchoring is important in cell biology is its high conservation among eukaryotic cells; indeed, it is found even in yeast and trypanosome. In 1993, using complementation of GPI-anchored protein deficient cell lines and expression cloning, Kinoshita and colleagues first isolated the cDNA of the *PIG-A* gene (Takeda et al 1993; Miyata et al 1993). *PIG-A* is a housekeeping gene located on the short arm of the X chromosome (Xp22.1); the organization of the genomic gene was described in 1994 (Bessler et al 1994). The *PIG-A* gene, in combination with at least two other proteins, encodes an enzyme essential to transfer N-acetyl glucosamine to phosphatidyl inositol; this is the very first step of the GPI-anchor biosynthesis (Armostrong et al 1992; Hirose et al 1992; Takahashi et al 1993). GPI-deficient cell lines showing defects in any of the various metabolic steps have been produced by experimental mutagenesis (Kinoshita et al 1995); however, the study of PNH has shown, at the very beginning surprisingly, that the same early step is impaired in all patients, and all patients have a mutation in the *PIG-A* gene (Takeda et al 1993, Luzzatto et al 1997, Nafa et al 1995). The present explanation for this finding is that among the various genes involved in the GPI-anchor synthesis, *PIG-A* may be the only one that is X-linked (Almeida et al 2009). As a consequence, a single mutation in that gene will produce an abnormal cell in either sex: males have only one allele and females have only one functional allele (as result of X-chromosome inactivation). Although females have two *PIG-A* alleles, only half of the mutation will occur in the functional X; thus, the risk of having the disease is the same in both genders. Since a defect causing a metabolic block is generally recessive, it is very unlikely (although not impossible) that a double mutation targeting both alleles of an autosomal gene in the same cell may occur in vivo. In keeping with this assumption, quite recently two kindreds harboring a mutation in the *PIG-M* gene were described (hence, with the genetic lesion inherited, not acquired). Indeed, all affected members did not develop PNH, but presented a quite distinct clinical syndrome characterized by a partial GPI deficiency associated with a propensity to thrombosis and seizures, in the absence of significant hemolysis (Almeida et al 2006).

3.2 *PIG-A* mutations in PNH

Direct sequencing of the *PIG-A* gene has demonstrated distinct mutations in all PNH patients (Luzzatto et al 2000; Nishimura et al 1999); in most cases, each patient has a single mutation (even if distinct *PIG-A* mutated clones may co-exist in some patients) and mutations are unique to each patient (private mutations). These mutations can be found in all blood lineages, consistent with a genetic lesion occurring in hematopoietic stem cell(s) (Takeda et al 1993; Endo et al 1995). All types of mutations have been observed (Nafa et al 1995; Nafa et al 1998): small deletions or insertions producing frameshift (the most frequent), nucleotide substitutions resulting in stop codon, large deletions, missense mutations causing amino acids substitutions or new sites for alternative splicing. No particular clustering of mutations has emerged, even if most of the mutations occur in exon 2, probably because it is the largest. If we compare the type of mutations found in PNH with those found in G6PD deficiency -- another (this time inherited) X-linked disorder of a housekeeping gene -- a clear discrepancy is evident. In PNH, a vast majority of mutations have extremely severe functional consequences, (i.e., production of truncated proteins, leading to a complete GPI deficiency – the PNH type III phenotype), whereas missense mutations are rare (usually resulting in the PNH type II phenotype); in G6PD deficiency almost all mutations are missense, leading to single amino acid substitutions with conserved (although possibly altered) function. Two considerations may be relevant to this discrepancy: i. in inherited disorders, mutations in a housekeeping gene may be lethal, and thus have been selected to allow residual functional activity; by contrast, null mutations can be seen if they are somatically acquired, because they do not affect organ development and pertains only to a small fraction of somatic cells, which may survive albeit with some functional abnormality; ii. if missense mutations in PNH are rare, it means that the gene must be seriously damaged for leading to a clonal expansion. Indeed, the rare missense mutations found in PNH patients are associated with a marked reduction of GPI-linked proteins, indicating that they usually have affected either mRNA stability or protein function, or both. Remarkably, different types of mutations may account for different cell phenotypes in PNH patients, especially when the erythrocytes are considered. In fact, RBCs harboring a mutation leading to the complete inactivation of the *PIG-A* gene product will unequivocally show a complete deficiency of all GPI-APs from their surface (the so-called PNH type III phenotype). In contrast, mutations leading to partial inactivation of the *PIG-A* gene (for instance missence mutations) may lead to a partial deficiency of GPI-APs, known as the PNH type II phenotype. Of note, this biochemical finding has direct functional consequences; in fact, as discussed later on, type II and type III erythrocytes have a quite distinct susceptibility to complement-mediated lysis (Rosse & Dacie 1966). Quite surprisingly, some PNH patients may harbor at the same time type II and type III cells, suggesting that distinct *PIG-A* mutated HSCs may expand concomitantly (Endo et al 1995; Nafa et al 1998). Indeed, even phenotypically identical PNH cells may carry distinct *PIG-A* genotypes (Endo et al 1995, Nishimura et al 1997), suggesting that the functional phenotype rather than the specific genetic defect may play a major role in the development of the disease (Luzzatto et al 1997), as discussed below.

4. Pathophysiology

4.1 The dual pathophysiology theory

PNH develops through a somatic mutation in the *PIG-A* gene occurring in HSC(s), which originate progeny mature blood cells uniquely lacking of all GPI-APs from their surface.

PNH is therefore an acquired genetic blood disorder, that cannot be transmitted to the progeny; however, the *PIG-A* mutation is likely insufficient to cause the disease and additional events are thought to be involved (Rotoli & Luzzatto 1989).

4.1.1 The *PIG-A* mutation is not sufficient for the development of clinical PNH

A number of observations support the idea that the *PIG-A* mutation itself is necessary, but not sufficient to cause PNH. In fact, the expansion of PNH cells over normal hematopoiesis remains a key step to develop the disease phenotype. These observations include both findings from tentative animal models of PNH, as well as findings from human individuals, with or without PNH.

Murine models of PNH. In order to explore experimentally the causal relationship between the *PIG*-A mutation and the development of PNH, murine models have been generated in the last few years to recapitulate human PNH (Rosti 2002). Initially, a complete knockout animal has been attempted, but it could not be produced due to fetal loss, demonstrating that *pig-a* is necessary for embryogenesis (Kawagoe et al 1996). Thus, a different strategy was devised, aiming to inactivate the mouse *pig-a* gene directly in embryonic stem (ES) cells, using the conventional knock-out gene targeting technique. Preliminary *in vitro* studies demonstrated that *pig-a* deficient ES cells were able to differentiate into mature cells of various hematopoietic lineages, thus showing that *pig-a* is not necessary for the differentiation and maturation of hematopoietic progenitors (Rosti et al 1997). However, when this approach was challenged *in vivo*, using chimeras obtained by inserting *pig-a* knocked out ES cells in early embryonic development, only a few chimeras survived (pointing out, once again, the pivotal role of the GPI-anchor for embryonic development), showing a low proportion of GPI-deficient blood cells at birth, which subsequently decreased with aging (Tremml et al 1999). These data support the theory that there was no absolute growth advantage for *pig-a* mutated cells as compared to normal cells coexisting in the same organism. Notably, the generation of a mouse model showing *in vivo* expansion of *pig-a* mutated hematopoiesis, thus better mimicking the human PNH disease, required a more sophisticated experimental approach (Keller et al 2001; Jasinski et al 2001). This included a conditional inactivation of the murine *pig-a* gene implemented using Cre recombinase and its specific recombination sites loxP; when the Cre/loxP system was targeted to the hematopoietic stem cells or the erythroid/megakaryocytic lineage using tissue-specific c-FES and GATA-1 regulatory sequences, respectively, the generation of mice having almost 100% of red cells with the PNH phenotype was obtained. However, even these mice do not really mimic the disease phenotype seen in humans, because PNH hematopoiesis tends to decrease over time (Jasinski et al 2001). Indeed, the conclusion from murine models is that the *pig-a* mutation is not sufficient itself to sustain the expansion of PNH-like hematopoiesis over time, suggesting the presence of additional causal factors.

PIG-A mutations in human individuals. PIG-A mutation may be identified in affected cells from all PNH patients, demonstrating a clear etiological role in the development of PNH. However, it is not true that all individuals who undergo inactivating mutations in the *PIG-A* gene develop clinical PNH. In fact, it has been shown that a few blood cells harboring the PNH phenotype (namely, a complete or partial deficiency in all GPI-APs) may be detected even in normal individuals, at a frequency of 10 to 50 cells per million (Araten et al 1999). This was possible thanks to an ultra-sensitive flow cytometry analysis (see above, diagnosis of PNH) of large numbers of circulating granulocytes or erythrocytes obtained from healthy subjects. When these phenotypically abnormal cells were selected and studied at the genetic level, they revealed themselves to be clonal, and to carry specific *PIG-A* mutations (as demonstrated by a nested PCR technique) undistinguishable from those identified in PNH patients (Araten et al 1999). This clearly demonstrated that, *in vivo*, a *PIG-A* mutation was not sufficient to cause the disease, for at least two different reasons. First, to sustain clonal expansion, such mutations have to occur in multipotent HSC, while in most cases they statistically could pertain to cells without self-renewal capability, such as differentiated blood cells or committed hematopoietic progenitors. Second, a *PIG-A* mutation, even when occurring in a HSC, could simply confers a biological phenotype (the GPI deficiency) that requires additional, *PIG-A*-independent, conditions for further clonal expansion leading to the disease. The latter view is also supported by the observation that, at least in some patients, PNH hematopoiesis may include more than one abnormal clone. This was initially postulated based on the differential susceptibility of erythrocyte population to complement lysis (Rosse & Dacie 1966; Rotoli et al 1984), as subsequently demonstrated by flow cytometry (van der Schoot et al 1990), and finally confirmed by *PIG-A* sequencing (Endo et al 1996; Nishimura et al 1997)). In keeping, the expansion of distinct clones carrying the same, albeit molecularly heterogeneous, functional defect seems to suggest an expansion based on non-stochastic processes, such as selection, rather than a random process. This is also supported by the observation that relapse of PNH may be sustained by clones harboring *PIG-A* mutations different from those identified at diagnosis (Nafa et al 1998).

4.1.2 Clonal expansion of the *PIG-A* mutated clone(s) and development of clinical PNH
This background raised the hypothesis of a dual pathophysiology for PNH: the *PIG-A* mutation is not sufficient to cause the disease, and requires a second, independent event (Rotoli & Luzzatto 1989). This theory is also known as the "relative advantage" (Luzzatto et al 1997) or "escape" theory (Young & Maciejewski 2000). According to this view, a mutation in the *PIG-A* gene might be a fairly common phenomenon, with no major biological consequences, because in physiological conditions the mutated cell has no reason for expanding in the presence of a vast majority of normal cells. In fact, no intrinsic proliferative advantage has been demonstrated in PNH hematopoietic progenitors in comparison to normal ones (Araten et al 2002). However, additional factors may alter this equilibrium, creating the conditions for the expansion of PNH clone(s), and possibly leading to the occurrence of a single *PIG-A* mutated stem cell sustaining hematopoiesis even for the rest of the patient's life (Nishimura et al 2002; Nishimura et al 2004). The nature of such second event(s) can be of various origin, and distinct pathways -- not necessarily mutually exclusive -- have been postulated.

An immune-mediated damage of hematopoiesis sparing PNH cells. The well-accepted theory of PNH pathophysiology claims that such second event is a change in the microenvironment of hematopoiesis, leading to the selective expansion of the *PIG-A* mutated cells. It is quite accepted that such external factor, which does not affect the intrinsic features of the *PIG-A* mutated cells, is an (auto)-immune attack against hematopoiesis. Several clinical and experimental observations support the presence of such auto-immune attack in PNH; they include the well-known clinical overlap between PNH and aplastic anemia (AA, which is in most cases immune-mediated) (Lewis & Dacie 1967), as well as the direct demonstration of immune abnormalities in PNH patients. All these observations are discussed later on in this chapter. Indeed, normal and PNH cells are not different in terms of growth or survival, but PNH cells could be spared by immune-mediated damage, finally resulting in a progressive consumption of normal hematopoiesis, with relative expansion of PNH hematopoiesis (Rotoli & Luzzatto 1989; Luzzatto et al 1997; Young & Maciejewski 2000). This was confirmed by gene expression profiling performed in normal and PNH HSCs: when CD34+ cells from PNH patients were separated according to the presence or absence of GPI-APs on their surface, distinct patterns of gene expression were identified. In fact, phenotypically normal (GPI-AP positive) CD34+ cells harbored diffuse abnormalities of their transcriptome, with over-expression of genes involved in apoptosis and immune activity, paralleling the findings seen in CD34+ cells of AA patients. By contrast, phenotypically abnormal PNH CD34+ (GPI-AP negative) showed a gene expression profiling closer to that obtained in CD34+ cells from healthy individuals (Chen et al 2005). Notably, normal and PNH CD34+ cells did not show any difference in the genes involved in growth or proliferation, rather suggesting the presence of sublethal extrinsic damage in phenotypically normal HSCs but not in their *PIG-A* mutated counterpart. Indeed, PNH cells ultimately expand as a result of a selective pressure that acts negatively on normal hematopoiesis; however, the molecular reasons underlying the "escape" still remain elusive. Contradictory data have been produced on a putative differential sensitivity to inhibitory stimuli between normal and PNH cells; susceptibility to apoptosis has been reported to be increased, normal or decreased in different models. It has been shown that human cell lines carrying the *PIG-A* mutation are less susceptible to NK-mediated killing compared to their normal counterpart (Nagakura et al 2002). In a more sophisticated model, GPI-deficient cells were not able to induce primary and secondary stimulation of both antigen-specific and alloreactive T cells, providing experimental support to the hypothesis that the PNH clone could inefficiently interact with the immune system (Murakami et al 2002). Indeed, the actual mechanisms causing the escape may include the absence of specific GPI-APs directly targeted by effector immune cells, or a protection due to the absence of important molecules involved in cell-cell interaction (e.g., accessory molecules). Alternatively, a broader impaired sensitivity to common effector mechanisms may be hypothesized, possibly due to the lack of GPI-APs or to non specific structural changes of the raft structure in the outer surface. Remarkably, the observation that patients with a B-cell lymphoproliferative disorder treated by alemtuzumab may develop expansion of GPI-deficient (PNH-like) T cells indirectly confirms the escape theory. Alemtuzumab is a monoclonal antibody that kills lymphocytes targeting the GPI-linked protein CD52; after treatment, CD52-negative lymphocytes may be found, which also lack all other GPI-APs. Once such lymphocytes are cloned, mutations in the *PIG-A* gene can be demonstrated; interestingly, the same mutation can be found also in a few cells from pre-treatment blood samples. In most cases these expansions are self-limiting and transient, and GPI-deficient T-cells gradually disappear after alemtuzumab discontinuation. Thus, this model elucidates most features of the PNH pathogenesis: the pre-existence of *PIG-A* mutated cells, their expansion only in the presence of a selective pressure negatively acting on normal cells (mutated cells are intrinsically resistant to alemtuzumab due to the absence of CD52), and the gradual disappearance of the mutated clone once the selective mechanism has been removed (Hertestein et al 2005). It has to be remarked that none of these alemtuzumab-treated patients developed PNH, because the expansion of GPI-AP deficient clones includes only mature lymphocytes and not multipotent HSCs (alemtuzumab does not kill HSC or hematopoietic progenitors, because CD52 expression is restricted to the lymphoid cells).

Additional mutations conferring growing advantage. The selective advantage of the *PIG-A* mutated clone could also be explained by a second (or a pre-existing) mutation of the aberrant clone, which confers an absolute growth advantage. The most striking evidence supporting this theory is the observation that a few PNH patients may harbor, in the *PIG-A* mutated clone, an additional concomitant genetic lesion in the chromosome 12. This lesion was identified in a mutation in the 3′ of the *HMGA2* gene, which leads to HMGA2 over-expression and subsequent proliferative advantage (Inoue et al 2006). However, this mutation has not been found in larger series of PNH patients, making the pathogenic role of this lesion questionable. Clonal dominance of the PNH clone may also be due to other, still unknown, additional mutation(s) of the *PIG-A* mutated cells, possibly secondary to an intrinsic genetic instability of the abnormal clone. However, recent data exclude that *PIG-A* mutated cells have any increase in genetic instability. In fact, using the *PIG-A* itself as sentinel gene, the intrinsic rate of somatic mutation in PNH cells did not differ from that of normal cells, and it was remarkable less than that of cells with known genetic instability (i.e., Fanconi Anemia cells) (Araten et al 2007). Thus, these data argue against the possibility that PNH can be due to either a pre-existing genetic instability favoring the *PIG-A* mutation, or to a genetic instability secondary to the *PIG-A* mutation itself, which could predispose to additional genetic events necessary for PNH development. This is also supported, *in vivo*, by the clinical observation that malignant evolution in PNH patients is extremely rare, even if possible (Krause 1983; Devine et al 1987a); karyotypic abnormalities can been found in a few PNH patients, but in most cases they are transient and do not lead to leukemic transformation (Araten et al 2001). Remarkably, both MDS and truly leukemic cells not necessarily come from the *PIG-A* mutated clone; in fact, even more frequently they arise from the non-PNH, normal, residual hematopoiesis (van Kamp et al 1994; Araten et al 2001). Thus, the malignant evolution seems not related to any intrinsic feature secondary to the *PIG-A* mutation, but rather to the underlying bone marrow disorder, possibly including even clonal dominance itself.

The neutral evolution theory. More recently, a third possibility has been postulated, that even the expansion of the *PIG-A* mutated HSC could be a simple stochastic phenomenon, not requiring any additional event; this theory has been described as the "neutral evolution" hypothesis. According to the mathematic model provided by Dingli (Dingli et al 2008), given the stochastic nature of hematopoiesis (Notaro & Luzzatto et al 2010), a *PIG-A* mutation may randomly occur within the active HSCs pool, which in adults comprises about 400 cells, each replicating, on average, once per year. Subsequently, the expansion of the mutant clone may simply reflect the stochastic dominance of a few HSC, regardless of any functional feature (either absolute or conditional growth advantage), which may lead to a PNH clone size large enough to cause the disease. According to the authors, this model would fit the actual (expected) incidence of PNH (Hill et al 2006c). The chances that a single clone (even carrying a neutral mutation like the *PIG-A*) overcomes residual hematopoiesis increases with oligoclonal hematopoiesis, reconciling the model with the observation that clinical PNH mostly develop in patients with an underlying bone marrow failure.

4.2 Hematopoiesis in PNH patients
4.2.1 Marrow failure and PNH
As discussed later on, anemia is a typical presentation of PNH; however, cytopenias involving other blood lineages are also common in PNH patients. Cytopenia in these patients is mainly due to impaired production by the bone marrow, as confirmed by the

reduction in hematopoietic progenitors assessed by culture assays. In fact, it has been demonstrated that bone marrow from PNH patients show a significant reduction in all lineage-committed progenitors (CFU-E, BFU-E, CFU-GM, CFU-GEMM) (Rotoli et al 1984; Maciejewski et al 1997) , as well as in stem cells/multi-potent progenitors (LTC-IC) (Maciejewski et al 1997). This was demonstrated in all PNH patients, regardless of their clinical presentation (see disease classification) (Parker et al 2005); namely, a subclinical marrow failure can be detected even in patients with hypercellular bone marrow. The functional impairment of the bone marrow may become clinically evident in a fraction of patients (at least one third), leading to mild cytopenia up to clinically significant bone marrow failure, seen as aplastic anemia (AA) (Lewis & Dacie 1967). In fact, many PNH patients may sooner or later develop frank aplastic anemia during the course of their disease (Hillmen et al 1995; Sociè et al 1996; De Latour et al 2008); conversely, AA patients may also develop PNH. Indeed, a substantial fraction of AA patients (up to 40%) may have detectable PNH clone (Nissen et al 1999; Mukhina et al 2001; Sugimori et al 2006; Scheinberg et al 2010), in most cases not large enough to cause evident hemolysis; however, the size of the PNH clone may vary over time, possibly leading to clinical PNH. Thus, PNH and AA are closely embedded (Dameshek 1967), and should be considered as different presentations of the same disorder rather than independent conditions. Furthermore, regardless of its clinical presentation, PNH must be considered by definition a bone marrow disorder because of its impairment of hematopoiesis, which is both quantitative (clinical or subclinical) and qualitative (the aberrant phenotype stems from the *PIG-A* mutated HSC). To some extent, PNH could be considered an attempt of the body to prevent the development of AA by rescuing hematopoiesis with PNH cells (Rotoli & Luzzatto 1989); in fact, the PNH clone ensures some mature blood cells, even if it leads to specific consequences secondary to the abnormality of the PNH cells (i.e., hemolysis and thrombophilia).

4.2.2 Immune derangement in PNH patients

Given the clinical overlap between PNH and AA, it is reasonable to hypothesize that pathogenic mechanisms involved in AA may also play a pivotal role in PNH, representing the additional factor required for developing clinical PNH once a *PIG-A* mutation has occurred (without any specific chronologic order). The immunological mechanisms in idiopathic AA play a pivotal role in damaging the hematopoietic compartment, leading to HSC pool consumption or to functional impairment and subsequent pancytopenia (Young & Maciejewski 2000; Young et al 2006). A number of experimental observations supports the presence of an anti-hematopoiesis immune attack, although the target antigens are still undefined, as are the mechanisms leading to the breach in immune tolerance. Unknown triggers of autoimmunity induce a cellular immune response resulting in a preferential expansion of specific T cell clones that may damage the hematopoietic progenitors, directly or through indirect mechanisms, such as the production of inhibitory cytokines. Stem cell damage can be mediated by cytokine-transduced inhibition (mostly type I cytokines, such as interferon-γ and tumor necrosis factor-α), or by direct cell-mediated killing due to cytotoxic lymphocytes (CTLs) (reviewed in Young et al 2006). Such mechanisms, which may attack innocent bystander cells in addition to the primary target cells, ultimately result in apoptosis, the main key mechanism of HSC damage. Circulating and marrow CTLs have been demonstrated in vivo in AA patients, and their inhibitory effect on hematopoiesis has been documented in vitro (reviewed in Young et al 2006); this cellular immune response has been dissected at the molecular level through the identification of in vivo-dominant T cell clonotypes, which are evidence of a pathogenic antigen-driven immune response (Risitano et al 2004). Since in PNH a similar antigen-driven immune response targeting marrow tissue may be postulated, investigators have evaluated the same pathways of the immune system for possible abnormalities. As for AA, evidence of immune derangement in PNH has been produced, mostly pointing out the pivotal role of cell-mediated immunity. In fact, oligoclonality of the T cell pool has been reported (Karadimitris et al 2000), and immunodominant pathogenic CTL clones may be detected in most PNH patients (Risitano et al 2004; Plasilova et al 2004). Notably, immunodominant T-cell clones identified in PNH patients may share highly homologous T-cell receptor beta (TCR-beta) sequences, and additional closely related sub-dominant T-cell clones may be identified, consistent with an antigen-driven public immune response (Gargiulo et al 2007). The observation that recurrent or highly homologous TCR-beta sequences may be identified regardless of the individual patient's HLA background (in contrast with what is seen in AA) (Risitano et al 2004), may also suggest that a non-peptidic triggering antigen may be involved, possibly related to the GPI-anchor itself (Gargiulo et al 2007). Functionally, these pathogenic T cells harbor an effector, cytotoxic phenotype, characterized by expression of CD8 and CD57. These effector lymphocytes also show an imbalance in the expression of the activating and inhibitory surface receptors; in fact, they tend to over-express the activating isoforms of inhibiting superfamily receptors, which elicit a powerful cytolytic activity (Poggi et al 2005). Notably, in some PNH patients these CTL clonal populations may expand to represent a subclinical (Risitano et al 2005) or even clinically meaningful LGL proliferations (Karadimitris et al 2001).

4.3 Hemolysis in PNH patients
4.3.1 The complement system

The complement system is a key component of innate immunity, that has evolved to recognize both exogenous pathogenic microorganisms as well as injured self tissues, and to amplify adaptive immunity (Müller-Eberhard 1988; Holers 2008). The complement system encompasses distinct functional pathways with unique mechanisms of activation, which then all merge into a common final effector mechanism -- the cytolytic membrane attack complex (MAC). Thus, initiation of complement activation may occur along three different pathways – classical, alternative or lectin – which independently lead to activation of C3 and C5 convertases. While the classical and the lectin pathways require specific triggers to be activated, usually infectious agents, it has been known for decades that the complement alternative pathway (CAP) exhibits low-grade continuous activation due to spontaneous hydrolysis of C3 (the so-called tick-over phenomenon) (Pangburn et al 1981; Pangburn & Müller-Eberhard 1983). In addition, some components of the CAP constitute an amplification mechanism (the so called CAP amplification loop), which amplifies complement activation regardless of the specific pathway that initially generates the first C3b molecule. Fine mechanisms have evolved to control the complement system, including membrane-bound proteins (complement receptor 1 [CR1], membrane cofactor protein [MCP], and the membrane proteins CD55 and CD59) as well as fluid-phase components, including complement factor I (FI) and factor H (FH). Among these, CD55 and CD59 are of pivotal importance in PNH, given that they are normally expressed on blood cells through the GPI-anchor (Medof et al 1986).

4.3.2 Complement regulatory proteins and PNH erythrocytes

CD55, also known as Decay Accelerating Factor (DAF), is a 70-kd protein first isolated in 1969 (Hoffman 1969) and subsequently purified in 1982 (Nicholson-Weller et al 1982) which inhibits the formation and the stability of C3 convertase (both C3bBb and C4b2a) (Nicholson-Weller 1992). Historically, CD55 was the first complement regulator reported to be absent on PNH erythrocytes (Pangburn et al 1983(a); Pangburn et al 1983(b); Nicholson-Weller et al 1983) possibly accounting for the increased susceptibility of PNH erythrocytes to complement mediated lysis. However, further studies suggested that factors other than CD55 should also be involved, possibly acting downstream on the complement cascade (Medof et al 1987; Shin et al 1986). Subsequently, CD59 (also known as Membrane Inhibitor of Reactive Lysis , MIRL) was identified as an additional complement inhibitor expressed on normal erythrocytes, while PNH erythrocytes were demonstrated deficient in CD59 (Holguin et al 1989(a)). CD59 interferes with the terminal effector complement, blocking the incorporation of C9 onto the C5b-C8 complex, forming the membrane attack complex (MAC) (Meri et al 1990). Thus, independently from CD59 the lack of CD50 may explain complement-mediated hemolysis of PNH erythrocytes (Holguin et al 1989(b)). The hierarchical contribution of CD55 and CD59 to hemolysis suggests that CD59 is the key molecule which, if absent, leads to lysis (Wilcox et al 1991); in contrast, redundant mechanisms (including CD59 itself) usually overcome the isolated deficiency of CD55 (Holguin et al 1992). This is also confirmed by clinical observations: in fact, patients carrying the so-called Inab phenotype (an isolated CD55 deficiency, with normal CD59 expression) do not suffer from hemolysis (Telen & Green 1989; Merry et al 1992) whereas anecdotic cases of CD59 deficiency lead to a clinical phenotype undistinguishable from PNH (Yamashina et al 1990; Motoyama et al 1992).

4.3.3 Increased susceptibility of PNH erythrocytes to complement-mediated lysis in vitro and in vivo

It is intelligible that the deficiency of the complement regulatory proteins CD55 and CD59 renders PNH erythrocytes susceptible to uncontrolled complement activation and subsequent lysis.

In vitro. The very initial studies on PNH performed by Dr. Ham associated the hemolysis observed in PNH patients with an intrinsic susceptibility of red cells to complement activation *in vitro* (Ham 1937; Ham & Dingle 1939). In fact, the acidified serum assay (also known as the Ham test) – where the acidification activates the complement through the alternative pathway - became the standard technique for the diagnosis of PNH. The abnormality resulted intrinsic to patient erythrocytes, given that hemolysis occurs regardless of the origin of serum, while sera from patients do not result into the lysis of erythrocytes from normal individuals. This assumption was also confirmed in cross-transfusion studies (Rosse 1971). Since these initial studies it was evident that not all the erythrocytes drawn from a patient had the same susceptibility to complement-mediated lysis, making the point that all patients presented a mosaicism of normal and affected erythrocytes. Rosse and Dacie clearly elucidated that in erythrocytes obtained from PNH patients three different phenotypes could be identified, differing in their sensitivity to complement-mediated lysis *in vitro* (Rosse & Dacie 1966; Rosse 1973) . The first phenotype had a normal (equal to that of erythrocytes from healthy individuals) sensitivity to complement, while abnormal cells could have a dramatic hypersensitivity to complement-mediated lysis (15-25 times the normal one), or just a moderate hypersentivity (3-5 times normal). These phenotypes are referred as PNH type I, type III and type II, respectively (Rosse & Dacie 1966; Rosse 1973); now we know that they correspond to a normal expression of GPI-APs (type I), or to a complete (type III) or partial (type II) deficiency of GPI-APs, as documented by flow cytometry (van der Schoot et al 1990). Notably, PNH patients may have either PNH type II or type III only, or may harbor a combination of both phenotypes. As anticipated, the proportion of the specific phenotype shapes the clinical manifestations of an individual patients (especially the extent of hemolysis), and may vary greatly not only among patients, but even in the same patient during the course of the disease.

In vivo. The *in vivo* consequence of the hypersensitivity of PNH erythrocyte to complement activation accounts for the most obvious manifestation of PNH, namely intravascular hemolysis and subsequent hemoglobinuria. Indeed, it is well known that PNH erythrocytes chronically undergo intravascular hemolysis in PNH patients *in vivo*, with a lifespan reduced to 10% compared to normal RBCs. This chronic hemolysis likely results from steady-state complement activation, due to the low-grade spontaneous C3 tick-over leads to chronic CAP activation on the PNH erythrocyte surface (Pangburn et al 1981; Pangburh & Müller-Eberhard 1983). It should be reiterated that both the initial complement activation and the down-stream effector mechanisms are uncontrolled on PNH erythrocytes. Specifically, the lack of CD55 impairs the regulation of C3 convertases (regardless the triggering pathway – classical or alternative) (Mold et al 1990), leading to increased C3 activation and further progression along the subsequent steps of the complement cascade. Thus on PNH erythrocytes -- due to the lack of CD55 -- the complement cascade activated by the CAP continues through to MAC assembly, finally coming to lysis for the lack of CD59. In this view, PNH can be considered mostly a CAP-mediated disease (Holers 2008); in real life, this physiological low-level complement activation is greatly amplified during inflammatory or infectious diseases. Indeed, overt hemolysis and paroxysms of PNH patients likely results from a specific triggering action on the complement cascade, which may occur along each of the three distinct complement pathways. There are no data demonstrating which is the complement pathway activated in specific conditions *in vivo* (i.e. infections); however one may speculate that all the three pathways may co-operate, with a possible hierarchical dominance of the CAP, given its capability to amplify any complement activation regardless the initial triggering pathway.

4.4 Thrombophilia and PNH
In addition to hemolytic anemia and bone marrow failure, thrombophilia is the third typical manifestation of PNH; however, in contrast to the other two, much less is known about its pathophysiology. A number of possible mechanisms have been hypothesized, and some pieces of evidence have been provided, although the final mechanism remains speculative, possibly because it can be multifactorial. The clinical observation that thrombotic complications are more common in patients with larger PNH clones (Hall et al 2003; Grünewald et al 2003; Moyo et al 2004) and greater hemolysis may suggest that the pathogenic mechanism could be in some way embedded with complement activation (Markiewski et al 2007) and hemolysis itself. At least four distinct (but not mutually exclusive) mechanisms can be hypothesized. First, uncontrolled complement regulation on

platelet surface might lead to platelet activation and aggregation, enhancing clot formation (Gralnick et al 1995; Louwes et al 2001). Second, thrombophilia may directly results from hemolysis, due to the build-up of cell-free plasma hemoglobin released by the erythrocytes. This may occur through the ability of free hemoglobin to scavenge nitric oxide from plasma, blocking its inhibitory action on platelet aggregation and adhesion to endothelium, as well as its regulatory effect on vessel wall tone (Schafer et al 2004; Rother et al 2005). An other mechanism by which hemolysis might lead to thrombophilia includes the generation of procoagulant particles. In fact, microvesicles are known to be released in PNH patients upon hemolysis and complement activation from RBCs (Hugel et al 1999), WBCs (monocytes) and platelets, (Wiedmer et al 1993; Simak et al 2004) and even from the endothelium. However, even if their procoagulant action is commonly accepted (van Beers et al 2009), their specific role in the pathophysiology of thromboembolisms in PNH is not yet proven. The fourth possible mechanism of thrombophilia in PNH might be an impairment of the fibrinolytic system, due to the lack of membrane-bound urokinase-type plasminogen activator receptor (uPAR) -- which is GPI-linked, and to the excess of its soluble form (Ninomiya et al 1997; Sloand et al 2006).

5. Clinical features

PNH is characterized by a unique triad of clinical features: intravascular hemolysis, thromboembolic events and cytopenia (Dunn et al 2000; Parker & Ware 2003; Notaro & Luzzatto 2003). However, not all three manifestations are presents in all the patients, and the individual presentation of each patient may greatly vary according to the most dominant signs and symptoms. Thus, many investigators have tried to classify PNH according to the most typical clinical presentations; however, distinct categories are hard to define for a disease with such an unpredictable presentation and evolution.

5.1 Classification

The most adopted classification of PNH was proposed by the International PNH Interest Group in 2005 (Parker et al 2005), whereby PNH patients are grouped according to the presence of hemolysys and of an underlying bone marrow disorder. Accordingly, three distinct subtypes are identified: i. classic PNH, characterized by hemolysis without other marrow disorder (i.e., hemolytic PNH patients without relevant cytopenia); ii. PNH in the setting of another bone marrow disorder, characterized by hemolysis associated with an underlying marrow disorder, usually AA or MDS (i.e., hemolytic PNH patients with cytopenia; AA or MDS may be concomitant or have preceded PNH); iii. subclinical PNH, characterized by the presence of PNH cells in the absence of any clinical or laboratory sign of hemolysis, in the setting of other hematological disorders (i.e., AA or MDS patients with GPI-AP deficient cells, but not clinical PNH). This classification does not completely take into account that, by definition, PNH carries an underlying bone marrow disorder, and as a result most PNH patients have cytopenia or some signs of marrow failure. In fact, a recent registry study (de Latour et al 2008) made the point that many PNH patients do not fit either one of the two major categories, and a fourth subgroup has been included (intermediate PNH, characterized by hemolysis and mild cytopenia not qualifying for the diagnosis of AA). However, even this classification seems to fail the goal of identifying patient subgroups with distinct clinical outcome (de Latour et al 2008). Some other groups have used in the past a different classification (Notaro & Luzzatto 2003), where the category of AA/PNH patients is restricted to those with concomitant severe AA and clinically meaningful hemolysis, who require more intensive care and are supposed to have a worse prognosis. According to this classification, classic PNH patients are further grouped into hyperplastic and hypoplastic (based on peripheral counts and bone marrow analysis), AA/PNH patients are only those with severe marrow failure and concomitant clinically relevant hemolysis, whereas subclinical PNH patients are characterized by small PNH clone(s) (even with minimal signs of hemolysis) associated with either AA or thromboembolic disease (the latter are very rare cases with a clinical PNH that does not include relevant hemolysis).

5.2 Hemolysis

Hemolysis is the most typical manifestation of PNH, which by definition affects all patients with clinical PNH. However, the extent of hemolysis varies among patients, according to size of the PNH clone(s), type of PNH erythrocytes (type II versus type III), and possibly the level of complement activation (which may vary according to specific medical conditions or patient-specific features). Typically, hemolysis is chronic (secondary to the low-level spontaneous complement activation), with possible exacerbations (the paroxysms) consequent to a massive complement activation, often in association with infections or other triggering events. Hemolysis of PNH erythrocytes occurs in the vessels (intravascular hemolysis), and leads to a number of clinical consequences. The most evident sign to the patient is the hemoglobinuria, with the emission of dark urine, whose aspect is commonly defined as "*marsala wine*" or coke-like, according to the Country of origin of the observer and/or the time of the report (Parker 2002) . The color of urine is not constant over time, with the most typical dark urine often seen in the morning (hence the name "*paroxysmal nocturnal hemoglobinuria*"); however, the patient's urine mostly range from dark yellow to orange and dark red, with very rapid variations during the day. Even if nocturnal CO_2 retention has been hypothesized as possible cause of plasma pH fall and subsequent complement activation (Ham 1937), the reasons underlying nocturnal exacerbation of hemolysis are not yet fully understood (unless first-morning hyperconcentrated urine is not by itself an explanation for evident hemoglobinuria). The typical biochemical marker of hemolysis is the increase in lactate dehydrogenase (LDH), which may be as high as tenfold the upper normal value; additional intra-erythrocytary components may also increase, such as aminotransferases (especially the alanine one). As in other hemolytic disorders, unconjugated bilirubin levels may increase, even up to frank jaundice; compensatory erythropoiesis is usually demonstrated by very high reticulocyte counts, even if the latter value greatly depends upon the underlying marrow function (patients with hyperproliferative PNH may show even 300000-400000 cell x 10^9/L, while those with AA/PNH usually have less than 60000 cell x 10^9/L). Secondary iron deficiency may appear as a consequence of perpetual iron loss through urine. Clinically, the main consequence of continuous hemolysis is the development of anemia, and possibly other related symptoms such as asthenia and weakness. The extent of anemia is very heterogeneous among patients, also depending on other factors such as compensatory erythropoiesis (which may be impaired in patients with more severe marrow failure) or even iron/vitamin deficiency. As a result, anemia may be severe in some patients and requiring frequent transfusions, or well-compensated in other cases, even with normal-like hemoglobin levels. Furthermore, anemia may greatly vary even in the clinical course of an individual patients, with sudden worsening or unexpected improvements in the absence of any known reason; anecdotic cases showing spontaneous remission of the disease have also been reported (Hillmen et al 1995; Sociè et al 1996; de Latour et al 2008). In addition to anemia, it is now accepted that hemolysis may induce by itself specific disabling symptoms. This is usually seen in concomitance with the typical "paroxysms" of PNH, which are massive hemolytic crises often triggered by specific conditions (e.g., infections, surgery). These disabling symptoms include malaise and fatigue, with possible painful crises; the latter are quite typical, and mostly involve the abdomen, mimicking an acute abdomen. Some patients also report lumbar or sub-sternal pain, headache, dysphagia (both painful and difficult swallowing) and erectile dysfunction (Rother et al 2005). PNH paroxysms are irregular and unpredictable in individual patients, although most show a quite regular recurrence in the long run period. However, some of these hemolysis-related symptoms (especially malaise and fatigue exceeding those expected based on the low hemoglobin level) can be also seen as a consequence of chronic hemolysis. All these symptoms, which significantly impact patient well-being , are thought to be due to smooth muscle dystonia secondary to local nitric oxide (NO) consumption by plasma free-hemoglobin (Rosse 2000, Moyo et al 2004, Rother et al 2005).

5.3 Bone marrow failure

The second key clinical feature of PNH is cytopenia; in contrast to erythrocytes, PNH granulocytes and paltelets have anormal lifespan *in vivo* (Brubaker et al 1977; Devine et al 1987b); as discussed above, an underlying marrow disorder is embedded in the dual pathophysiology of the disease and with PNH clone expansion (Rotoli & Luzzatto 1989). Thus, some degree of marrow failure is common or even expected in PNH patients, ranging from mild cytopenias to severe aplastic anemia (Dunn et al 2000; Parker & Ware 2003; Notaro and Luzzatto 2003), and it may qualify for distinct disease categories (Parker et al 2005). Remarkably, the specific picture of each individual patient may change during the course of the disease, with patients initially presenting with normal marrow function and subsequently developing more severe marrow failure, as well as patients initially diagnosed with aplastic anemia subsequently developing frank hemolytic PNH (Tichelli et al 1992; Scheinberg et al 2010). Bone marrow failure usually becomes evident because of neutropenia and thrombocytopenia; however, it has to be remarked that marrow failure may also contribute to anemia in PNH patients. In fact, many PNH patients have a reticulocyte count that is inadequate to the hemoglobin level (iron deficiency may also contribute to that). The proportion of PNH patients with marrow failure ranges from 30 to 70% in different series, possibly because of heterogeneous definitions of bone marrow failure itself. The most homogeneous data from the French registry indicate that over 430 PNH patients 26% presented with normal counts (neutrophils > 1.5×10^9/L, platelets > 120×10^9/L) at diagnosis, 52% were classified as AA/PNH (with at least two of the following: Hb < 10gr/dL, neutrophils < 1.0×10^9/L, platelets > 80×10^9/L) and the remaining 22% as intermediate PNH (de Latour et al 2008).

5.4 Thrombophilia

The third typical manifestation of PNH is thrombophilia, with thrombosis developing in about 40% of all patients; accordingly, PNH is the medical condition with the higher risk of thrombosis. Unfortunately, as the underlying pathogenic mechanisms are not fully understood, thromboses are largely unpredictable in PNH patients, even if according to most series they generally develop in patients with large clones and massive hemolysis (Hall et al 2003; Moyo et al 2004). The thrombotic risk is peculiar to each patient, possibly as a result of additional independent (environmental or genetic) risk factors that may shape the individual predisposition to thrombosis. For instance, inherited polymorphisms such as Factor V Leiden mutation and the 677 C>T methylenetetrahydrofolate reductase gene variant (as well as other polymorphisms leading to hyperhomocysteinemia) may have a relevant role, although this has not been proven so far (Nafa et al 1996). However, this concept has in someway been confirmed by the observation that the thrombotic risk is different in PNH patients with specific ethnicity; in fact, Asian patients have a lower incidence of thrombosis (Nishimura et al 2004), while Afro-Americans and Latin-Americans seem to have an increased incidence (Araten et al 2005). Thrombosis of PNH is quite unique, because it mostly occurs at venous sites which are unusual for other non-PNH-related thrombosis. Intra-abdominal veins are the most frequent sites, followed by cerebral and limb veins; other possible sites include dermal veins, the lungs – with pulmonary embolus - and the artheries – leading to arterial thrombosis. Thrombotic disease may be life-threatening and is the main cause of death for PNH patients (Hillmen et al 1995; Socie et al 1996; de Latour et al 2008). Typical severe presentations of thrombotic PNH include hepatic venous (Budd-Chiari syndrome) (Hoekstra et al 2009), portal, mesenteric, and renal vein thrombosis. Usually patients are asymptomatic, until clinical manifestations appear, especially pain; other signs and symptoms are specific according to the vessel involved (e.g., ascites, varices and splenomegaly in hepatic/portal thrombosis, or stroke in cerebral vein thrombosis). Unfortunately, pain is not a useful symptom by itself, because it may also be due to vessel wall dystonia or to a transient ischemic attack (especially of the intestine) rather than to true thrombosis. However, a thrombotic episode has to be suspected in all PNH patients with obscure pain, even when it may mimic acute abdomen; ultra sound scan and magnetic resonance imaging (especially angiography) are useful to rule out these dangerous complications. Recurrence after the first episode and/or development of chronic thrombotic disease is typical of PNH (Hillmen et al 1995; Socie et al 1996; de Latour et al 2008; Audebert et al 2005; Moyo et al 2004); this is especially common in the setting of the Budd-Chiari syndrome, when the thrombotic process initially affects small veins, and then progressively involves large hepatic veins, with the development of life-threatening manifestations like variceal bleeding, jaundice, ascitis and liver failure. At this stage, liver regenerative nodules may also appear, which may erroneously suggest the presence of hepatocellular carcinoma. Thrombosis of other splancnic vein may usually lead to secondary ischemia and infarction, possibly leading to gangrene of the peripheral organ. Even if thromboses in PNH are unpredictable, recent data suggest that some biochemical parameters may work as surrogate markers of overt thrombophilia in PNH. They include D-dimers and other plasma markers of coagulation pathway activation, reactive fibrinolysis and endothelial cell activation (Helley et al 2010). However, their use has not been validated yet.

5.5 Other clinical manifestations

Renal failure. Both acute and chronic renal failure have been described in PNH patients (Nair et al 2008). Acute renal insufficiency is usually seen in concomitance with hemolytic crisis, as a result of massive hemoglobinuria. This condition is usually self-limiting and tends to recover spontaneously in a few days after the resolution of the crisis, although specific interventions (even dialysis) may be needed in the acute phase. Chronic kidney disease (CKD) has also been reported; in a recent paper the incidence of clinically relevant CKD was estimated in the range of 20% (Hillmen et al 2010), but these data have not been confirmed by other groups (nor in previous large retrospective studies) (Hillmen et al 1995; Socie et al 1996; de Latour et al 2008). Pathophysiologically, CKD might be related to microthrombi of the renal vessels, as well as to renal cortex siderosis, which can be easily demonstrated in PNH patients by magnetic resonance imaging.

Infections. Infectious complications are common in PNH patients; they mostly pertain to cases with concomitant marrow failure, as a direct consequence of neutropenia. However, they could also be related to some functional impairment of PNH neuthrophils and monocytes, and especially of their oxidative response - which is necessary for microorganism destruction - as documented by some *in vitro* data (Cacciapuoti et al 2007).

Pulmonary hypertension. Pulmonary hypertension (PH) has also been reported as possible complication of PNH by a single group (Hill et al 2006b); however, the clinical relevance of this observation remains to be confirmed in larger studies.

5.6 Pregnancy

Pregnancy is a specific issue which deserves an appropriate discussion in the setting of PNH. In fact, pregnancy in PNH certainly carries a high risk of complications for both mother and fetus. The main cause of complications is thrombophilia, which obviously worsen during pregnancy, and may lead to any of the thrombotic presentations described above. Additional risks may be related to suboptimal hemoglobin levels that hamper normal fetal development, as well as to cytopenia secondary to marrow failure, which may lead to infectious and hemorrhagic complications. It has to be remarked that, as for AA, pregnancy rarely causes worsening or recurrence of underlying bone marrow failure. A recent review (Fieni et al 2006) collecting 43 patients reported between 1965 and 2005 estimated the range of maternal and fetal mortality to 11.6% and 7.2%, respectively, which is quite lower than what previously thought. All the deaths were due to thrombotic complications, including fetal loss secondary to placental vein thrombosis; no case of fetal malformation was reported. Other major maternal complications included hemorrhage and infections; the most common fetal complication was pre-term delivery due to maternal complications (including placental vein thrombosis). On the other hand, pregnancies with successful outcome in the absence of any complication have lso been described. Thus, caution should be advised in counseling PNH women about a possible pregnancy, for both maternal and fetal risk. Regardless of the absolute contraindication to pregnancy (which could be re-discussed in the era of new treatment strategies), pregnancy in PNH remains a high-risk medical condition which requires an experienced caring team.

6. Natural history

The natural history of PNH is quite unpredictable, given the very heterogeneous disease presentation and evolution. In fact, some patients may live with the disease for decades, without major complications, whereas some others present with life-threatening medical complications, which in any case may develop at any moment during the course of the disease. Thus, the evolution and outcome of an individual patient is largely unpredictable.

Despite the rarity of the disease, some information from large series is available, although it might suffer from possible selection biases (e.g., exclusion of patients with early death due to dramatic presentation, such as lethal thrombosis) (Hillmen et al 1995; Socie et al 1996; de Latour et al 2008). Median survival was estimated above 10 years in the past decade in two independent series, with one fourth of patients surviving longer than 25 years (Hillmen et al 1995; Sociè et al 1996); more recently, the update of the French registry has revealed a median survival of about 22 years from diagnosis (de Latour et al 2008). Notably, these changes in median survival refer to the years before the introduction of the anti-complement therapy, and survival improvement was time-dependent (10-year survival was 63%, 76% and 92% according to diagnosis before 1995, 1995-2005 and after 2005, respectively), suggesting a relevant improvement in supportive care. Survival does not differ according to disease category: in fact, 10-year overall survival was 75%, 82% and 74% in classic PNH, intermediate PNH and AA/PNH, respectively. The main causes of death were thrombosis (cerebral thrombosis 25%, Budd-Chiari 23% - expressed as percentage of all deaths) and infectious complications (25%); they were both major causes of morbidity too. Even if PNH is not a malignant disease, progression to myelodysplastic syndrome and acute leukemia was observed with a 10-year cumulative incidence of 3.8%, which is similar to previous series (Hillmen et al 1995; Sociè et al 1996; Fujioka & Asai 1989) and to that reported for AA patients. Thrombosis developed in about 50% of classic PNH and 30% of intermediate PNH or AA/PNH patients; marrow failure developed in about 25% of classic and intermediate PNH patients. In the whole series, thrombosis was the main negative prognostic factor, followed by development of by- or pan-cytopenia, lower hemoglobin levels and previous diagnosis. Thrombosis affected long-term survival in all disease categories, including AA/PNH; risk factors for the development of thrombosis included thrombosis at diagnosis, old age, transfusion and lack of immunosuppressive treatment, and PNH clone size. Recurrent infections affected up to 40% of patients, representing the second main clinical complications of PNH; hemorrhage was an other relevant complication, especially in thrombocytopenic patients. Thus, even if most PNH patients may have a quite long life expectancy, the course of their disease may be stormy, with frequent hospitalizations, possible comorbidities and subsequent impaired quality of life. On the other hand, some patients may experience an indolent course, without major complications; a few PNH patients may also undergo spontaneous clinical remission of their disease, which can be estimated in about 5% (de Latour et al 2008) (even if an older study reported up to 15%, possibly due to definition bias) (Hillmen et al 1995). It has to be underlined that these data on the natural history of the disease might significantly change in the current era of effective anti-PNH treatment, mainly eculizumab or even bone marrow transplantation.

7. Diagnosis

PNH has to be suspected in patients showing mild to severe anemia with moderate reticulocytosis, elevated serum LDH and possibly mild jaundice, with negative Coombs test; all these clues suggest a non-immune hemolytic anemia. The occurrence of dark urine and urinary hemosiderin, both evidence of intravascular hemolysis, strongly support the suspect of PNH; haptoglobin is usually very low or undetectable. Additional signs to be considered are the presence of mild to severe leuko-thrombocytopenia and/or a history of thromboembolic events of unknown origin, including cerebrovascular accidents. In specific conditions, PNH may be considered even in the absence of clinically evident hemolytic anemia, such as in patients with AA or those showing recurrent thromboembolic events in the absence of documented risk factors; all these patients may deserve a careful screening for PNH. Diagnostic tests for PNH have much changed in the past three decades: the Ham test, which was the diagnostic test until the 1980s, has been completely replaced by flow cytometry.

The Ham test

Historically, the Ham test, also known as acidified serum assay, was since its identification in the 1930s the best test to diagnose PNH. Indeed, even the pathophysiological definition of PNH is based on the increased susceptibility of affected erythrocytes to complement mediated lysis (Rosse & Dacie 1966; Rosse 1991). The Ham test is an *in vitro* assay which employs this unique feature of PNH erythrocytes, testing the lysis in sera where the complement cascade (and specifically the complement alternative pathway) has been activated by pH lowering (by the addition of HCl). In these conditions, erythrocytes from PNH patients show a substantial lysis, which may vary according to the proportion of affected (*PIG-A* mutated) cells and to the type of mutation (type II versus type II PNH). Hemolysis occurs in both autologous and ABO-matched sera; as a control, lysis does not occur if the serum has been inactivated at 56° C (which inactivates some complement components), or when erythrocytes from healthy individuals are tested. In experienced hands, the test is relatively simple, and quite specific; however, its sensitivity is limited, with a threshold of about 5-10% PNH erythrocytes required for a definitive diagnosis. Other lysis assays exist, such as the sucrose lysis (or sugar water test); they exploit reduced ionic strength rather than acidification-based complement activation. However, their sensitivity and specificity for PNH are worse than those of the Ham test, and false positive may be common in other inherited hemolytic conditions. Obviously, all these lysis assays may only detect the presence of PNH erythrocytes, but cannot be utilized to detect cells with a PNH phenotype within any other blood lineage.

Flow cytometry

At present the diagnosis of PNH is based on flow cytometry analysis of blood cells (Parker et al 2005; Richards et al 2002); the high sensitivity and specificity of this analysis has made the Ham and similar tests obsolete. In fact, fluorochrome-conjugated monoclonal antibodies specific to several GPI-APs expressed on the various blood cell lineages are available for routine testing; thus, simultaneous multi-parameter analysis allows accurate detection of GPI-AP deficient cell populations, measuring their extent within each blood lineage (erythrocytes, granulocytes, monocytes and lymphocytes). By this technique, one or two erythrocyte populations with abnormal expression of GPI-APs may be found in PNH patients: one completely lacking GPI-AP expression (type III PNH cells), and another characterized by GPI-AP faint (dim) expression (type II PNH cells). These findings match the observation initially made by Dr. Rosse, demonstrating the presence of distinct subpopulations of erythrocytes with different sensitivity to complement-mediated lysis (Rosse & Dacie 1966); as discussed above, this may also imply that different populations may be genetically different. The demonstration of GPI-AP deficient populations is easy for all cell lineage, even if discrimination between type II and type III PNH cells is more difficult for white blood cells; antibodies specific for GPI-APs selectively expressed by specific cell lineage may render the test more sensitive and specific. Different panels of monoclonal antibodies have been proposed by different groups (Richards et al 2000;

Borowitz et al 2010); they usually include CD55 and CD59 for erythrocytes, CD66b, CD66c and CD24 for granulocytes, CD14 or CD48 for monocytes, CD48 or CD59 for lymphocytes. A counter-staining for gating strategies on specific blood cell populations may be included; in fact, a complete testing for PNH includes the analysis of erythrocytes, granulocytes, monocytes, and possibly lymphocytes (even if they are usually minimally affected, because most of them are long-living cells sustained by peripheral homeostasis). Platelets are usually not tested for PNH phenotype, due to the difficulty to separate normal platelets from PNHs (Maciejewski et al 1996; Vu et al 1996). The simultaneous absence of different GPI-linked proteins on the same cells validates the specificity of the test; as far as the sensitivity is concerned, flow cytometry analysis in experienced hands may detect even very small PNH clones (below 1% in routine testing, (Borowitz et al 2010) up to 0.01% in ultra-sensitive analysis for research purpose) (Araten et al 1999; Sugimori et al 2006). More recently, the novel fluorescent reagent aerolysin (FLAER), which specifically binds to the GPI anchor, showed even greater sensitivity for the detection of small PNH cell population, up to 0.01% as a single marker (Brodsky et al 2000; Sutherland et al 2007). FLAER can be easily combined with other monoclonal antibodies for a comprehensive and simultaneous study of all blood leukocytes. However, given that FLAER requires to be processed by proteolytic enzymes expressed on leucocyte surface, it cannot be utilized detect PNH erythrocytes or platelets.

Molecular studies

Molecular studies on DNA or mRNA, aimed to identify the specific causative mutation within the *PIG-A* gene, are usually considered superfluous rather than confirmatory. In fact, they do not add any clinically informative data and can even be somewhat misleading. Indeed, a false negative result may occur, especially when mononuclear cells are used as nucleid acid source (proportion of PNH lymphocytes are minimal in the majority of patients), or in case of some intronic mutations; on the other hand, false positive results may also occur due to the intrinsic sensitivity of the technique. Notably, molecular studies do not deliver the most relevant information as flow cytometry-based assay, which is the exact proportion of affected GPI-deficient (thus *PIG-A* mutated) cells. Thus, molecular testing is not recommended for the diagnosis of PNH.

Blood

The blood film is usually not very informative in PNH patients. Red blood cells are usually macrocytic due to reticulocytosis (which can be demonstrated by vital dyes), but cell size may greatly vary. Polychromatophilic or even nucleated erythrocytes may be present as a result of compensatory erythropoiesis. Microcytic hypocromic erythrocytes may also be present, because of the secondary iron deficiency; red cell fragments may be observed, especially in concomitance with thrombotic complications. Leukocytes do not show any abnormality, even if neutropenia is commonly seen in patients with AA/PNH; thrombocytopenia is also quite frequent.

Coombs test

The differential diagnosis of PNH includes all other hemolytic conditions; thus, the Coombs test should be performed as initial assay. By definition, the Coombs test is negative in PNH, as it is a non-immune hemolytic anemia. However, it has to be remarked that a positive Coombs test may result from allo-immunization secondary to transfusion. More recently, it has been shown that a C3-only positive Coombs test may develop in most PNH patients on eculizumab treatment (Risitano et al 2009a); this finding is not due to any antibody, but rather it derives from mechanistic reasons that will be discussed later on.

Bone marrow

The bone marrow pattern may be significantly different according to the presentation of the disease. In fact, patients with classic PNH may present with hyperproliferative bone marrow, and markedly increased erythropoiesis; however, due to the underlying bone marrow disorder, they may also present normal or even reduced marrow cellularity. The latter pattern is typical in AA/PNH patients, where cellularity is below 30%, as assessed by threphine biopsy. Commonly, morphological abnormalities may be observed, sometimes leading to the misdiagnosis of MDS; it has to be underlined that in most cases such abnormalities are not specific and simply reflect the stressed erythropoiesis. Additional tests can be performed on bone marrow specimens. Cytogenetic studies may occasionally reveal karyotypic abnormalities, which may occur in either PNH or normal cells; however, they do not necessarily carry a bad prognosis as for MDS (Araten et al 2001). Flow cytometry may be used to rule out leukemic transformation; given that surface expression of most GPI-APs undergoes changes during differentiation and maturation, bone marrow flow cytometry is not recommended for the diagnosis of PNH.

Urine

Even a macroscopic observation of urine may be a useful tool for the diagnosis of PNH; in fact, eye-evident hemoglobinuria may be one of the clinical presentations. Plasma free hemoglobin secondary to intravascular hemolysis depletes haptoglobin; as a result, free hemoglobin is continuously present in the glomerular filtrate. The excess hemoglobin is partially reabsorbed in the proximal tubule, and the iron stored as intracellular ferritin granules easily detected in the urine cast by appropriate iron (Perl's) staining – as hemosiderin granules. Hemosiderinuria is constantly present in all hemolytic PNH patients (even in the absence of hemoglobinuria, which fluctuates according to the concomitant hemolysis), thus it still represents an easy test to support the initial suspect of PNH.

Other instrumental studies

The management of PNH patients may require many other laboratory and instrumental studies useful to investigate the evolution of the disease and its possible complications. They especially include all the techniques useful to assess the presence of possible thrombosis; according to the specific sites, the most useful are computed tomography or magnetic resonance based, (for the cerebral and sometimes the hepatic districts), or ultra-sound based (for the abdomen and limbs). Specific angiographic studies are always helpful, especially once a thrombotic episode has been demonstrated (and always for the assessment of the cerebral district), to better assess the extent of the clot and its evolution. All these studies should be performed without delay, at diagnosis and/or in the presence of specific symptoms.

8. Treatment

The treatment of PNH is driven by the specific disease presentations (Brodsky 2009; Luzzatto et al 2011); however, in most cases treatment is essentially supportive, aiming at living with the disease with the least clinical burden. Thus, the main goals of PNH treatment includes the control of anemia and possibly of hemolysis; in patients with either marrow failure or thrombosis additional specific treatments are needed. Given the chronic course of PNH, an other major goal is the prevention of possible complications, mainly thrombosis and infections, to ensure long-term survival. More recently, etiological treatments for PNH have become available with the introduction of the first anti-complement agent, the anti-complement component 5 (C5) eculizumab. Finally, the only curative option for PNH is allogeneic stem cell transplantation.

8.1 Supportive therapies

The supportive treatment of PNH aims to control the main clinical manifestations of the disease; thus, it can be split according to specific manifestation – hemolysis and subsequent anemia, bone marrow failure and thrombocytopenia.

8.1.1 Management of hemolysis and anemia

Hemolysis and subsequent anemia are the hallmarks of PNH, affect most PNH patients and often require specific treatment. Unfortunately, until the new millennium there was no specific option for controlling hemolysis. Steroids were broadly used as chronic administration or for acute hemolytic crises, without any proof of efficacy. Indeed, some investigators claimed that steroids are useful in controlling chronic complement-mediated hemolysis (Issaragrisil et al 1987; Bourantas 1994) and, even more, paroxysmal crises likely interfering with complement activation and/or the underlying conditions (i.e., inflammation) triggering the complement cascade; however, so far no mechanism of action has been provided. It has been suggested that steroids might ameliorate patient well-being even in the absence of any direct control of hemolysis (Parker et al 2005); in particular, they may be effective in improving the symptoms associated with paroxysmal crises, such as dysphagia and abdominal pain, although this effect in most cases may result from the self-limiting behavior of the paroxysms. However, a continuous use of steroids is discouraged in PNH patients, given the long-term toxicity of chronic steroidal therapy; a short-term use in presence of the paroxysms is not harmful but likely useless. Androgens have been utilized as well, with limited benefit (Harrington et al 1997); however, given their potential utility in stimulating erythropoiesis and especially megakaryocytopoiesis (Katayama et al 2001), they are primarily indicated in the presence of marrow impairment rather than to control hemolysis (see below). Once again, a risk-to-benefit evaluation should be specifically made for all individual cases, given that liver toxicity, virilizing action and other side effects have to be considered; in addition, some concerns about a potential increase in the Budd-Chiari syndrome have been raised by some physicians (Parker et al 2005). Regardless of the possibility to block hemolysis, in many patients anemia leads to clinically relevant symptoms requiring specific interventions. As remarked in the pathophysiology section, anemia of PNH patients is someway multi-factorial; thus, if the main contributor (hemolysis) cannot be affected, one may try to interfere with the additional mechanisms to improve hemoglobin levels. Besides hemolysis, the main factor affecting hemoglobin level is the bone marrow function, especially its capability to adequately compensate the ongoing hemolysis. By definition, erythropoiesis is usually impaired in patients with AA/PNH syndrome, who may require specific treatments (see below); however, ineffective erythropoiesis is commonly seen even in classic PNH patients. Given the perpetual hemosiderinuria, iron deficiency is common in PNH patients (Luzzatto et al 2011), and simple iron supplementation may increase hemoglobin levels in many patients. Similarly, vitamin B12 and folate supplementation are usually indicated to sustain the compensatory erythropoiesis secondary to hemolysis (Luzzatto et al 2011). Erythroid stimulating agents, essentially recombinant erythropoietin, may also help enhance erythropoiesis (Stebler et al 1990; Bourantas et 1994), especially in cases showing inadequate production of endogenous erythropoietin (McMullin et al 1996). Paradoxically, all these strategies may be of limited clinical benefit, because of the increased hemolysis (and hemolysis-related symptoms) resulting from the production of PNH erythrocytes susceptible to complement-mediated lysis. Notwithstanding these interventions, moderate to severe anemia may develop in a substantial proportion of PNH patients, for whom transfusions are the main strategy to control anemia. RBC transfusions are given to PNH patients according to their hemoglobin level; as for other chronic anemic patients, transfusions should be administered to maintain hemoglobin levels above 8 gr/dL. Transfusions transiently improve anemia-related symptoms, as well as hemolysis-related symptoms (the production of PNH erythrocytes temporarily decreases by effect of the higher hemoglobin levels). Remarkably, in contrast to other transfusion-dependent patients, iron overload is usually not a transfusion-related complication in PNH, given the massive iron loss through urine; this may change in PNH patients receiving transfusions during eculizumab treatment (Risitano et al, 2009b). However, as in other transfusion-dependent patients, refractoriness to transfusion may develop, mostly due to allo-sensitization. Refractoriness to transfusions was considered a severe complication requiring alternative treatment – even stem cell transplantation; however, nowadays it is not necessarily a severe complication, given the availability of the anti-complement treatment by eculizumab. Eculizumab has also dramatically changed the management of hemolysis for all PNH patients with meaningful hemolysis, as discussed later on.

8.1.2 Management of marrow failure

The management of marrow failure in PNH patients is the same as for AA patients, and represents the main challenge for physicians dealing with the treatment of this condition (Risitano 2011). Indeed, in addition to supportive strategies such as anti-infectious, anti-thrombotic and anti-hemorrhagic prophylaxis and/or treatment, etiologic therapies can also be attempted. According to the pathogenic mechanisms and the dual hypothesis described above, an immune-mediated inhibition of hematopoiesis is postulated in PNH, similar to that demonstrated in AA. Thus, immunosuppressive strategies have been reasonably utilized in PNH patients, even if large prospective studies are lacking. Cyclosporine A has led some improvement in a few series (Schubert et al 1997; Stoppa et al 1996; van Kamp et al 1995). More intensive regimens (as those recommended in severe AA) using the anti-thymocyte globulin associated with high dose prednisone and cyclosporin A have also been exploited; however, the available results are quite heterogeneous (Tichelli et al 1992; Sanchez-Valle et al 1993). Alternative immunosuppressive agents such as cyclophosphamide (Brodsky et al 2010) or the anti-CD52 monoclonal antibody alemtuzumab (Risitano et al 2010a) may be an alternative option (as salvage treatment); in the setting of alemtuzumab-based treatment, there is no concern over the potential selection risk for PNH hematopoiesis, given that the GPI-linked CD52 is not expressed on HSCs. Regardless of the specific immunosuppressive regimen, when this etiological treatment leads to an improvement of the underlying bone marrow impairment, usually normal (non-

PNH) hematopoiesis may be restored, possibly resulting in a progressive dilution (or even extinction) of the PNH clone. However, some patients may continue to have remarkable hemolysis due to the persistence of the PNH clone(s). In addition to the immunosuppressive therapy, it has to be pointed out that marrow failure represents the main indication to allogeneic stem cell transplantation for PNH patients; in fact, all young PNH patients with bone marrow failure should be considered for transplantation if they have a HLA-matched donor (Luzzatto et al 2011), or even if they have an unrelated donor (later in their disease course). Indeed, marrow failure of PNH patients has to be treated as aplastic anemia by either immunosuppression or allogeneic stem cell transplantation, regardless of the presence of the PNH clone(s) (Risitano 2011).

8.1.3 Management of thrombophilia

The management of the propensity to develop thrombosis is the hottest issue in PNH, since this complication represents the first cause of death. Unfortunately, there are no controlled prospective clinical trials concerning either primary and secondary thrombosis prophylaxis, or acute treatment of the event. The issue of primary prophylaxis is controversial, and no consensus exists; some physicians advocate the use of warfarin for all newly diagnosed PNH patients, while others do not use any prophylaxis. Both approaches are reasonable, given the unpredictability of thromboembolic events and the lack of evidence supporting any of these strategies; possible benefits are counterbalanced by the risk of hemorrhage from warfarin therapy, which may be considerable in PNH patients with low platelet count. Given that up to two thirds of PNH patients may never develop any thrombosis during the course of their disease, some physicians consider unacceptable to risk hemorrhagic complications (especially in those who are thrombocytopenic); this perception is strengthened by the fact that current primary prophylaxis is not necessarily protective in all patients (de Latour et al 2008; Luzzatto et al 2011). A reasonable compromise may be the adoption of primary prophylaxis for patients at higher risk of thrombosis, which can be identified by the presence of additional inherited (e.g., ethnicity, factor V Leiden) or acquired (e.g., lupus anti-coagulant, pregnancy) risk factors for thrombosis. A single group reported that prophylaxis by warfarin in patients with WBC PNH clones larger than 50% resulted in a very low incidence of thromboembolic events compared to historical controls (Hall et al 2003); however, hemorrhagic complications (even fatal) were also observed, and these date need to be confirmed in larger, possibly prospective studies. To data, there is no experience with newer and possibly more manageable agents, such as thrombin inhibitors, which might play a major role in the future. In contrast, as far as secondary prophylaxis is concerned, there is general agreement that all PNH patients experiencing any thromboembolic event should remain life-long on anticoagulants; however, even in this setting, no consensus exists about the best strategy. Low-molecular-weight heparin, as well as warfarin at different therapeutic ranges, are both utilized, with some physicians even considering the addition of anti-platelet agents; most physicians start with heparin, and subsequently shift to warfarin. However, despite the extended prophylaxis, recurrence of thrombosis (either as new events or progression of the existing ones) is frequent and affects the survival of PNH patients (Audebert et al 2005; de Latour et al 2008). Moreover, life-threatening hemorrhagic events are quite frequent in this cohort of patients, mostly when concomitant thrombocytopenia is present (Hall et al 2003, Moyo et al 2004). Finally, the management of an acute thromboembolic disease may require an intensive therapy similar to that for myocardial infarct; in addition to anti-coagulants at therapeutical doses, fibrinolytic therapies using tissue plasminogen activator have been exploited, showing efficient clearance of the thrombus in individual cases (McCullin et al 1994; Hauser et al 2003; Sholar & Bell 1985; Araten et al 2010). As for hemolytic anemia, the management of thrombophilia has substantially changed with the introduction of eculizumab.

8.2 Anti-complement treatment
8.2.1 Eculizumab: A humanized anti-complement component 5 monoclonal antibody
Eculizumab (h5G1.1-mAb, Soliris®, Alexion Pharmaceuticals) is a humanized monoclonal antibody (mAb) (Rother et al 2007) derived from the murine anti-human C5 mAb; it specifically binds the terminal complement component 5, thereby inhibiting its cleavage to C5a and C5b (Matis & Rollins 1995). Thus, eculizumab blocks the formation of MAC, the terminal effector mechanism leading to intravascular hemolysis of PNH erythcocytes. The blockade of the complement cascade at the level of C5 does not affect early complement components, preserving pivotal functions such as clearance of immune complexes and microorganisms (Matis and Rollins 1995). Eculizumab was initially investigated in patients suffering from other complement-mediated disorders; however, PNH appeared the best candidate disease to benefit from eculizumab treatment. In fact, eculizumab may compensate for the absence of CD59 on PNH erythrocytes, preventing their lysis upon complement activation (which is also uncontrolled given the absence of CD55). Eculizumab is administered intravenously, thus its bioavailability is 100%; its estimated half-life is 271 hours. Eculizumab therapy was designed to rapidly reach pharmacodynamic levels using an induction regimen, followed by a maintenance dosage schedule aiming to avoid concentration drops below the plasma level of 35 µg/mL (Hillmen et al 2006), which is the threshold level for pharmacodymanic effectiveness (based on *in vitro* data). In all PNH studies eculizumab has been administered intravenously as 4 weekly doses of 600 mg (induction regimen), followed by 900 mg doses every other week (maintenance regimen), starting 1 week after induction (week 5); this is the standard schedule, approved by the FDA for the treatment of hemolysis in PNH patients.

8.2.2 Safety and efficacy of eculizumab
Eculizumab and intravascular hemolysis: efficacy from the registration studies. The management of hemolysis of PNH, which was palliative until 2000, has dramatically changed with the availability of eculizumab (Brodsky 2009; Luzzatto et al 2011). In the last few years eculizumab has been extensively investigated for the treatment of hemolysis in patients with transfusion-dependent PNH. Safety and efficacy of eculizumab were initially established in a phase II pilot study (Hillmen et al 2004) as well as in two phase III clinical studies (TRIUMPH and SHEPHERD) (Hillmen et al 2006; Brodsky et al 2008), and subsequently were confirmed in a common open-label Extension study (Hillmen et al 2007). All patients receiving eculizumab were vaccinated against *Neisseria Meningiditis* at least two weeks before starting treatment. After the initial pilot study, which provided the proof-of-principle of effective blockade of intravascular hemolysis in eleven heavily transfused PNH patients (Hillmen et al 2004), eculizumab was tested in a double-blind, placebo-controlled, multinational randomized trial which enrolled 86 patients (Hillmen et al 2006). The eligibility criteria included at least 4 red cell transfusions in the previous 12 months, a PNH

type III erythrocyte population ≥10%, platelets ≥100 x 10^9/L, and lactate dehydrogenase (LDH) ≥1.5 times the upper limit of normal (Hillmen et al 2006). Treatment with eculizumab resulted in a dramatic reduction of intravascular hemolysis, as measured by LDH, leading to hemoglobin stabilization and transfusion independence in about half the patients. Control of intravascular hemolysis was achieved in all patients, and even cases who still required transfusions showed a reduction of their transfusional needs. The effects of eculizumab on hemolysis were evident after the first administration, and lasted for the whole study period. Compared to placebo, eculizumab significantly improved fatigue and quality of life, as measured by validated questionnaires (Hillmen et al 2006). These data were confirmed in the open-label phase III study SHEPHERD, which included a broader PNH population (minimum pretreatment transfusion requirement was one, and minimum platelet count requirement was 30 x 10^9/L) (Brodsky et al 2008). In the 96 patients enrolled in the study, treatment with eculizumab resulted in an almost complete control of intravascular hemolysis, regardless of the pretreatment transfusion requirement, with transfusion independence achieved in half the patients, and significant improvement in fatigue and quality of life (Brodsky et al 2008). The subsequent open-label Extension study enrolled a total of 187 patients who had previously completed one of the parent clinical trials (Hillmen et al 2007). The Extension study confirmed the efficacy and safety of eculizumab with a longer follow up, confirming that the effects of eculizumab treatment on intravascular hemolysis were retained over time (Hillmen et al 2007).

Eculizumab and thrombophilia. The Extension study included as a secondary endpoint the assessment of thrombotic risk in PNH patients chronically receiving eculizumab treatment, by looking to the incidence of thromboembolic events in the pretreatment and treatment periods in the same patients (Hillmen et al 2007). The rate of thromboembolism decreased from 7.37 to 1.07 events/100 patient-years after eculizumab treatment, with a 85% relative reduction. This reduction was preserved even in patients on anticoagulants, suggesting that eculizumab may be the most effective agent to prevent thromboembolisms in PNH patients (Hillmen et al 2007). Whether eculizumab exerts its effect on thrombophilia of PNH directly, or through the blockade of intravascular hemolysis (e.g., by reduction of NO consumption or reduced release of procoagulant microvesicles), it is still unknown. Recently, it has been reported that eculizumab treatment results in a significant decrease in the plasma markers of coagulation pathway activation, reactive fibrinolysis and endothelial cell activation (Helley et al 2010). This finding suggests that the pathophysiology of thrombosis in PNH may involve multiple pathways, and that the triggering events possibly affected by eculizumab have not been yet identified. However, if the protective effect of eculizumab on the thromboembolic risk are confirmed in a long-term period, it is reasonable to anticipate that eculizumab may result in an improvement of survival of PNH patients. Such effect on survival has been recently shown in a limited cohort of patients (Kelly et al 2011).

Eculizumab and PNH: any additional benefit? More recently, it has been reported that eculizumab may lead to additional beneficial effects for PNH patients. As stated before, by inhibiting intravascular hemolysis eculizumab controls all hemolysis-related symptoms, including painful crisis, dysphagia and erectile dysfunction (Hill et al 2005). In addition, by counteracting NO consumption, eculizumab might reduce the risk of pulmonary hypertension (PH) (Hill et al 2010b). This conclusion was mainly derived from the 50% reduction of N-terminal pro-brain natriuretic peptide (NT-proBNP), which was elevated at baseline in about 50% of PNH patients. Unfortunately this study does not include a direct estimation of pulmonary artery pressure by doppler echocardiography, making it uncertain as to whether these PNH patients exhibited clinically relevant PH. However, even if NT-proBNP can be considered a non-invasive marker for PH, possibly reflecting increased pulmonary vascular resistance and right ventricular dysfunction, it is usually utilized as prognostic marker in patients with proven diagnosis of PH. In another study, eculizumab appeared to improve renal function of PNH patients, as measured by estimated glomerular filtration rate (eGFR), preventing possible CKD (Hillmen et al 2010). The authors report that before treatment a fraction of PNH patients may have decreased eGFR, qualifying for stage 3-5 CKD (about 20%); eculizumab treatment resulted in an improvement of eGFR, and reduced the risk of major clinical kidney events. Nevertheless, PH and CKD are not commonly described in PNH patients (de Latour et al 2008); therefore, the real clinical impact of these finding has to be assessed in appropriate studies.

Eculizumab and pregnancy. Most hematologists try to dissuade PNH women from pursuing pregnancy, due to both maternal and fetal risk of complications, mainly secondary to thrombosis. Since eculizumab has became available, three pregnancies have been reported in women on this agent all through the gestation period; all of them had healthy newborns, without any maternal complication (Kelly et al 2010; Marasca et al 2010). Thus, even if eculizumab is formally not indicated in PNH pregnant women, and indeed the label for eculizumab classifies it as a pregnancy class C drug, common sense suggests that eculizumab be not automatically withdrawn in the case of pregnancy, giving careful consideration to the need to control the major causes of both maternal and fetal morbidity (intravascular hemolysis and subsequent anemia, and thrombophilia). It is still a matter of debate whether these data are sufficient to change our current counseling, allowing highly motivated PNH women to start pregnancy during eculizumab treatment.

Safety and tolerability of eculizumab treatment. The safety profile of eculizumab was assessed in the six studies involving PNH patients (Hillmen et al 2006; Brodsky et al 2008; Hillmen et al 2007), as well as on eleven studies utilizing eculizumab for different indications; the cumulative exposure was 147.44 and 492.20 patient-years in the two populations, respectively. Three deaths were reported in the PNH studies, all related to the underlying disease in two cases (one cerebral vascular accident and one progression to chronic myelomonocytic leukemia) and to an unrelated accident in the third (cerebral herniation). The main concern was a putative increased risk of infections, mostly by encapsulated bacteria, namely *Neisseria Spp.* Given the occurrence of a single case of meningitis by *Neisseria meningitidis* in the initial non-PNH cohort, all patients exposed to eculizumab were vaccinated against *Neisseria meningitidis* using a polyvalent vaccine. In addition, all patients received a warning on meningitis and infectious symptoms, as well as a rescue antibiotic prescription. No case of meningitis has been documented among the 195 PNH patients receiving eculizumab in the clinical trials; however, three patients developed a *Neisseria meningitidis* infection (possibly from *N. meningitidis* groups not covered by the prescribed vaccine), with sepsis in two cases. None of these patients developed meningitis or other complications, and all recovered promptly as a result of early diagnosis and treatment. The incidence of serious adverse events was similar in eculizumab-treated patients and in those receiving the placebo within the TRIUMPH trial; furthermore, none of the serious adverse events was considered as possibly, probably or definitely related to eculizumab. The overall rate of infectious events did not increase compared to the placebo group; however, herpes simplex and some other site-specific infections (nasopharyngitis, upper respiratory tract infection, urinary tract infection and sinusitis) appeared to be more frequent within the eculizumab-treated population. However, in all cases the intensity was mild and the clinical resolution prompt. The occurrence of immunogenity was assessed, and was demonstrated to be very infrequent, if at all present, and without consequence on drug efficacy. In summary, the treatment with eculizumab is safe and well-tolerated for the treatment of PNH, with negligible side effects (Hillmen et al 2006). Long-term treatment has not shown any deviation from this safety profile, as confirmed by post-marketing experience; however, anti-meningococcal vaccination and warning for symptoms of meningitis remains mandatory.

8.2.3 Emerging observations during treatment with eculizumab

C3-mediated extravascular hemolysis during eculizumab treatment. Since the introduction of eculizumab in 2005, growing evidence suggests that its effect on MAC inhibition may unmask a biologically relevant and potentially pathogenic role for the early phases of the complement cascade. We have recently documented that a novel, clinically significant finding may appear in PNH patients receiving eculizumab, accounting for some portion of residual anemia and heterogeneous hematological benefit from treatment (Risitano et al 2009a). In fact, while basically all patients achieve normal or almost normal LDH levels (pointing out an adequate control of intravascular hemolysis), only about a third reach a hemoglobin value above 11 gr/dL). In contrast, the remaining patients on eculizumab continue to exhibit moderate to severe (transfusion-dependent) anemia, in about equal proportions. In our initial series of 56 PNH patients, we have demonstrated by flow cytometry that all the 41 PNH patients on eculizumab harbored C3 fragments bound to a substantial portion of their PNH erythrocytes (while none of the untreated patients did) (Risitano et al 2009a). Our data were confirmed in an independent series by an other group that exploited a direct antiglobulin test using C3d-specific anti-sera (Hill et al 2010a). We concluded that membrane-bound C3 fragments work as opsonins on PNH erythrocytes, resulting in their entrapment by reticuloendothelial cells through specific C3 receptors and subsequent extravascular hemolysis (Risitano et al 2009a; Luzzatto et al 2010). This mechanism is supported by persistent reticulocytosis, hyperbilirubinemia and anemia in patients on eculizumab, and was also confirmed by an *in vivo* erythrocyte survival study by ^{51}Cr labeling (which showed reduced survival and hepatosplenic ^{51}Cr uptake) (Risitano et al 2009a).

The complement cascade regulation during eculizumab treatment. Pathophysiologically, it is clear that such a mechanism becomes evident only when eculizumab prevents MAC-mediated hemolysis, allowing longer survival of PNH erythrocytes, which continue to suffer from uncontrolled C3 convertase activation and C3 fragment deposition due to CD55 deficiency (Luzzatto et al 2010; Risitano et al 2011). Indeed, CAP is physiologically in a state of continuous activation because spontaneous (low-grade) hydrolysis of an internal thioester bond of C3 generates a C3b-like molecule, $C3(H_2O)$; nascent $C3(H_2O)$ is able to recruit factor B in forming (in the fluid phase) an unstable pro-C3 convertase. Once cleaved by factor D (generating $C3(H_2O)Bb$), this complex will in turn cleave additional C3 molecules to generate C3b, which binds predominantly to glycophorin A and activate (now in a membrane-bound phase) the CAP amplification loop (Parker et al 1982; Pangburn et al 1983c; Müller-Eberhard 1988; Risitano et al 2011). On PNH erythrocytes, the lack of CD55 will allow this process (which is self-limiting on normal cells) to continue, leading to progressive CAP-mediated amplification, even in the presence of eculizumab (which acts downstream). The reasons why only a fraction of PNH erythrocytes has membrane-bound C3, and why the proportion varies among patients, are not fully understood. Nevertheless, *in vitro* data support the concept that PNH erythrocytes are all susceptible to C3 deposition once exposed to conditions causing complement activation (Sica et al 2010). We have hypothesized that inter-individual differences in other physiological inhibitors (such as CR1 , complement FH and complement FI) may modulate the complement activation in a patient-specific fashion, leading to distinct patterns of C3 deposition. In addition, even more complex factors may drive the subsequent fate of C3-bound PNH erythrocytes; in fact, some patients may harbor large proportion of C3-bound PNH erythrocytes, without showing a clinically relevant extravascular hemolysis (Risitano et al 2010b). At the moment, there is yet no ability to predict before starting eculizumab which patients will develop C3-mediated extravascular hemolysis.

Current strategies to overcome C3-mediated extravascular hemolysis. C3 opsonization of PNH erythrocytes is a common phenomenon for PNH patients treated with eculizumab, even if the subsequent extravascular hemolysis may remain limited or well-compensated in most cases (Luzzatto et al 2010). However, additional therapeutic strategies are needed for patients developing a clinically relevant C3-mediated extravascular hemolysis, because they may continue to require frequent red cell transfusions, possibly developing subsequent iron overload (Risitano et al 2009a). We reported a patient managed by splenectomy (Risitano et al 2008), who achieved a substantial improvement of hemoglobin level without any medical complication; however, many physicians raise the concern that this approach may carry an increased life-long risk of infections (Brodsky 2009). In addition, the risk of intra- or peri-operatory complications (especially thrombosis, or hemorrhage in thrombocytopenic patients) might also argue against this therapeutic option. Very recently a group reported a single case where steroids were beneficial in controlling C3-mediated extravascular hemolysis (Berzuini et al 2010). To best of our knowledge, this observation has not been confirmed in a larger series, and the well known side effects of long-term steroid use should advise against the use of steroids in PNH patients on eculizumab (Risitano et al 2010b). In some patients, the use of recombinant erythropoietin has proven beneficial by increasing compensatory erythropoiesis (Hill et al 2007).

A look into the future of complement inhibition. The emergence of experimental and clinical evidence for CAP-initiated and C3 fragment-mediated extravascular hemolysis suggests that new treatment strategies appropriately targeting the early phases of the complement cascade should be assessed. The ideal agent should prevent the early phase of complement activation on PNH cells and defuse the amplification mechanisms (e.g., the CAP amplification loop). A systemic blockade of C3 activation through all pathways by monoclonal antibodies (similar to the anti-C5 eculizumab) could be considered (e.g., by anti-C3 monoclonal antobiïodies) (Lindorfer et al 2010); however this approach may carry the risk of infectious and autoimmune complications secondary to a complete switching off of the complement system at this point. A novel candidate agent has been designed by creating a recombinant fusion protein between two endogenous complement-related proteins, complement factor H (FH) and complement receptor 2 (CR2). FH is a physiological complement inhibitor that modulates the initial CAP activation in the fluid phase by preventing C3 convertase activity and by promoting C3b inactivation into iC3b (Whaley et al 1976). Indeed, FH defuses the CAP amplification loop, and it has been demonstrated protective from lysis for PNH erythrocytes *in vitro* (Ferreira & Pangburn 2007). In the aim to deliver FH activity locally at the site of complement activation, FH was fused with the iC3b/C3d-binding domain of CR2. The resulting CR2-FH fusion protein has shown a dramatic inhibition of hemolysis of PNH erythrocytes *in vitro* (Risitano et al 2009c), and further investigations are currently under way. A phase I clinical trial has just started to enroll PNH patients (Alexion Pharmaceuticals, personal communication). Once these or other next generation complement inhibitors proceed to clinical development, then we can determine whether such targeted inhibition should be additional or alternative to eculizumab. Indeed, the adequate control of C3, or both C3 and C5 activation on PNH red cells might make the downstream blockade by eculizumab redundant.

8.3 Hematopoietic stem cell transplantation

Cell therapy (insertion of molecules on the outer surface of blood cells) (Hill et al 2006a) and gene therapy (insertion of a functional *PIG-A* gene in early hematopoietic progenitors) have been hypothesized in the past as a curative approach for PNH. However, they seem unfeasible or even inappropriate; in fact, if the escape theory is correct, the gene therapy approach may not result in clinical benefit in PNH, since a repair of the damaged cell should result in cell destruction, as is believed to occur for normal hematopoiesis in PNH patients. The only curative strategy for PNH is allogeneic hematopoietic stem cell transplantation (SCT); SCT has been exploited since the late '80, and has proven effective in eradicating the abnormal PNH clone possibly leading to definitive cure of PNH, even if morbidity and mortality remain a major limitation. Most reports in the literature refer to single cases or small series from single-institutions (Bemba et al 1999, Raiola et al 2000; Saso et al 1999), while large prospective studies are lacking. In an overview, Parker et al (Parker et al 2005) collected data from 67 patients transplanted from different types of donors (syngeneic, sibling or HLA-identical unrelated) and using different types of conditioning (myeloablative or reduced-intensity). The results from the entire group showed a 75% long-term survival, which is quite higher than that reported in individual series (55-100%), likely as a result of a reporting bias. Data from two large registry studies are also available. The International Bone Marrow Transplant Registry reported 57 consecutive SCT performed for PNH (16 AA/PNH) between 1978 and 1995 (Matos-Fernandez et al 2009), showing a 2-year survival of 56% in 48 HLA-identical sibling transplants (the median follow-up was 44 months). The incidence of grade II or more severe acute GvHD was 34%, and that of chronic GvHD of 33%; graft failure (n=7) and infections (n=3) were the most common causes of treatment failure. An other retrospective study from the Italian Transplant Group (GITMO) on 26 PNH patients (4 AA/PNH) transplanted between 1998 and 2006 showed a 57& survival rate at 10 years. Acute and chronic GvHD were 42% (grade III-IV 12%) and 50% (extensive 16%), respectively (Santarone et al 2010). Given these results, guidelines for SCT in PNH are hard to define; the most difficult task today is to identify PNH patients who could benefit from HSCT (Brodsly 2010). At the moment, the main indication for SCT in PNH patients is an underlying bone marrow failure; as for AA patients, SCT may be performed as first-line therapy in the presence of an HLA-identical sibling donor, or in case of treatment failure in patients with an HLA-matched unrelated donor (Risitano 2011). The patient's age largely drives the choice of treatment, given that transplant-related mortality and morbidity increase with age. Refractoriness to transfusions and life-threatening thrombosis were also indications to SCT in the past, but nowadays they rather represent indications to anti-complement treatment, with the exception of Countries where eculizumab is not available (yet). However, SCT remains a worthy second-line therapy for the few patients not achieving a good response to eculizumab. As for AA, SCT (regardless of the type of donor, sibling or unrelated donor) is the treatment of choice for PNH patients developing a clonal evolution to MDS or even AML. The Working Party for Severe Aplastic Anemia of the European Bone Marrow Transplantation Group, together with the French PNH Registry, are currently running a retrospective studies comparing the outcome of all BMT performed in Europe with the natural history of PNH (in the pre-eculizumab era). Likely the results from this study will guide future treatment strategies for PNH patients, according to specific disease presentation and complications. A number of questions remain open in the setting of SCT for PNH, to improve the clinical outcome: the most relevant is the choice of the conditioning regimen. Based on available data, AA/PNH patients should be treated as non-PNH AA patients; thus, the conditioning should be cyclophosphamide/ATG for sibling transplants, and fludarabine-based RIC for unrelated transplants (to be performed as in case of failure of IST) (Bacigalupo et al 2010). In contrast, classic, non-hypoplastic, PNH patients receiving SCT should benefit from myeloablative conditioning (e.g., busulphan-based) (Raiola et al 2000); however, RIC regimens (fludarabine-based) (Takahashi et al 2004) may be appropriate for patients who are older or who present with relevant comorbidities.

9. Conclusion

PNH has attracted the efforts of several generations of investigators in the last three decades for its biological and clinical uniqueness. While the '80s unraveled the GPI-anchor and the functional defect of the PNH clone, and the '90s revealed the *PIG-A* gene and its role in the pathophysiology of the disease, this new century brought forth innovative therapeutic approaches. Thanks to current treatment options, we are finally able to change the natural history of PNH, possibly giving back to PNH patients a normal-like life expectancy, in addition to a significant reduction of disease manifestations and improvement in their quality of life. As often occurs in medicine, thanks to these novel treatments we are also improving our biological knowledge of the disease and of current treatments. Thus, the scientific community has already accepted the next challenge: utilize these recent insights to develop novel targeted treatment strategies, for further improvement of current management of PNH patients.

10. Acknowledgments

I am grateful to Professor Bruno Rotoli who handed down to myself his devotion to PNH patients and PNH science; this chapter mostly stems from his long-lasting thoughtful teachings. I also thank Dr. Rosario Notaro, Professor Lucio Luzzatto, Dr. Jaroslaw Maciejewski and Dr. Neal Young for their contribution to my knowledge of PNH.

11. References

[1] Almeida AM, Murakami Y, Layton DM, et al. Hypomorphic promoter mutation in PIGM causes inherited glycosylphosphatidylinositol deficiency. Nat Med. 2006; 12:846-51.

[2] Almeida A, Layton M & Karadimitris A. Inherited glycosylphosphatidyl inositol deficiency: a treatable CDG. Biochim Biophys Acta. 2009; 1792:874-80.

[3] Araten DJ, Nafa K, Pakdeesuwan K, et al. Clonal populations of hematopoietic cells with paroxysmal nocturnal hemoglobinuria genotype and phenotype are present in normal individuals. Proc Natl Acad Sci U S A. 1999; 96:5209-5214.

[4] Araten DJ, Swirsky D, Karadimitris A, et al. Cytogenetic and morphological abnormalities in paroxysmal nocturnal haemoglobinuria. Br J Haematol. 2001; 115:360-8.

[5] Araten DJ, Bessler M, McKenzie S, et al. Dynamics of hematopoiesis in paroxysmal nocturnal hemoglobinuria (PNH): no evidence for intrinsic growth advantage of PNH clones. Leukemia. 2002; 16:2243-8.

[6] Araten DJ, Thaler HT & Luzzatto L. High incidence of thrombosis in African-American and Latin-American patients with Paroxysmal Nocturnal Haemoglobinuria. Thromb Haemost. 2005; 93:88-91.

[7] Araten DJ & Luzzatto L. The mutation rate in PIG-A is normal in patients with paroxysmal nocturnal hemoglobinuria (PNH). Blood. 2006; 108:734-6.

[8] Araten DJ, Notaro R, Thaler H, et al. Thrombolytic therapy for reversal of thrombosis in paroxysmal nocturnal hemoglobinuria. Blood. 2010; 116:1721(a).

[9] Armstrong C, Schubert J, Ueda E, et al. Affected paroxysmal nocturnal hemoglobinuria T lymphocytes harbor a common defect in assembly of N-acetyl-D-glucosamine inositol phospholipid corresponding to that in class A Thy-1- murine lymphoma mutants. J Biol Chem. 1999; 267:25347-51.

[10] Audebert HJ, Planck J, Eisenburg M, et al. Cerebral ischemic infarction in paroxysmal nocturnal hemoglobinuria report of 2 cases and updated review of 7 previously published patients. J Neurol. 2005; 252:1379-86.

[11] Bacigalupo A, Socie' G, Lanino E, et al; Severe Aplastic Anemia Working Party of the European Group for Blood and Marrow Transplantation. Fludarabine, cyclophosphamide, antithymocyte globulin, with or without low dose total body irradiation, for alternative donor transplants, in acquired severe aplastic anemia: a retrospective study from the EBMT-SAA working party. Haematologica. 2010; 95: 976-82.

[12] Bemba M, Guardiola P, Gardret L et al. Bone marrow transplantation for paroxysmal nocturnal haemoglobinuria. Br J Haematol. 1999; 105 :366-368.

[13] Berzuini A, Montanelli F & Prati D. Hemolytic anemia after eculizumab in paroxysmal nocturnal hemoglobinuria. N Engl J Med. 2010; 363:993-4.

[14] Bessler M, Hillmen P, Longo L, et al. Genomic organization of the X-linked gene (PIG-A) that is mutated in paroxysmal nocturnal haemoglobinuria and of a related autosomal pseudogene mapped to 12q21. Hum Mol Genet. 1994; 3:751-7.

[15] Borowitz MJ, Craig FE, Digiuseppe JA, et al; Clinical Cytometry Society. Guidelines for the diagnosis and monitoring of paroxysmal nocturnal hemoglobinuria and related disorders by flow cytometry. Cytometry B Clin Cytom. 2010; 78:211-30.

[16] Bourantas K. High-dose recombinant erythropoietin and low-dose corticosteroids for treatment of anemia in paroxysmal nocturnal hemoglobinuria. Acta Haematol. 1994; 91-62-5.

[17] Brodsky RA, Mukhina GL, Li S, et al. Improved detection and characterization of paroxysmal nocturnal hemoglobinuria using fluorescent aerolysin. Am J Clin Pathol. 2000; 114:459-66.

[18] Brodsky RA, Young NS, Antonioli E, et al. Multicenter phase III study of the complement inhibitor eculizumab for the treatment of patients with paroxysmal nocturnal hemoglobinuria. Blood. 2008; 114:1840-47.

[19] Brodsky RA. How I treat paroxysmal nocturnal hemoglobinuria. Blood. 2009; 113:6522-7.

[20] Brodsky RA, Chen AR, Dorr D, et al. High-dose cyclophosphamide for severe aplastic anemia: long-term follow-up. Blood. 2010; 115:2136-41.

[21] Brodsky RA. Stem cell transplantation for paroxysmal nocturnal hemoglobinuria. Haematologica. 2010; 95:855-6.

[22] Brubaker LH, Essig LJ & Mengel CE. Neutrophil life span in paroxysmal nocturnal hemoglobinuria. Blood. 1977; 50:657-62.

[23] Cacciapuoti C, Terrazzano G, Barone L, et al. Glycosyl-phosphatidyl-inositol-defective granulocytes from paroxysmal nocturnal haemoglobinuria patients show increased bacterial ingestion but reduced respiratory burst induction. Am J Hematol. 2007; 82:98-107.

[24] Chen G, Zeng W, Maciejewski JP, et al. Differential gene expression in hematopoietic progenitors from paroxysmal nocturnal hemoglobinuria patients reveals an apoptosis/immune response in 'normal' phenotype cells. Leukemia. 2005; 19:862-8.

[25] Crosby WH. Paroxysmal nocturnal hemoglobinuria; a classic description by Paul Strübling in 1882, and a bibliography of the disease. Blood. 1951; 63:270-84.

[26] Dameshek W. Riddle: what do aplastic anemia, paroxysmal nocturnal hemoglobinuria (PNH) and "hypoplastic" leukemia have in common? Blood. 1967; 30:251-254.

[27] de Latour RP, Mary JY, Salanoubat C, et al; French Association of Young Hematologists. Paroxysmal nocturnal hemoglobinuria: natural history of disease subcategories. Blood. 2008; 112:3099-106.

[28] Devine DV, Siegel RS & Rosse WF. Interactions of the platelets in paroxysmal nocturnal hemoglobinuria with complement. Relationship to defects in the regulation of complement and to platelet survival in vivo. J Clin Invest. 1987a; 79:131-7.

[29] Devine DV, Gluck WL, Rosse WF, et al. Acute myeloblastic leukemia in paroxysmal nocturnal hemoglobinuria. Evidence of evolution from the abnormal paroxysmal nocturnal hemoglobinuria clone. J Clin Invest. 1987b; 79:314-7.

[30] Dingli D, Luzzatto L & Pacheco JM. Neutral evolution in paroxysmal nocturnal hemoglobinuria. Proc Natl Acad Sci U S A. 2008; 105:18496-500.

[31] Dunn DE, Liu JM & Young NS. 2000. Paroxysmal nocturnal hemoglobinuria. In: Young NS (ed). Bone Marrow Failure Syndromes. Philadelphia: W.B. Saunders Company. p 99-121.

[32] Endo M, Ware RE, Vreeke TM, et al. Molecular basis of the heterogeneity of expression of glycosyl phosphatidylinositol anchored proteins in paroxysmal nocturnal hemoglobinuria. Blood. 1996; 87:2546-57.

[33] Enneking J. Eine neue form intermittierender Haemoglobinurie (Haemoglobinuria paroxysmalis nocturna). Klin. Wehnschr. 1928. 7: 2045.

[34] Ferreira VP & Pangburn MK. Factor H mediated cell surface protection from complement is critical for the survival of PNH erythrocytes. Blood. 2007; 15;110:1290-2.

[35] Fieni S, Bonfanti L, Gramellini D, et al. Clinical management of paroxysmal nocturnal hemoglobinuria in pregnancy: a case report and updated review. Obstet Gynecol Surv. 2006; 61:593-601.

[36] Fujioka S & Asai T. Prognostic features of paroxysmal nocturnal hemoglobinuria in Japan. Nihon Ketsueki Gakkai Zasshi. 1989; 52:1386-94.

[37] Gargiulo L, Lastraioli S, Cerruti G, et al. Highly homologous T-cell receptor beta sequences support a common target for autoreactive T cells in most patients with paroxysmal nocturnal hemoglobinuria. Blood.2007; 109:5036-42.

[38] Gralnick HR, Vail M, McKeown LP, et al. Activated platelets in paroxysmal nocturnal haemoglobinuria. Br J Haematol. 1995; 91:697-702.

[39] Grünewald M, Siegemund A, Grünewald A, et al. Plasmatic coagulation and fibrinolytic system alterations in PNH: relation to clone size. Blood Coagul Fibrinolysis. 2003; 14:685-95.

[40] Ham TH. Chronic hemolytic anemia with paroxysmal nocturnal hemoglobinuria. A study of mechanism of hemolysis to acid-base equilibrium. N Engl J Med. 1937; 217:915-917.

[41] Ham TH & Dingle JH. Studies on the destruction of red blood cells. II. Chronic hemolytic anemia with paroxysmal nocturnal hemoglobinuria: certain immunological aspects of the hemolytic mechanism with special reference to serum complement. J Clin Invest. 1939; 18:657-672.

[42] Hall C, Richards S & Hillmen P. Primary prophylaxis with warfarin prevents thrombosis in paroxysmal nocturnal hemoglobinuria (PNH). Blood. 2003; 102:3587-91.

[43] Harrington WJ Sr, Kolodny R, Horstmann LL et al. Danazol for paroxysmal nocturnal hemoglobinuria. Am J Hematol. 1997; 54:149-54.

[44] Hauser AC, Brichta A, Pabinger-Fasching I, et al. Fibrinolytic therapy with rt-PA in a patient with paroxysmal nocturnal hemoglobinuria and Budd-Chiari syndrome. Ann Hematol. 2003; 82:299-302.

[45] Helley D, de Latour RP, Porcher R, et al; French Society of Hematology. Evaluation of hemostasis and endothelial function in patients with paroxysmal nocturnal hemoglobinuria receiving eculizumab. Haematologica. 2010; 95:574-81.

[46] Hertenstein B, Wagner B, Bunjes D, et al. Emergence of CD52-, phosphatidylinositolglycan-anchor-deficient T lymphocytes after in vivo application of Campath-1H for refractory B-cell non-Hodgkin lymphoma. Blood. 1995; 86:1487-1492.

[47] Hill A, Rother RP & Hillmen P. Improvement in the symptoms of smooth muscle dystonia during eculizumab therapy in paroxysmal nocturnal hemoglobinuria. Haematologica. 2005; 90:ECR40.

[48] Hill A, Ridley SH, Esser D, et al. Protection of erythrocytes from human complement-mediated lysis by membrane-targeted recombinant soluble CD59: a new approach to PNH therapy. Blood. 2006a; 107:2131-7.

[49] Hill A, Wang X, Sapsford RJ, et al. Nitric oxide consumption and pulmonary hypertension in patients with paroxysmal nocturnal hemoglobinuria. Blood. 2006b; 108:305a.

[50] Hill A et al. The incidence and prevalence of Paroxysmal Nocturnal Hemoglobinuria (PNH) and survival of patients in Yorkshire. Blood 2006c; 108:985a.

[51] Hill A, Richards SJ, Rother RP, et al. Erythropoietin treatment during complement inhibition with eculizumab in a patient with paroxysmal nocturnal hemoglobinuria. Haematologica. 2007; 92:ECR14.

[52] Hill A, Rother RP, Arnold L, et al. Eculizumab prevents intravascular hemolysis in patients with paroxysmal nocturnal hemoglobinuria and unmasks low-level extravascular hemolysis occurring through C3 opsonization. Haematologica. 2010a; 95,567-573.

[53] Hill A, Rother RP, Wang X, et al. Effect of eculizumab on haemolysis-associated nitric oxide depletion, dyspnoea, and measures of pulmonary hypertension in patients with paroxysmal nocturnal haemoglobinuria. Br J Haematol. 2010b; 149:414-25.

[54] Hillmen P, Lewis SM, Bessler M, et al. Natural history of paroxysmal nocturnal hemoglobinuria. N Engl J Med. 1995; 333:1253-1258.

[55] Hillmen P, Hall C, Marsh JC, et al. Effect of eculizumab on hemolysis and transfusion requirements in patients with paroxysmal nocturnal hemoglobinuria. N Engl J Med. 2004; 350:552-559.

[56] Hillmen P, Young NS, Schubert J, et al. The complement inhibitor eculizumab in paroxysmal nocturnal hemoglobinuria. N Engl J Med. 2006; 355:1233-43.

[57] Hillmen P, Muus P, Duhrsen U, et al. Effect of the complement inhibitor eculizumab on thromboembolism in patients with paroxysmal nocturnal hemoglobinuria. Blood. 2007; 110:4123-8.

[58] Hillmen P, Elebute M, Kelly R, et al. Long-term effect of the complement inhibitor eculizumab on kidney function in patients with paroxysmal nocturnal hemoglobinuria. Am J Hematol. 2010; 85:553-9.

[59] Hirose S, Ravi L, Prince GM, et al. Synthesis of mannosylglucosaminylinositol phospholipids in normal but not paroxysmal nocturnal hemoglobinuria cells. Proc Natl Acad Sci U S A. 1992; 89:6025-9.

[60] Hoekstra J, Leebeek FW, Plessier A, et al. Paroxysmal nocturnal hemoglobinuria in Budd-Chiari Syndrome: findings from a cohort study. Journal of hepatology. 2009; 51:696-706.

[61] Hoffman EM. Inhibition of complement by a substance isolated from human erythrocytes. I. Extraction from human erythrocyte stromata. Immunochemistry. 1969; 6:391-403.

[62] Holers VM. The spectrum of complement alternative pathway-mediated diseases. Immunol Rev. 2008; 223:300-16.

[63] Holguin MH, Fredrick LR, Bernshaw NJ, et al. Isolation and characterization of a membrane protein from normal human erythrocytes that inhibits reactive lysis of the erythrocytes of paroxysmal nocturnal hemoglobinuria. J Clin Invest. 1989; 84:7-17.

[64] Holguin MH, Wilcox LA, Bernshaw NJ, et al. Relationship between the membrane inhibitor of reactive lysis and the erythrocyte phenotypes of paroxysmal nocturnal hemoglobinuria. J Clin Invest. 1989; 84:1387-94.

[65] Holguin MH, Wilcox LA, Bernshaw NJ, et al. Erythrocyte membrane inhibitor of reactive lysis: effects of phosphatidylinositol-specific phospholipase C on the isolated and cell-associated protein. Blood. 1990; 75:284-9.

[66] Holguin MH, Martin CB, Bernshaw NJ, et al. Analysis of the effects of activation of the alternative pathway of complement on erythrocytes with an isolated deficiency of decay accelerating factor. J Immunol. 1992; 148:498-502.

[67] Hugel B, Socié G, Vu T, et al. Elevated levels of circulating procoagulant microparticles in patients with paroxysmal nocturnal hemoglobinuria and aplastic anemia. Blood. 1999; 93:3451-6.

[68] Inoue N, Izui-Sarumaru T, Murakami Y, et al. Molecular basis of clonal expansion of hematopoiesis in 2 patients with paroxysmal nocturnal hemoglobinuria (PNH). Blood. 2006; 108:4232-6.

[69] Issaragrisil S, Piankijagum A & Tang.Naitrisorana Y. Corticosteroid therapy in paroxysmal nocturnal hemoglobinuria. Am J Hemato. 1987; 25:77-83.

[70] Jasinski M, Keller P, Fujiwara Y, et al. GATA1-Cre mediates Piga gene inactivation in the erythroid/megakaryocytic lineage and leads to circulating red cells with a partial deficiency in glycosyl phosphatidylinositol-linked proteins (paroxysmal nocturnal hemoglobinuria type II cells). Blood. 2001 ; 98:2248-2255.

[71] Karadimitris A, Manavalan JS, Thaler HT, et al. Abnormal T-cell repertoire is consistent with immune process underlying the pathogenesis of paroxysmal nocturnal hemoglobinuria. Blood. 2001; 96:2613-262.

[72] Karadimitris A, Li K, Notaro R, et al. Association of clonal T-cell large granular lymphocyte disease and paroxysmal nocturnal haemoglobinuria (PNH): further evidence for a pathogenetic link between T cells, aplastic anaemia and PNH. Br J Haematol. 2001; 115:1010-4.

[73] Katayama Y, Hiramatsu Y & Kohriyama H. Monitoring of Cd59 expression in paroxysmal nocturnal hemoglobinuria treated with danazol. Am J Hematol. 2001; 68:280-3.

[74] Kawagoe K, Kitamura D, Okabe M, et al. Glycosylphosphatidylinositol-anchor-deficient mice: implications for clonal dominance of mutant cells in paroxysmal nocturnal hemoglobinuria. Blood. 1996; 87:3600-6.

[75] Keller P, Payne JL, Tremml G, et al. FES-Cre targets phosphatidylinositol glycan class A (PIGA) inactivation to hematopoietic stem cells in the bone marrow. J Exp Med. 2001; 194:581-589.

[76] Kelly RJ, Hill A, Arnold LM, et al. Long-term treatment with eculizumab in paroxysmal nocturnal hemoglobinuria: sustained efficacy and improved survival. Blood. 2011;117:6786-92.

[77] Kelly R, Arnold L, Richards S, et al. The management of pregnancy in paroxysmal nocturnal haemoglobinuria on long term eculizumab. Br J Haematol. 2010; 149:446-450.

[78] Krause JR. Paroxysmal nocturnal hemoglobinuria and acute non-lymphocytic leukemia. A report of three cases exhibiting different cytologic types. Cancer. 1983; 51:2078-82.

[79] Kinoshita T, Medof ME, Silber R, et al. Distribution of decay-accelerating factor in the peripheral blood of normal individuals and patients with paroxysmal nocturnal hemoglobinuria. J Exp Med. 1985; 162:75-92.

[80] Kunstling TR & Rosse WF. Erythrocyte acetylcholinesterase deficiency in paroxysmal nocturnal hemoglobinuria (PNH). A comparison of the complement-sensitive and insensitive populations. Blood. 1969; 33:607-16.

[81] Lewis SM & Dacie JV. The aplastic anaemia--paroxysmal nocturnal haemoglobinuria syndrome. Br J Haematol. 1967; 13:236-51.

[82] Lindorfer MA, Pawluczkowycz AW, Peek EM, et al. A novel approach to preventing the hemolysis of paroxysmal nocturnal hemoglobinuria: both complement-mediated cytolysis and C3 deposition are blocked by a monoclonal antibody specific for the alternative pathway of complement. Blood. 2010; 115:2283-91.

[83] Louwes H, Vellenga E & de Wolf JT. Abnormal platelet adhesion on abdominal vessels in asymptomatic patients with paroxysmal nocturnal hemoglobinuria. Ann Hematol. 2001; 80:573-6.

[84] Luzzatto L, Bessler M & Rotoli B. Somatic mutations in paroxysmal nocturnal hemoglobinuria: a blessing in disguise? Cell. 1997; 88:1-4.

[85] Luzzatto L & Nafa G. Genetics of PNH. 2000. In: Young NS, Moss J (ed). Paroxysmal nocturnal hemoglobinuria and the glycosylphosphatidylinositol-linked proteins. Sa Diego: Academic Press. p 21-47.

[86] Luzzatto L & Notaro R. 2003. Paroxysmal nocturnal hemoglobinuria. In Handin RI, Lux SE, Stossel TP (eds): Blood, principles and practice of hematology (2nd ed.). Philadelphia, PA (USA), Lippincot Williams & Wilkins; p 319-34.

[87] Luzzatto L, Risitano AM & Notaro R. Paroxysmal nocturnal hemoglobinuria and eculizumab. Haematologica. 2010; 95:523-6.

[88] Luzzatto L, Gianfaldoni G & Notaro R. Management of paroxysmal nocturnal haemoglobinuria: a personal view. Br J Haematol. 2011; 153:709-20.

[89] Luzzatto L & Notaro R. Biological basis of paroxysmal nocturnal hemoglobinuria. Hematology education: the educational program for the annual congress of European Hematology Association. 2010;222-227.

[90] Maciejewski JP, Sloand EM, Sato T, et al. Impaired hematopoiesis in paroxysmal nocturnal hemoglobinuria/aplastic anemia is not associated with a selective proliferative defect in the glycosylphosphatidylinositol-anchored protein-deficient clone. Blood. 1997; 89:1173-81.

[91] Maciejewski JP, Young NS, Yu M, et al. Analysis of the expression of glycosylphosphatidylinositol anchored proteins on platelets from patients with paroxysmal nocturnal hemoglobinuria. Thromb Res. 1996; 83:433-47.

[92] Mahoney JF, Urakaze M, Hall S, et al. Defective glycosylphosphatidylinositol anchor synthesis in paroxysmal nocturnal hemoglobinuria granulocytes. Blood. 1992; 79:1400-3.

[93] Marasca R, Coluccio V, Santachiara R, et al. Pregnancy in PNH: another eculizumab baby. Br J Haematol. 2010; 150:707-708.

[94] Marchiafava E & Nazari A. Nuovo contributo allo studio degli itteri emolotici cronici. Policlinico, (sez. med.). 1911. 18: 241.

[95] Markiewski MM, Nilsson B, Ekdahl KN, et al. Complement and coagulation: strangers or partners in crime? Trends in immunology. 2007; 28:184-92.

[96] Matis LA & Rollins SA. Complement-specific antibodies: designing novel anti-inflammatories. Nat Med. 1995; 1:839-42.

[97] Matos-Fernandez NA, Abou Mourad YR, Caceres W, et al. Current status of allogeneic hematopoietic stem cell transplantation for paroxysmal nocturnal hemoglobinuria. Biol Blood Marrow Transplant. 2009; 15:656-61.

[98] McMullin MF, Hillmen P, Elder GE, et al. Serum erythropoietin level in paroxysmal nocturnal hemoglobinuria: implications for therapy. Br J Haematol. 1996; 92:815-7.

[99] McMullin MF, Hillmen P, Jackson J, et al. Tissue plasminogen activator for hepatic vein thrombosis in paroxysmal nocturnal haemoglobinuria. J Intern Med. 1994; 235:85-9.

[100] Medof ME, Walter EI, Roberts WL, et al. Decay accelerating factor of complement is anchored to cells by a C-terminal glycolipid. Biochemistry. 1986; 25:6740-7.

[101] Medof ME, Gottlieb A, Kinoshita T, et al. Relationship between decay accelerating factor deficiency, diminished acetylcholinesterase activity, and defective terminal

complement pathway restriction in paroxysmal nocturnal hemoglobinuria erythrocytes. J Clin Invest. 1987; 80:165-74.

[102] Meri S, Morgan BP, Davies A, et al. Human protectin (CD59), an 18,000-20,000 MW complement lysis restricting factor, inhibits C5b-8 catalysed insertion of C9 into lipid bilayers. Immunology. 1990; 71:1-9.

[103] Merry AH, Rawlinson VI, Uchikawa M, et al. Studies on the sensitivity to complement-mediated lysis of erythrocytes (Inab phenotype) with a deficiency of DAF (decay accelerating factor). Br J Haematol. 1989; 73:248-53.

[104] Micheli N. Anemia emolitica cronica con emosiderinuria perpetua. Policlinico, (sez. prat.). 1928; 35:2574.

[105] Miyata T, Takeda J, Iida Y, et al. The cloning of PIG-A, a component in the early step of GPI-anchor biosynthesis. Science. 1993; 259:1318-1320.

[106] Motoyama N, Okada N, Yamashina M, et al. Paroxysmal nocturnal hemoglobinuria due to hereditary nucleotide deletion in the HRF20 (CD59) gene. Eur J Immunol. 1992; 22:2669-73.

[107] Mold C, Walter EI, Medof ME. The influence of membrane components on regulation of alternative pathway activation by decay-accelerating factor. J Immunol. 1990; 145:3836-41.

[108] Moyo VM, Mukhina GL, Garrett ES, et al. Natural history of paroxysmal nocturnal haemoglobinuria using modern diagnostic assays. Br J Haematol. 2004; 126:133-8.

[109] Mukhina GL, Buckley JT, Barber JP, et al. Multilineage glycosylphosphatidylinositol anchor-deficient haematopoiesis in untreated aplastic anaemia. Br J Haematol. 2001; 115:476-82.

[110] Müller-Eberhard HJ. Molecular organization and function of the complement system. Annu Rev Biochem. 1988; 57:321-47.

[111] Murakami Y, Kosaka H, Maeda Y, et al. Inefficient response of T lymphocytes to glycosylphosphatidylinositol anchor-negative cells: implications for paroxysmal nocturnal hemoglobinuria. Blood. 2002; 100:4116-4122.

[112] Muus P, Szer J, Schrezenmeier H, et al. Evaluation of Paroxysmal Nocturnal Hemoglobinuria Disease Burden: The Patient's Perspective. A Report From the International PNH Registry. Blood. 2010; 116:1525a.

[113] Nagakura S, Ishihara S, Dunn DE, et al. Decreased susceptibility of leukemic cells with PIG-A mutation to natural killer cells in vitro. Blood. 2002; 100:1031-1037.

[114] Nafa K, Mason PJ, Hillmen P, et al. Mutations in the PIG-A gene causing paroxysmal nocturnal hemoglobinuria are mainly of the frameshift type. Blood. 1995; 86:4650-5.

[115] Nafa K, Bessler M, Castro-Malaspina H, et al. The spectrum of somatic mutations in the PIG-A gene in paroxysmal nocturnal hemoglobinuria includes large deletions and small duplications. Blood Cells Mol Dis. 1998a; 24:370-84.

[116] Nafa K, Bessler M, Deeg HJ, et al. New somatic mutation in the PIG-A gene emerges at relapse of paroxysmal nocturnal hemoglobinuria. Blood.1998b; 92:3422-7.

[117] Nafa K, Bessler M, Mason P, et al. Factor V Leiden mutation investigated by amplification created restriction enzyme site (ACRES) in PNH patients with and without thrombosis. Haematologica. 1996; 81:540-2.

[118] Nakakuma H, Nagakura S, Iwamoto N, et al. Paroxysmal nocturnal hemoglobinuria clone in bone marrow of patients with pancytopenia. Blood. 1995; 85:1371-6.

[119] Nair RK, Khaira A, Sharma A, et al. Spectrum of renal involvement in paroxysmal nocturnal hemoglobinuria: report of three cases and a brief review of the literature. Int Urol Nephrol. 2008; 40:471-5.

[120] Nicholson-Weller A, Burge J, Fearon DT, et al. Isolation of a human erythrocyte membrane glycoprotein with decay-accelerating activity for C3 convertases of the complement system. J Immunol. 1982; 129:184-9.

[121] Nicholson-Weller A, March JP, Rosenfeld SI, et al. Affected erythrocytes of patients with paroxysmal nocturnal hemoglobinuria are deficient in the complement regulatory protein, decay accelerating factor. Proc Natl Acad Sci U S A. 1983; 80:5066-70.

[122] Nicholson-Weller A. Decay accelerating factor (CD55). Curr Top Microbiol Immunol. 1992; 178:7-30.

[123] Ninomiya H, Hasegawa Y, Nagasawa T, et al. Excess soluble urokinase-type plasminogen activator receptor in the plasma of patients with paroxysmal nocturnal hemoglobinuria inhibits cell-associated fibrinolytic activity. Int J Hematol. 1997; 65:285-91.

[124] Nishimura J, Inoue N, Wada H, et al. A patient with paroxysmal nocturnal hemoglobinuria bearing four independent PIG-A mutant clones. Blood. 1997; 89:3470-6.

[125] Nishimura J, Murakami Y, Kinoshita T. Paroxysmal nocturnal hemoglobinuria: An acquired genetic disease. Am J Hematol. 1999; 62:175-82.

[126] Nishimura Ji J, Hirota T, Kanakura Y, et al. Long-term support of hematopoiesis by a single stem cell clone in patients with paroxysmal nocturnal hemoglobinuria. Blood. 2002; 99:2748-2751.

[127] Nishimura J, Kanakura Y, Ware RE, et al. Clinical course and flow cytometric analysis of paroxysmal nocturnal hemoglobinuria in the United States and Japan. Medicine (Baltimore). 2004; 83:193-207.

[128] Nissen C, Tichelli A, Gratwohl A, et al. High incidence of transiently appearing complement-sensitive bone marrow precursor cells in patients with severe aplastic anemia--A possible role of high endogenous IL-2 in their suppression. Acta Haematol. 1999; 101:165-72.

[129] Oni BS, Osunkoya BO & Luzzatto L. Paroxysmal nocturnal hemoglobinuria: evidence for monoclonal origin of abnormal red cells. Blood. 1970; 36:145-152.

[130] Orphanet. Paroxysmal Nocturnal Hemoglobinuria. 1-12-2004. Ref Type: Internet Communication

[131] Pangburn MK, Schreiber RD & Müller-Eberhard HJ. Formation of the initial C3 convertase of the alternative complement pathway. Acquisition of C3b-like activities by spontaneous hydrolysis of the putative thioester in native C3. J Exp Med. 1981; 154:856-67.

[132] Pangburn MK, Schreiber RD, Trombold JS, et al. Paroxysmal nocturnal hemoglobinuria: deficiency in factor H-like functions of the abnormal erythrocytes. J Exp Med. 1983a; 157:1971-80.

[133] Pangburn MK & Müller-Eberhard HJ. Initiation of the alternative complement pathway due to spontaneous hydrolysis of the thioester of C3. Ann N Y Acad Sci. 1983; 421:291-8.

[134] Pangburn MK, Schreiber RD & Müller-Eberhard HJ. Deficiency of an erythrocyte membrane protein with complement regulatory activity in paroxysmal nocturnal hemoglobinuria. Proc Natl Acad Sci U S A. 1983b; 80:5430-4.

[135] Pangburn MK, Schreiber RD & Müller-Eberhard HJ. C3b deposition during activation of the alternative complement pathway and the effect of deposition on the activating surface. J Immunol. 1983c; 131:1930-5.

[136] Parker CJ, Baker PJ & Rosse WF. Increased enzymatic activity of the alternative pathway convertase when bound to the erythrocytes of paroxysmal nocturnal hemoglobinuria. J Clin Invest. 1982; 69:337-46.

[137] Parker CJ. Historical aspects of paroxysmal nocturnal hemoglobinuria; "defining the disease". Br J Haematol. 2002; 117:3-22.

[138] Parker CJ & Ware RE. 2003. Paroxysmal nocturnal hemoglobinuria. In: Greer J et al (ed). Wintrobe's clinical hematology – 11th ed. Philadelphia: Lippincott Williams & Wilkins. p 1203-1221.

[139] Parker C, Omine M, Richards S, et al; International PNH Interest Group. Diagnosis and management of paroxysmal nocturnal hemoglobinuria. Blood. 2005; 106:3699-709.

[140] Parker C. Eculizumab for paroxysmal nocturnal haemoglobinuria. Lancet. 2009; 373:759-67.

[141] Plasilova M, Risitano AM, O'Keefe CL, et al. Shared and individual specificities of immunodominant cytotoxic T cell clones in Paroxysmal Nocturnal Hemoglobinuria as determined by molecular analysis. Exp Hematol. 2004; 32:261-269.

[142] Poggi A, Negrini S, Zocchi MR, et al. Patients with paroxysmal nocturnal hemoglobinuria have a high frequency of peripheral-blood T cells expressing activating isoforms of inhibiting superfamily receptors. Blood. 2005; 106:2399-408.

[143] Pramoonjago P, Pakdeesuwan K, Siripanyaphinyo U, et al. Genotypic, immunophenotypic and clinical features of Thai patients with paroxysmal nocturnal haemoglobinuria. Br J Haematol.1999; 105:497-504.

[144] Raiola AM, Van Lint MT, Lamparelli T, et al. Bone marrow transplantation for paroxysmal nocturnal hemoglobinuria. Haematologica. 2000; 85:59-62.

[145] Richards SJ, Rawstron AC, Hillmen P. Application of flow cytometry to the diagnosis of paroxysmal nocturnal hemoglobinuria. Cytometry. 2000; 42:223-33.

[146] Risitano AM, Maciejewski JP, Green S, et al. In vivo dominant immune responses in aplastic anemia patients: molecular tracking of putatively pathogenic T cells by TCRβ-CDR3 sequencing. Lancet. 2004 ; 364:353-363.

[147] Risitano AM, Maciejewski JP, Muranski P, et al. Large granular lymphocyte (LGL)-like clonal expansions in paroxysmal nocturnal hemoglobinuria (PNH) patients. Leukemia. 2005; 19:217-22.

[148] Risitano AM, Marando L, Seneca E, et al. Hemoglobin normalization after splenectomy in a paroxysmal nocturnal hemoglobinuria patient treated by eculizumab. Blood. 2008; 112:449-51.

[149] Risitano AM, Notaro R, Marando L, et al. Complement fraction 3 binding on erythrocytes as additional mechanism of disease in paroxysmal nocturnal hemoglobinuria patients treated by eculizumab. Blood. 2009a; 113:4094-100.

[150] Risitano AM, Seneca E, Marando L, et al. From Renal Siderosis Due to Perpetual Hemosiderinuria to Possible Liver Overload Due to Extravascular Hemolysis: Changes in Iron Metabolism in Paroxysmal Nocturnal Hemoglobinuria (PNH) Patients on Eculizumab. Blood. 2009b; 114:4031a.

[151] Risitano AM, Holers VM & Rotoli B. TT30, a Novel Regulator of the Complement Alternative Pathway (CAP), Inhibits Hemolysis of Paroxysmal Nocturnal Hemoglobinuria (PNH) Erythrocytes and Prevents Upstream C3 Binding On Their Surface in An in Vitro Model. Blood. 2009c; 114:158a.

[152] Risitano AM, Selleri C, Serio B, et al; Working Party Severe Aplastic Anaemia (WPSAA) of the European Group for Blood and Marrow Transplantation (EBMT). Alemtuzumab is safe and effective as immunosuppressive treatment for aplastic anaemia and single-lineage marrow failure: a pilot study and a survey from the EBMT WPSAA. British Journal of Haematology. 2010a; 148, 791-6.

[153] Risitano AM, Notaro R, Luzzatto L, et al. Paroxysmal Nocturnal Hemoglobinuria: Hemolysis Before and After Eculizumab. New Engl J Med. 2010b; 363:2270-2.

[154] Risitano AM. Immunosuppressive therapies in the management of immune-mediated marrow failures in adults: where we stand and where we are going. Br J Haematol. 2011; 152:127-40.

[155] Risitano AM, Perna F & Selleri C. Achievements and limitations of complement inhibition by eculizumab in paroxysmal nocturnal hemoglobinuria: the role of complement component 3. Mini Rev Med Chem. 2011; 11:528-35.

[156] Rosse WF & Dacie JV. Immune lysis of normal human and paroxysmal nocturnal hemoglobinuria (PNH) red blood cells. I. The sensitivity of PNH red cells to lysis by complement and specific antibody. J Clin Invest. 1966; 45:736-748.

[157] Rosse WF. The life-span of complement-sensitive and –insensitive red cells in paroxysmal nocturnal hemoglobinuria. Blood. 1971; 37:556-562.

[158] Rosse WF. Variations in the red cells in paroxysmal nocturnal haemoglobinuria. Br J Haematol. 1973; 24:327-342.

[159] Rosse WF. Dr Ham's test revisited. Blood. 1991; 78:547-550.

[160] Rosse WF. Epidemiology of PNH. Lancet 1996; 348:560.

[161] Rosti V, Tremml G, Soares V, et al. Murine embryonic stem cells without pig-a gene activity are competent for hematopoiesis with the PNH phenotype but not for clonal expansion. J Clin Invest. 1997; 100:1028-1036.

[162] Rosti V. Murine models of paroxysmal nocturnal hemoglobinuria. Ann N Y Acad Sci. 2002; 963:290-6.

[163] Rother RP, Bell L, Hillmen P, et al. The clinical sequelae of intravascular hemolysis and extracellular plasma hemoglobin: a novel mechanism of human disease. JAMA. 2005; 293:1653-62.

[164] Rother RP, Rollins SA, Mojcik CF, et al. Discovery and development of the complement inhibitor eculizumab for the treatment of paroxysmal nocturnal hemoglobinuria. Nat Biotechnol. 2007; 25:1256-64.

[165] Rotoli B, Robledo R & Luzzatto L. Decreased number of circulating BFU-Es in paroxysmal nocturnal hemoglobinuria. Blood. 1982; 60:157-9.

[166] Rotoli B, Robledo R, Scarpato N, et al. Two populations of erythroid cell progenitors in paroxysmal nocturnal hemoglobinuria. Blood. 1984; 64:847-851.

[167] Rotoli B & Luzzatto L. Paroxysmal nocturnal haemoglobinuria. Baillieres Clin Haematol 1989; 2:113-138.

[168] Sanchez-Valle E, Morales-Polanco MR, Gomez-Morales E, et al. Treatment of paroxysmal nocturnal hemoglobinuria with antilymphocyte globulin. Rev Invest Clin. 1993; 45:457-461.

[169] Santarone S, Bacigalupo A, Risitano AM, et al. Hematopoietic stem cell transplantation for paroxysmal nocturnal hemoglobinuria: long-term results of a retrospective study on behalf of the Gruppo Italiano Trapianto Midollo Osseo (GITMO). Haematologica. 2010; 95:983-8.

[170] Saso R, Marsh J, Cevreska L, et al. Bone marrow transplants for paroxysmal nocturnal haemoglobinuria. Br J Haematol. 1999; 104:392-396.

[171] Schafer A, Wiesmann F, Neubauer S, et al. Rapid regulation of platelet activation in vivo by nitric oxide. Circulation. 2004; 109:1819-22.

[172] Scheinberg P, Marte M, Nunez O, et al. Paroxysmal nocturnal hemoglobinuria clones in severe aplastic anemia patients treated with horse anti-thymocyte globulin plus cyclosporine. Haematologica. 2010; 95:1075-80.

[173] Schubert J, Scholz C, Geissler RG, et al. G-CSF and cyclosporin induce an increase of normal cells in hypoplastic paroxysmal nocturnal hemoglobinuria. Ann Hematol. 1997; 74:225-30.

[174] Selvaraj P, Rosse WF, Silber R, et al. The major Fc receptor in blood has a phosphatidylinositol anchor and is deficient in paroxysmal nocturnal haemoglobinuria. Nature. 1988; 333:565-7.

[175] Shin ML, Hänsch G, Hu VW, et al. Membrane factors responsible for homologous species restriction of complement-mediated lysis: evidence for a factor other than DAF operating at the stage of C8 and C9. J Immunol. 1986; 136:1777-82.

[176] Sholar PW & Bell WR. Thrombolytic therapy for inferior vena cava thrombosis in paroxysmal nocturnal hemoglobinuria. Ann Intern Med. 1985; 103:539-41.

[177] Sica M, Pascariello C, Rondelli T, et al. In vitro complement protein 5 (C5) blockade recapitulates the Complement protein 3 (C3) binding to GPI-negative erythrocytes observed in Paroxysmal Nocturnal Hemoglobinuria (PNH) patients on e.culizumab. Haematologica. 2010; 95(s2):196(a).

[178] Simak J, Holada K, Risitano AM, et al. Elevated counts of circulating endothelial membrane microparticles in paroxysmal nocturnal hemoglobinuria indicate inflammatory status and ongoing stimulation of vascular endothelium. Br J Hemat. 2004; 125:804-813.

[179] Sloand EM, Pfannes L, Scheinberg P, et al. Increased soluble urokinase plasminogen activator receptor (suPAR) is associated with thrombosis and inhibition of plasmin generation in paroxysmal nocturnal hemoglobinuria (PNH) patients. Exp Hematol. 2008; 36:1616-24.

[180] Socie G, Mary JY, de Gramont A, et al. Paroxysmal nocturnal haemoglobinuria: long-term follow-up and prognostic factors. French Society of Haematology. Lancet. 1996; 348:573-7.

[181] Stebler C, Tichelli A, Dazzi H, et al. High-dose recombinant human erythropoietin for treatment of anemia in myelodysplastic syndromes and paroxysmal nocturnal hemoglobinuria: a pilot study. Exp Hematol. 1990; 18:1204-8.

[182] Stoppa AM, Vey N, Sainty D, et al. Correction of aplastic anaemia complicating paroxysmal nocturnal haemoglobinuria: absence of eradication of the PNH clone and dependence of response on cyclosporin A administration. Br J Haematol. 1996; 93:42-4.

[183] Sugimori C, Chuhjo T, Feng X, et al. Minor population of CD55-CD59- blood cells predicts response to immunosuppressive therapy and prognosis in patients with aplastic anemia. Blood. 2006; 107:1308-14.

[184] Sutherland DR, Kuek N, Davidson J, et al. Diagnosing PNH with FLAER and multiparameter flow cytometry. Cytometry B Clin Cytom. 2007; 72:167-77.

[185] Takahashi M, Takeda J, Hirose S, et al. Deficient biosynthesis of N-acetylglucosaminyl-phosphatidylinositol, the first intermediate of glycosyl phosphatidylinositol anchor biosynthesis, in cell lines established from patients with paroxysmal nocturnal hemoglobinuria. J Exp Med. 1993; 177:517-21.

[186] Takahashi Y, McCoy JP Jr., Carvallo C, et al. In vitro and in vivo evidence of PNH cell sensitivity to immune attack after nonmyeloablative allogeneic hematopoietic cell transplantation. Blood. 2004; 103:1383-1390.

[187] Takeda J, Miyata T, Kawagoe K, et al. Deficiency of the GPI anchor caused by a somatic mutation of the PIG-A gene in paroxysmal nocturnal hemoglobinuria. Cell. 1993; 73:703-11.

[188] Takeda J & Kinoshita T. GPI-anchor biosynthesis. Trends Biochem Sci. 1995; 20:367-71.

[189] Telen MJ & Green AM. The Inab phenotype: characterization of the membrane protein and complement regulatory defect. Blood. 1989; 74:437-41.

[190] Tichelli A, Gratwohl A, Nissen C, et al. Morphology in patients with severe aplastic anemia treated with antilymphocyte globulin. Blood. 1992; 80:337-45.

[191] Tremml G, Dominguez C, Rosti V, et al. Increased sensitivity to complement and a decreased red blood cell life span in mice mosaic for a nonfunctional Piga gene. Blood. 1999; 94:2945-54.

[192] van Beers EJ, Schaap MC, Berckmans RJ, et al; CURAMA study group. Circulating erythrocyte-derived microparticles are associated with coagulation activation in sickle cell disease. Haematologica. 2009; 94:1513-9.

[193] van der Schoot CE, Huizinga TW, van 't Veer-Korthof ET, et al. Deficiency of glycosyl-phosphatidylinositol-linked membrane glycoproteins of leukocytes in paroxysmal nocturnal hemoglobinuria, description of a new diagnostic cytofluorometric assay. Blood. 1990; 76:1853-1859.

[194] van Kamp H, Smit JW, van den Berg E, et al. Myelodysplasia following paroxysmal nocturnal haemoglobinuria: evidence for the emergence of a separate clone. Br J Haematol. 1994; 87:399-400.

[195] van Kamp H, van Imhoff GW, de Wolf JT, et al. The effect of cyclosporine on haematological parameters in patients with paroxysmal nocturnal haemoglobinuria. Br J Haematol. 1995; 89:79-82.

[196] Vu T, Griscelli-Bennaceur A, Gluckman E, et al. Aplastic anaemia and paroxysmal nocturnal haemoglobinuria: a study of the GPI-anchored proteins on human platelets. Br J Haematol. 1996; 93:586-9.

[197] Ware RE, Hall SE & Rosse WF. Paroxysmal nocturnal hemoglobinuria with onset in childhood and adolescence. N Engl J Med. 1991; 325:991-996.

[198] Whaley K & Ruddy S. Modulation of the alternative complement pathway by β1H globulin. J Exp Med. 1976; 144:1147-63

[199] Wiedmer T, Hall SE, Ortel TL, et al. Complement-induced vesiculation and exposure of membrane prothrombinase sites in platelets of paroxysmal nocturnal hemoglobinuria. Blood. 1993; 82:1192-6.

[200] Wilcox LA, Ezzell JL, Bernshaw NJ, et al. Molecular basis of the enhanced susceptibility of the erythrocytes of paroxysmal nocturnal hemoglobinuria to hemolysis in acidified serum. Blood. 1991; 78:820-9.

[201] Yamashina M, Ueda E, Kinoshita T, et al. Inherited complete deficiency of 20-kilodalton homologous restriction factor (CD59) as a cause of paroxysmal nocturnal hemoglobinuria. N Engl J Med. 1990; 323:1184-9.

[202] Young NS & Maciejewski JP. Genetic and environmental effects in paroxysmal nocturnal hemoglobinuria: this little PIG-A goes "Why? Why? Why?". J Clin Invest. 2000; 106:637-641.

[203] Young NS, Calado RT & Scheinberg P. Current concepts in the pathophysiology and treatment of aplastic anemia. Blood. 2006; 108, 2509-19.

8

Elevated System Energy Expenditure in Sickle Cell Anemia

Chidi G. Osuagwu

Department of Biomedical Technology
Federal University of Technology, Owerri, Imo State
Nigeria

1. Introduction

In Sickle-cell Anemia (SCA), anergy (lack of metabolic energy) and elevated resting energy expenditure (REE) are commonly observed phenomena. The many systemic changes in Sickle-cell anemia are, therefore, associated with measurable changes in patterns of energy uptake, utilization and efficiency. Understanding the scientific basis of these structural and energy changes suggest mechanisms of possible amelioration.The structural and energy changes in sickle-cell anemia can be viewed at different levels: at the level of the whole person, as reflected in anergy and elevated resting energy expenditure. At the level of the whole blood tissue, as shown in lowered blood pH (high hydrogen ion, H^+, concentration). This is also associated with structural changes in polyhedral charge-packing of hydrogen and hydroxyl ions (octahedral charge-packing, which is the ideal is not achieved). At the specific organ level, this is shown in the elevated energy cost of kidney proton-dialysis. Because of this kidney disease is a major cause of death among sickle cell sufferers. The cellular level shows the disruption of the erythrocyte membrane itself. The anti-turbulence biconcave 'erythrocytoid' shape is changed to the sickle-shape, resulting to increased blood flow-turbulence. This overworks the heart; causing high heart disease rates among patients. At the molecular level, this results to, for example, the inability to metabolize the key energy-source molecule glucose. This results to, as well as inability to extract energy from glucose, glycation of hemoglobin. Glycated hemoglobin has poor oxygen-carrying power, compounding the problem of the little hemoglobin available. Also there are shifts in redox equilibriums, enzyme and metabolite concentrations and activities, and so on. All these result to extra-energy costs to try to restore system optimal state of efficiency and stability. All these, together, explain elevated resting energy expenditure in sickle cell disease.

Different researchers have, over the years, discovered that sufferers from sickle cell anemia (SCA) expend more energy maintaining the same mass of their bodies than normal people (Kopp-Hollihan *et al*, 1999; Borrel *et al*, 1998). Some have worked to establish more efficient measurements of the observed differences from normal (Buchowski *et al*, 2002). Others have worked on theories and experiments towards remediation (Bourre, 2006; Enwonwu, 1988). On the internet, there are sites actively publicizing high-energy foods they consider ideal for sickle cell sufferers (Sherry, 2011). In folk medicine in the African communities, where sickle anemia is common, easy to digest high-energy foods are usually recommended for sickle cell patients.

To appreciate why a sick body, such as that of the sufferers of sickle-cell anemia, would cost more energy to maintain, as reflected in the higher resting energy expenditure (REE), than normal people's, we have to, first, appreciate some simple rules, with respect to energy economy; that nature employs in the design of natural systems. The living system, including the human body, is the ideal natural energy-using system. The living system is energy-conservative; efficient, compared to any other known system, in nature.

The rule is that for a given system in nature there is a functionally ideal arrangement. This ideal or optimal (not perfect, but best possible) arrangement is most energy efficient. It offers the best stability (*stay-ability*) to the system. The human body is designed to operate at optimal conditions; where it is most bio-energetically efficient and stable. Stability in human terms means good health, less stress and pain, and long life. Sickness, generally, is a state of body-system displacement from the optimal conditions of function and is, therefore, energy costly. The fever (abnormally high body temperature) commonly associated with sick people results from the decrease in efficiency of body energy use.We recall that entropy, disorderly flow of system energy, increases with temperature. Such elevated basal body temperature (high metabolic entropy) is commonly found in sickle-cell anemia sufferers, particularly during crisis.

The following statement by the researcher Zora Rogers (2011) "Fever is a common presenting symptom in many manifestations of sickle cell disease" summarizes the situation. Heat loss (fever) is sign of wasting energy. That is why the sufferer, inspite of higher *Resting Metabolic Energy* (RME) utilization, suffers from anergy (a state of lack of energy). Much of the energy and nutrients, including ascorbic acid, the reducing metabolite glutathione, etc, consumed or produced by patients of this disease are wasted (Fakhri *et al*, 1991; Kiessling *et al*, 2000; Reid *et al*, 2006). They go into the dissipative chaos of entropy, instead of being organized as parts of stable system structures such as fat, healthy nerves and muscles, which SCA sufferers lack. In this sense sickle cell anemia is, literally, a wasting disease. Energy and structures are dissipated.

2. Some contributing factors to energy wastage in sickle cell anemia (SCA)

There are so many factors that contribute to systemic energy wastage in sickle cell anemia. Because of its dramatic manifestations as anemia, particularly during crisis, sickle cell disease is seen, primarily as an anemia. The catastrophic fall in red blood cell concentration; and the accompanying yellow eyes, caused by excess bilirubin (a by-product of hemoglobin breakdown) would easily identify the disease as of blood origin. This assumption is sustained by the direct link between hemoglobin and blood oxygen concentration on the one hand and body energy generation on the other. Anemia can, therefore, be thought of, equally, as low energy metabolism syndrome; and more so for a chronic condition like sickle cell anemia. The first major factor that leads to anergy in sickle cell anemia is inefficient glucose metabolism.

2.1 Inefficient glucose metabolism in sickle cell anemia

Glucose is the main fuel molecule of the human body. Some key body cells depend mostly or solely on glucose for energy metabolism. Two of these glucose-dependent body cells include the red blood cell (rbc) and nerve cells, including brain cells. It is clear that anybody in whose body system glucose metabolism is compromised is in trouble with the vital tissues and organs associated with these cells; blood system and nervous system. This happens to be the case in sickle cell anemia. In SCA hexose metabolism is deranged

(Osuagwu and Mbeyi, 2007). Table 1 below shows the consistent rise in blood glucose level from the normal genotype (HbAA), through the one-gene (HbAS) and double gene-dose (HbSS) to the crisis (HbSS-crisis) state. The diminishing capacity to utilize glucose is seen to be, inadequately, compensated by the consistently enhanced utilization of extra fructose, from one state to the other.The differences are statistically significant between the states (Osuagwu and Mbeyi, 2007). This implies that the issue of capacity to utilize glucose should, by itself, be considered seriously, in handling anemia cases. Part of the explanation for this is that glucose is activated with the high energy molecule adenosine-triphosphate (ATP) by phosphorylation, before it can go into a cell. In a person with anergy (lack of metabolic energy), such as SCA patients, there is a shortage of the ATP to phosphorylate glucose. Fructose that gets into cells by passive transport or facilitated diffusion is consumed, in partial compensation. Exhaustive depletion of fructose in SCA should, by itself, be of primary concern. This is because the basic metabolism of cells that depend mainly on fructose, such as spermatozoa, would be compromised in the sickle cell disease state. This could be a major explanation for the poor spermatozoa health; and infertility observed in sickle cell males. The number, motility and other indices of spermatozoa vitality are all poor in men with SCA (Osegbe et al, 1981).

Any measure to promote glucose uptake into the cell would be of much help to SCA sufferers. Administration of insulin to facilitate glucose uptake for sickle cell sufferers in crisis is a management measure that logically suggests itself.This should be systematically investigated. By facilitating trans-membrane glucose transport, this measure will also result to better fructose conservation; and better sperm health and fertility. This should help sickle cell males live better lives; and bear healthier children.

Sickle Cell State	Number of Subjects In Group	Plasma Glucose Level, mg/dl	Plasma Fructose Level, mg/dl
HbAA	35	70.10 ± 7.50	1.32 ± 0.08
HbAS	32	74.75 ± 6.20	1.25 ± 0.05
HbSS	34	78.59 ± 4.20	1.09 ± 0.05
HbSSc	33	84.80 ± 4.10	0.99 0.04

Table 1. Plasma Glucose and Fructose Levels in Sickle Cell States.

2.2 Deranged pyruvate metabolism

Another major cause of poor glucose metabolism in sickle cell anemia is the non-efficient utilization of the end product of glycolysis; pyruvate. Table 2 summarizes this condition. The critical step in the generation of most energy (ATP) and reducing power (NADH) for the whole system fails in sickle cell disease; See Fig 1. Fig1, Fig 2 and Table 2 help to explain both anergy and acidosis in sickle cell anemia.

Sickle Cell State	HbAA	HbAS	HbSS	HbSS-crisis
Lactate Level, mM-L^{-1}	0.74 ± 0.19	0.75 ± 0.23	27.60 ± 1.39	31.40 ± 2.56
Lactate ratio	1.00	1.01	37.30	42.43
Pyruvate Level, mM-L^{-1}	0.11 ± 0.02	0.11 ± 0.03	2.03 ± 0.05	2.08 ± 0.11
Pyruvate ratio	1.00	1.00	18.45	18.91
Lactate/pyruvate	7.01	7.02	13.60	15.07

Table 2. Lactate and pyruvate levels in different sickle cell states.

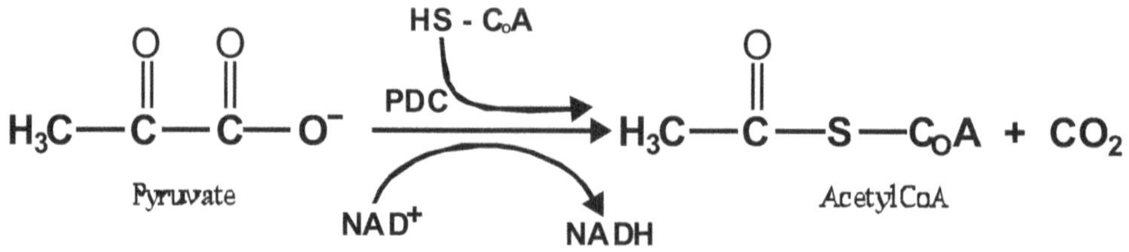

Fig. 1. Pyruvate dehydrogenase complex (PDC) links glycolysis to tissue respiration.

Pyruvate is the end-product of glycolysis and feedstock material for the production of Acetyl-CoA for the TCA cycle. If acetyl-CoA, the gate-substrate of the tricarboxylic acid (TCA) cycle is not generated, by successful pyruvate conversion, then most of the free energy stored in glucose cannot be extracted. This would, and does, result to anergy.

If reduced nicotinamide adenine dinucleotide (NADH) is not generated, there would be insufficient reducing power for the body system, down the electron transport chain; hyper-oxidation, excess free radicals, etc., will result. There is indeed observed hyper-oxidation and excess free radicals found in the body system of sickle cell patients, as theory indicated.

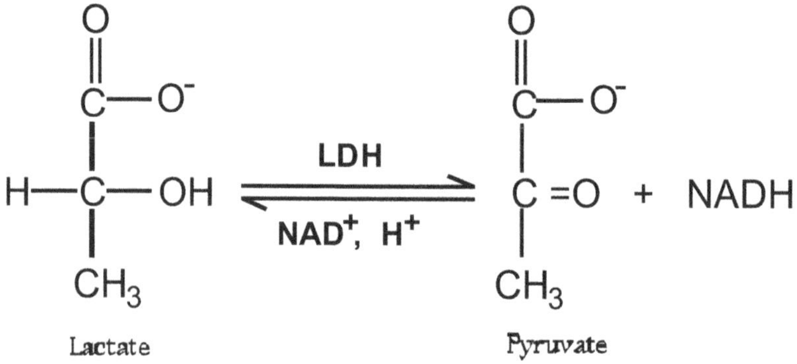

Fig. 2. Reversible oxidation of lactate to pyruvate.

If pyruvate accumulates, the equilibrium of Fig 2, which naturally favours the generation of lactate from pyruvate (Murray et al, 2006), will result to what is displayed in Table 2; a higher and higher ratio of lactate to pyruvate. Lactate acidosis will be the end result as observed in sickle cell patients. See Table 3. The data of Table 2 also best explains the dramatically different existential outcomes for single gene carriers (HbAS) as compared to double dose carriers (HbSS). The expression of the Sickle cell gene in relation to the pyruvate dehydrogenase complex is sigmoid (Osuagwu, 2009). Both the HbAA and HbAS values fall around the same point; which is why the HbAS, trait-carrier group, do not manifest the proportionate impact of the disease, as expected from theory. This suggests that the system-equilibrium mechanism of the HbAS is much better preserved than theory would suggest. But there is still an energy cost. The HbAS are not a hundred percent free of the pathological manifestation of the gene, as the popular notion suggests. They pay a smaller than expected energy price.

2.3 Energy cost of acidosis in SCA

A look at Fig 3 tells a simple story; the human body was designed by nature to be, overall, alkaline. The human body is by design an electron-rich system (alkaline). Food is a neutral substance that the human body can absorb, extract electrons (mostly as H· attached NAD⁺; NADH, etc) from. It then safely excretes the associated positive charges, particularly hydrogen ion, H⁺. As Fig 3 shows all the major body fluids are alkaline (electron-rich); all the excretory body fluids are acidic (hydrogen-ion rich).Part of the reason for this alkaline design is body energy economics. It is more efficient to extract energy from energy-rich molecules in an alkaline medium.

Consider the hydrolysis reaction that extracts energy from the key energy currency of the body adenosine triphosphate, ATP:

$$ATP^{4-} + H_2O \rightleftharpoons ADP^{3-} + HPO_4^{2-} + H^+ + Energy$$

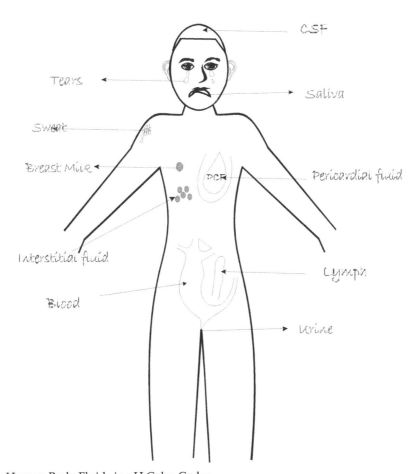

Fig. 3. Human Body Fluids in pH Color Codes.
Internal Body fluids are alkaline (blue); excretions are acidic (red); CSF = cerebro-spinal fluid.

A product of this reaction is the hydrogen ion, H^+, which gives acids their character. Le Chatellier's principle, on the self-restoring tendency of displaced equilibrium systems, teaches that ATP hydrolysis in acid medium would be resisted, because one of the products is an acid, H^+. To push ATP hydrolysis under such condition would in itself cost energy. In addition, the efficiency of the ATP hydrolyzing enzyme, ATPase, decreases with increasing acidity (Bronk, 1973). We know enzymes are denatured by acids, outside normal range of function. This implies extra energy cost and waste. On the other hand ATP hydrolysis would proceed rapidly in a more alkaline medium that would consume the produced H^+. The more alkaline the better; within physiological range. ATP hydrolysis is more efficient, yields more energy, in more alkaline medium (Manchester, 1980).

In recent times, there have been groups or movements, particularly via the internet, promoting the '*Alkaline Body*' as the ideal body. Their arguments are based on some of the points noted here. The problem with their position is they don't seem to realize that excess alkalinity of the body (alkalosis) is in itself a disease. The body is designed on the optimality principle. And human survival at beyond pH 7.65 is difficult.

2.4 Low blood pH in SCA

Table 3 shows clear tendency towards more acid body fluid, as the sickle-gene dose/state increases.Therefore the sickle cell sufferer's body consumes more ATP to do the same amount of, say, muscular work. The energy cost of extracting the same amounts of hydrogen ion, H^+, from blood into urine illustrates this point well. This data agrees with the theory outlined above.The more energy exerted to do the same amount of work, the more stress would be associated with it.

S/No	Genotype/State	n	Blood pH,	Urine pH,
1	HbAA = 0	42	7.39 ± 0.07	6.54 ± 0.15
2	HbAS = 1	42	7.35 ± 0.09	6.44 ± 3.15
3	HbSS = 2	42	7.32 ± 0.08	5.89 ± 0.39
4	HbSS-crisis = 3	42	7.15 ± 0.12	4.75 ± 0.46

Table 3. Sickle State, Blood and Urine pH.

2.4.1 Energy cost of kidney hydrogen ion dialysis in SCA

From the data of Table 3, the estimated enthalpies of dialysis, ΔH_d, for each of the four states are: HbAA = 1.96RT; HbAS = 2.10RT; HBSS = 3.29RT; HbSS-crisis = 5.53RT. The estimated entropies of dialysis $T\Delta S_d$, compared to the normal HbAA state are: HbAA = 0.00RT; HbAS = 0.14RT; HbSS = 1.34RT and HbSS-crisis = 3.57RT ($R = 8.31 Jmol^{-1} K^{-1}$ and T = 303K). This offers a bio-energetic explanation of why the kidney of the sickle cell disease sufferer, on average, fails at an early age; and is the top source of morbidity (Saborio and Scheinman, 1999; Osuagwu, 2007). The kidney hydrogen, H^+, dialysis energy expenditure gap between SCA sufferers and normal is so wide that it is somewhat surprising.

S/No	Genotype/State	n	ΔH_d	$T\Delta S_d$
1	HbAA = 0	42	1.96RT	0.00RT
2	HbAS = 1	42	2.10RT	0.14RT
3	HbSS = 2	42	3.29RT	1.34RT
4	HbSS-crisis = 3	42	5.53RT	3.57RT

Table 4. Indices of Energy Cost of KidneyHydrogen Ion DialysisIn SCA.

This data confirms that the stress, in this specific case of kidney proton dialysis, suffered by the HbAS individuals (7% more) compared HbSS-steady-state (68% more) and HbSS-crisis (182% more) for doing the same amount of system work compared to the HbAA, non-carrier individuals are high. In the specific case of HbSS-crisis, three times normal. This, among others, explains why resting energy expenditure of the SCA sufferer is high. This phenomenon, of disproportionate severity of gene expression in genotypic disease conditions, is likely to be observed in varying amounts in other genetic diseases. The explanation is likely due to interaction with other genes, which help buffer the effect of the defective gene. Also noteworthy is the general fact that a complex system under stress tends to self-conserve; and does so better the closer it is to ideal state, as HbAS is compared to HbSS. Any SCA anemia management measure that reduces hydrogen ion accumulation, or that can provide an alternative route for its excretion would be of major relief to the patient.

2.5 Energy cost of change in blood system charge-parking arrangement

Nature, always, prefers the optimal structure and associated energy expenditure in designs of system. One of these choices for optimality is in the packing of charges in living things (Osuagwu, 2010). The pH values we are familiar with represent ratios of hydrogen ions, H^+, and hydroxyl ions, OH^-, that can be packed together, with optimal stability.

Comparing the concentrations of hydroxyl and hydrogen ions in the bloods of normal (HbAA) and sickle sufferers at their measured pHs from Table 3 above reveals the data of Table 5. Similar charges repel and opposite charges attract each other. The most efficient way to arrange six hydroxyl ions to one hydrogen ion in the normal, HbAA, blood (pH = 7.39) would be as octahedron; the most efficient way to arrange four to one in HbSS blood (pH = 7.32) would be as tetrahedron (Fuller, 1975). The octahedral arrangement is the optimal considering, jointly, energy efficiency and stability. Any shift from this ideal is less efficient; and energy costly. This is one other way sickle cell sufferers pay a higher energy cost to try to maintain their body system. The stress wears their system down with time, faster than for normal people.

It has been noted that, generally, any shift from the ideal charge-packing arrangement would result to sickness (Osuagwu, 2007). Larger hydroxyl to hydrogen ratios, such as found in alkalosis is also troublesome; and disease-causing. The pH 7.65, which affords a hydroxyl to hydrogen ion ratio of 20: 1, is consistent with packing on the twenty vertices of the dodecahedron with the lone hydrogen ion at the centre of the structure, held in place by weak coordinate bonds to the surrounding hydroxyl ions. 20: 1 is the largest ratio consistent with life. Beyond that, death occurs.

	GENOTYPE	HbAA	HbSS
PARAMETER			
pH		7.39	7.32
$[H^+]$, mol-L^{-1}		$10^{-7.39}$	$10^{-7.32}$
pOH		6.61	6.68
$[OH^-]$, mol-L^{-1}		$10^{-6.61}$	$10^{-6.68}$
$[OH^-]/[H^+]$		$6.03 \approx 6$	$4.37 \approx 4$
Efficient –packing Structure		Octahedron	Tetrahedron

Table 5. Hydroxyl to Hydrogen ion Concentrations and Ratios Represented by Measured pH.

2.6 Energy cost of stresses on the erythrocyte

The red blood cell, erythrocyte, whose structural and physical collapse, sickling, has given the name to SCA is of special interest in accounting for the high energy expenditure in the disease state. Sickling, erythrocyte structural collapse, occurs because the cell is overwhelmed by stresses. Two such stresses are:

2.6.1 Erythrocyte and failure of glucose metabolism in SCA

What happens to a cell that depends solely on glucose if its metabolism fails? From significant data, some presented here, and published work (Osuagwu and Mbeyi, 2007), glucose metabolism is subnormal in SCA. But the erythrocyte, like the nerve cell, depends mostly on glucose for energy. SCA erythrocyte lacks the energy to maintain the integrity of its cell membrane (Osuagwu et al, 2008). This is a significant reason for SCA erythrocyte instability.

2.6.2 Excessive oxidative stress

An acidic medium is an oxidizing medium. The proton, H^+, is nature's unit oxidant. The acidic sickle cell sufferer's body-fluid, such as blood is, therefore, inherently oxidizing. Red blood cell that is embedded in this oxidizing medium, in this case the blood stream, becomes a victim. Its lipid, electron-rich membrane is oxidized; becomes rigid and breaks down.

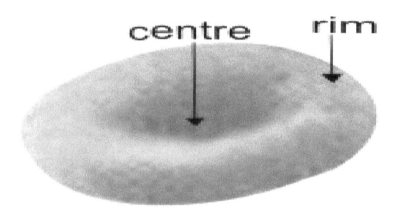

Fig. 4. Dimensions of the erythrocyte; ratios are powers of pi (3.14...).

The dimensions of the erythrocyte (Centre thickness: rim thickness: diameter: circumference) are fractal, sequential, powers of pi (π = 3.14...). This is the origin of the pi-discoid shape of the erythrocyte (Osuagwu, 2007).This pi-biconcave shape locates the greater part of the mass of the cell at the rim. This results to a very large moment of inertia; low angular momentum and great resistance to turbulence (Uzoigwe, 2006). This 'erthrocytoid' shape is the best to minimize frictional breakdown of the erythrocyte in the very viscid blood stream, through which it is propelled at great blood pressure, and speed, by the heart.Oxidative damage, by contributing to sickling, destroys this energy efficient pi-biconcave structure; increasing energy cost of blood-stream transport; and energy cost of forming new cells, with a rapid bone-marrow turnover. This is why sickle cell anemia also involves cardiovascular problems (Serjeant, 1974). Studies show that movement across the cell membrane is deranged; and the ion pumps that help maintain the trans-membrane concentration gradients consistent with life are compromised (see Table 6). It is observed that the concentration gradients of these cations deviate from the normal as the sickle condition intensifies.

Measure	HbAA	HbAS	HbSS	HbSS-c
No. of Subjects	62	62	62	62
Na^+, out, mmol/L	139.59 ± 2.89	139.05 ± 2.73	133.74 ± 2.44	109.02 ± 1.93
Na^+, in, mmol/L	15.42 ± 2.48	19.03 ± 3.25	20.64 ± 2.51	28.20 ± 1.69
$K_{eq}-Na^+(out/in)$	9.0525	7.3069	6.4797	3.8660
K^+, out, mmol/L	3.51 ± 0.33	4.05 ± 0.39	4.72 ± 0.42	5.52 ± 0.48
K^+, in, mmol/L	103.35 ± 4.49	97.91 ± 3.86	88.08 ± 3.80	83.94 ± 3.56
$K_{eq}-K^+(in/out)$	29.4444	24.1753	18.6610	15.2065
Ca^{2+}, out, mmol/L	8.48 ± 0.42	8.04 ± 0.11	7.90 ± 0.21	5.06 ± 0.32
Ca^{2+}, in, mmol/L	0.46 ± 0.09	0.58 ± 0.08	0.60 ± 0.70	2.30 ± 0.32
$K_{eq}-Ca^+(out/in)$	18.4348	13.8621	13.1667	2.2000

Table 6. Trans-membrane Cation Concentrations and Gradients, Keq, in Different Sickle cell States.

If the concentration of the potassium ions, K^+, which is more representative of the potential across the membrane, is looked at; it is observed that the energy to maintain the cell membrane integrity decreases as the sickle cell gene dosage increases. There is consistent drop in system-maintaining energy; as shown across the cell membrane.

Measure	HbAA	HbAS	HbSS	HbSS-c
No. subjects	62	62	62	62
Keq	29.44	24.18	18.66	15.21
$\Delta H_p, K^+; J$	8362.55 ± 35.00	7988.33 ± 253.66	7274.03 ± 229.12	6952.29 ± 211.49
Ratio	1.00	0.96	0.87	0.83

Table 7. Energy Decrease Across Cell Membrane as Sickle Cell Intensity Increases.

Because of this extra need for energy, the need for extra nutrients by the sickle cell sufferer has been known for a long time (Reed et al, 1987).

3. System energy wastage and sickle cell anemia management

The different points of energy wastage (high entropy) in sickle cell anemia, outlined above, have helped to explain the anergy (system lack of energy), instability and other symptoms of the disease. They also offer clues as to points and modes of possible intervention for disease management. They also offer the possibility of rationalizing existing interventions that appear effective. Inability to extract reducing power/hyper-oxidation from nutrients; the build-up of glucose, acidosis, the viscid blood and erythrocyte lysis, etc., are all issues that can be dealt with by rational intervention.

Diet or nutritional management is already well-established as a method of sickle cell disease management. But from the facts outlined here, one can see that intervention to improve glucose metabolism would be very helpful to the SCA patients. Also would dietary supplements that promote pyruvate metabolism; such as lipoic acid. Alkalinizing nutrients would be of overall good. But acid-forming nutrients would need to be taken with care; as are agents that support free-radical generation and propagation.

Special care would have to be taken in relation to the impact of any management strategy on the kidney. As observed the organ is under severe energy stress in the sickle cell patients' system.We learn from Fig 3 that sweat-inducing exercises would do some good to the SCA patients, as part of the excess acidity will be excreted that way; taken care not to over-do it and induce crisis.

Overall, the observed elevation in resting energy expenditure (REE) by the sickle cell disease sufferer can be understood in terms of known energy-related physiological, anatomical and biochemical processes. They can, therefore, be managed, for amelioration, from the careful consideration of these.

4. Summary

The observed elevation of basal energy expenditure in sickle cell anemia has been explained, in this work, in terms of established principles' of nature and bioenergetics. The genetic programme that results to sickle cell anemia appears to involve more than the genes coding for hemoglobin formation; and bone marrow metabolism. Energy metabolism is, critically, involved. And the derangements along the energy pathways have consequences that affect different levels of system function and integrity. It is shown that management of sickle cell anemia by intervention along the body's energy metabolism pathways can be helpful, in relieving the anergy (lack of energy) experienced by the sufferers of the disease. This can come about, for instance, by stabilizing erythrocyte cell membrane; minimizing blood turbulence, cell lysis and enhancing oxygen carrying capacity. The consumption of foods or supplements that supply reducing power, in the form of say ascorbic acid, glutathione or alkalinizing nutrients would be of help to the sickle cell sufferer in this regard. They would do this by free-radical-scavenging, reduction of acidity and the enhancement of ATP hydrolysis efficiency.

Enhancing glucose and pyruvate metabolism and hydrogen ion excretion, perhaps more than anything, would enhance the energy efficiency of the SCA blood system; lowering the resting energy expenditure. Achieving this would improve the energy status and general well-being of the sickle cell sufferer.

5. References

[1] Borel, MJ; Buchowski, MS; Turner, EA; Peeler, BB; Goldstein, RE and Flakoll, PJ. Alteration in Basal Nutrient Metabolism Increase Resting Energy Expenditure in Sickle Cell Disease. American Journal of Physiology: Endocrinology and Metabolism; Feb 1998; 274(2): 257-264.

[2] Bourre, JM; Effects of Nutrients (in Foods) on Structure and Function of the Nervous System: Update on the Dietary Requirement for Brain; Part I: Micronutrients. Journal of Nutrition in Health and Aging; 2006, Sept-Oct, 10 (5):377-85.

[3] Bronk, JR (1973). Chemical Biology, An Introduction to Biochemistry; The MacMillan Company, NY. p. 247.

[4] Buchowski, MS; Chen KW; Bryne D and Wang, WC. Equation to Estimate Resting Energy Expenditure in Adolescents with Sickle Cell Anemia. The American Journal of Clinical Nuitrition; Dec. 2002; 76(6):1335-1344.

[5] Enwonwu, CO 1988; Nutritional Support in Sickle Cell Anemia: Theoretical Considerations. Journal of National Medical Association; 1988, Feb; 80(2):139-44.

[6] Fakhri, ME; Aggarwal, SK; Gayoum, A and Sherrif, DS. Reduced Plasma Ascorbic Acid and Red Cell Glutathione Contents in Sickle Cell Disease- A Preliminary Report. Indian Journal of Biochemistry; 6(1): 47-50, 1991.

[7] Fuller, RB (1975). Synergetics. Macmillan Publishers, NY; p. 321.

[8] Kiessling, K; Roberts, N; Gibson, JS and Ellroy, JC. A Comparison in Normal Individuals and Sickle Cell Patients of Reduced Glutathione Precursors and their Transport between Plasma and Red Cells. Hematological Journal, 2000; 1(4): 243-249.

[9] Kopp-Hollihan, LE; van Loan, MD; Mentzer, WC and Heyman, MD; Elevated Resting Energy metabolism in Adolescents with Sickle Cell Anemia; Journal of American Dietetics Association; 1999, Feb 99(22):195-9.

[10] Manchester, KL; Free Energy, ATP Hydrolysis and Phosphorylation Potential. Biochemical Education; 8(3), 1980.

[11] Murray, R; Cramer, D; Mayes, P and Rodwell, V (2006). Glycolysis and the Oxidation of pyruvate. Harper Illustrated Biochemistry (27th edn). McGraw-Hill, NY.

[12] Osegbe, DN; Akinyanju, O and Amaku,EO; Fertility in males with sickle cell disease. Lancet; 318 (8241- 2): 275-276; August 1981.

[13] Osuagwu, CG and Mbeyi CU; Altered Plasma Hexose Sugar Metabolism in Sickle Cell Anemia. African Journal of Biotechnology; 1(3): pp 037-40; August, 2007.

[14] Osuagwu, CG. The Energy Cost of Kidney Proton Dialysis in Sickle Cell Anemia. African Journal of Biotechnology, 2007; 6 (2): 128-130.

[15] Osuagwu, CG. Polyhedral Charge-packing Model of Blood pH Changes in the Disease State. African Journal of Biotechnology, 2007; 6 (9): 1128-1131.

[16] Osuagwu, CG; Nwanjo, HU and Ajaegbu, VU. Decreased Erythrocyte Resting Membrane Potential in Sickle Cell Anaemia. Nigerian Journal of Biochemistry and molecular Biology, 2008; 24(2): 51.54.

[17] Osuagwu, CG. Turbulence: Erythrocyte Structure and Fluid-dynamic Pi (π) Designs. Journal of Medical Research and Technology, December 2007; 4 (2).

[18] Osuagwu, CG; Primary Pyruvate Acidosis in Sickle Cell Anaemia. Nigerian Journal of Biochemistry and Molecular Biology, 2009; 24 (2): 48-51

[19] Osuagwu, CG. Physiochemical Logics of Natural Selection of Biostructural Elements. Nigerian Journal of Biochemistry and Molecular biology, 2010; 25 (1): 73-76.

[20] Reed, OJ; Redding-Lallinger, R and Orringer, EP. Nutrition and Sickle Cell Disease. American Journal of Hematology, 1987; 24(4): 441-455.

[21] Reid, M; Badaloo, A; Forrester, T and Jahoor, F. In Vivo Rates of Erythrocytes Synthesis in Adults with Sickle Cell Disease. American Journal of Physiology, Endocrinology and Metabolism; 291: E73-E79; 2006.

[22] Rogers, ZR. Management of Fever in Sickle Cell Disease. *UptoDate*, June 10, 2011. UptoDate, Inc. www.uptodate.com.

[23] Saborio P and Scheinman, JI. Sickle Cell Nephropathy; Journal of the American Society of Nephrology, 1999; 10: 187-192.

[24] Serjeant, GR (1974). The Clinical Features of Sickle Cell Disease. North Holland Publishing Co, Amsterdam.

[25] Sherry, E. Foods High in Energy for Sickle Cell Anemia Patients. Livestrong.com; Demand Media Inc. (2011).

[26] Uzoigwe, C. The Human Erythrocyte Has Developed the Biconcave Shape to Optimize the Flow Property of Blood. Medical hypothesis, 2006; 7 (5):1159-1163.

An Emerging Face of Fanconi Anemia: Cancer

Sevgi Gözdaşoğlu
Ankara University
Turkey

1. Introduction

Fanconi anemia (FA) is a chromosomal instability syndrome characterized by various congenital malformations, progressive pancytopenia, chromosome breakage and predisposition to malignancy (Alter, 2003a). Autosomal recessive, FA is also inherited with X-linked inheritance reported in FA complementation group B (Meetei et al., 2004). FA pathway controls genomic stabilisation in mammalian cells and is referred to as FA pathway of antioncogenesis. Children with FA have a very high risk of developing acute myeloid leukemia (AML) and myelodysplastic syndrome (MDS). The incidence of AML in children with FA is 15.000 times that of children in the general population (Auerbach & Allen, 1991). Acute leukemia is the terminal event in about 5-20% of these cases (Ebell et al., 1989), MDS in about 5-10%, and solid tumors was held responsible in about 5-10% of the remaining cases. Patients with FA are at a high risk of developing solid tumors of the head, neck, esophagus, liver and female genitalia (Alter, 2003c, Rosenberg, Greene & Alter, 2003). In order to clarify the relationship between FA and cancer, the description of FA was recently updated as "an inherited genomic instability disorder, caused by mutations in genes regulating replication-dependent removal of interstrand DNA crosslinks" (Moldovan & D'Andrea, 2009). The research on the complex roles of FA proteins in repairing DNA improved our understanding of cancer biology. In this chapter, my main objective is twofold: to analyze clinical findings, diagnosis and hematological characteristics of FA, and to evaluate the relationship between FA pathway and cancer from the perspective of a pediatrician.

2. Fanconi anemia

FA is a familial pancytopenia associated with bone marrow hypoplasia and congenital malformations, originally discovered in three brothers by Fanconi in 1927 (Gözdaşoğlu et al., 1980). 2000 cases were reported in the literature between the years of 1927 and 2009 (Alter, 2011). FA should be considered a syndrome, not a disease due to its heterogeneity. The physical phenotype ranges from normal appearance to manifest congenital malformations, the hematological spectrum ranges from nominal values to those associated with severe aplastic anemia (Alter, 1993b). Clinical heterogeneity in FA follows from genetic heterogeneity. The heterozygote prevalence for FA is estimated to be 1 in 300 in the United States (Alter, 1993a). Homozygote frequency is estimated at 1-3 per million (Joenje et al., 1995). The male-female ratio of occurrence is 1.2:1 (Alter, 2003a). The age of diagnosis ranges from birth to 48 years with an average of 8 years. About 10-20% of families have consanguineous marriage (Alter, 1992).

2.1 Congenital abnormalities
Several congenital abnormalities may accompany this disorder such as skeletal abnormalities, hyperpigmentation, renal malformation, microcephaly, hypogonadism and mental and growth retardations (Gözdaşoğlu et al., 1980; Akar & Gözdaşoğlu, 1984). Among skeletal system anomalies, radial ray defects such as hypoplasia of the thumb and the radius are observed most (Figures 1, 2, 3). In addition to congenital hip dislocations, scoliosis, vertebral anomalies, cafe-au-lait spots, diffuse hyperpigmentation and hypopigmentation are frequent. A short stature is prominent in more than half of the cases in utero and following birth. The median height is about 50 percentile in the patients, which can be related to growth hormone deficiency or hypothyroidism. Mycrophtalmia, microcephaly and deafness may be observed, renal anomalies such as unilateral and renal aplasia, renal hypoplasia, horse-shoe kidney and double ureter may be encountered in about a third of the cases. Boys have genital anomalies as hypogenitalia, undescended testis and hypospadias. Girls have uterus anomalies. There have been reports of gastrointestinal defects such as esophageal, duodenal atresia, imperforated anus, tracheo-esophageal fistula, cardiac defects such as patent ductus arteriosus, ventricular septal defect, pulmonary stenosis, aortic stenosis, aortic coarctation, central nervous system anomalies such as hydrocephalus and absence of septum pellucidum (Alter, 2003b; Kwee & Kuyt, 1989; Smith et al., 1989). The FA phenotype can vary within family members; a report of four FA cases within two related consanguineous families who all had the same FANCA mutation demonstrated a wide variation in birth weight, skin pigmentation and the severity of skeletal, renal and genital abnormalities (Koç et al., 1999). Approximately 25-40% of the FA patients in the International Fanconi Anemia Registry (IFAR) do not exhibit any major malformation (Alter, 2003a).

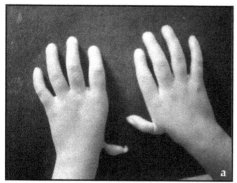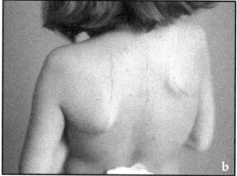

Fig. 1. a) The picture of a 6-year-old girl with Fanconi anemia showing hypoplastic and proximally placed rudimentary thumbs, clinodactyly. b) Sprengel deformity and scoliosis.

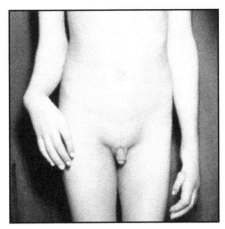

Fig. 2. The picture of a 10-year-old boy with aplastic anemia showing the absence of radius and thumb on the right hand, hypoplastic thumb on the left hand and hypogenitalismus.

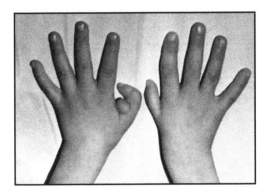

Fig. 3. Bifid left thumb and proximally placed right thumb.

2.2 Hematologic abnormalities

In homozygote FA, the most prominent finding is hematologic disorders. The blood count at birth is mostly normal and macrocytosis is generally the first sign of FA. This is followed by thrombocytopenia and anemia. Pancytopenia develops typically at 5-10 years of age, median at seven years (birth to 31 years) (Butturini et al., 1994). IFAR defined hematologic abnormality as hemoglobin level below 10 g/dL, absolute neutrophil count below $1x10^9$/L or platelet count below 100 x 10^9/L (Alter et al., 2003a). On retrospective analysis of 145 FA patients, some congenital anomalies were seen to carry a potential risk of the development of bone marrow failure. The risk of bone marrow failure in those with radius anomaly is 5.5 times more than those without. The presence of abnormal head, deafness, developmental delay, cardiopulmonary abnormality and abnormal kidney, also kown as 5-item congenital abnormality, increase the risk of bone marrow failure (Rosenberg et al., 2004).

Hematologic disorders are the first sign of FA in young adults not exhibiting any congenital anomalies. Stress erythropoesis exists in FA with characteristics of macrocytosis, increased HbF and the antigen *i* (Table 1). These characteristics may also be found in the anemia free siblings of FA patients (Alter, 2003a). Aspiration from bone marrow reveals marked depression or absence of hematopoietic cells and replacement by fatty tissue containing reticulum cells, lymphocytes, plasma cells and usually tissue mast cells. Nucleated red cells are also decreased in number and they may display megaloblastic features (Fig. 4). Bone marrow biopsy is essential for diagnosis (Lanzkowsky, 1999). In a study based on data from 388 cases with FA, actuarial risk of developing hematopoietic abnormalities was 98% by the age of 40 (Butturini et al., 1994).

Stress erythropoesis
- macrocytosis
- Hb F ↑
- Antigen i

Trombocytopenia, anemia
Pancytopenia median age: 7 years (5-10 years)
Bone marrow failure in radius aplasia; 5.5 ↑

Table 1. Hematological findings in FA.

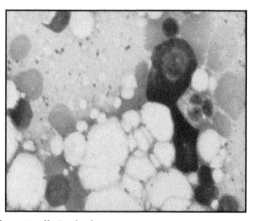

Fig. 4. Fatty tissue and mast cells in the bone marrow.

The most striking feature of FA cells is an increased spontaneous chromosomal instability. Diepoxybutane (DEB) test remains a classical test for diagnosis, involving the detection of chromosomal breaks, gaps, rearrangements, radials, exchange and endoreduplications in peripheral lymphocytes following culturing with clastogenic agents (such as DEB or mitomycin-C) (Fig. 5a, b) (Auerbach et al., 1981). FA homozygotes have a mean of 8.96 breaks per cell in the DEB test according to the IFAR (Alter, 2003a).

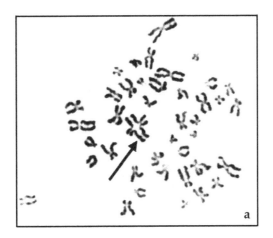

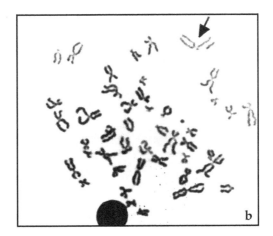

Fig. 5. a) Chromosomal structure abnormalities in the patient with FA. Arrow indicates typical quadriradial chromosome. b) Cytogenetic abnormalities in the metaphase plaque. Arrow indicates chromatid breaks and fragmentation.

Interpretation of the results of DEB test may be complicated by mosaicism. Approximately 25% of patients with FA have evidence of spontaneously occurring mosaicism as manifest by the presence of two subpopulations of lymphocytes, one of which is hypersensitive to cross-linking agents while the other behaves normally in response to these agents. Mosaicism might be associated with a relatively mild hematological course (Lo Ten Foe et al., 1997). DEB test gives a false negative for these patients. DEB testing to establish the diagnosis could be performed on an alternative cell type, such as skin fibroblasts (Alter & Kupfer, 2011). Although DEB test is of crucial importance in the diagnosis of FA, it should be also noted that molecular genetic diagnostic methods have also started to be used in the identification of this disorder.

2.3 Cellular disorders and hematopoiesis

Patients with FA generally develop some degree of bone marrow dysfunction ranging from mild asymptomatic cytopenias in any lineage to severe aplastic anemia, MDS or AML. The absence of marrow failure does not rule out FA (Shimamura, 2003). A number of cytokines are critical in the control and regulation of cellular homeostasis in bone marrow. Several cellular disorders associated with FA were reported in a large number of studies. FA cells have important phenotypic abnormalities related to hematopoiesis as shown in Table 2.

Sensitivity to cross- linking agents
Prolongation of G2 phases of cell cycles
Sensitivity to oxygen
Sensitivity to ionized radiation
Overproduction of tumor necrosis factor-α
Direct defects in DNA repair:
-   Accumulation of DNA adducts
-   Defect in repair DNA cross links
Genomic instability
-   Spontaneous chromosome breakage
-   Hypermutability
Increased apoptosis
Defective p53 induction
Intrinsic stem cell defect
Decreased colony growth

Table 2. Cellular disorders in FA (From Lanzkowsky, P. Manual of Pediatric Hematology and Oncology 1999).

Defective hematopoiesis in FA was shown by the investigation of in vitro bone marrow cell cultures. Interleukin (IL)-6 and granulocyte macrophage-colony stimulating factor expression reduced in many patients with FA (Stark et al., 1993). In another research, the overproduction of tumor necrosis factor-α in FA was also reported (Schultz & Shahidi, 1993). On the other hand, these patients have increased loss of telomere signals compared with controls (Hanson et al., 2001). Abnormal telomere metabolism might play a role in the evoluation of bone marrow failure and malignant transformation in FA (Li et al., 2003). The cytokine changes, increased apoptosis and telomere shortening play a significant role in the microenvironment of bone marrow and the regulation of cellular homeostasis (Fig. 6). Bone marrow failure occurs at a median age of 7 years. Hematopoietic tissue is particularly sensitive to DNA damage caused by radiation or cytotoxic drugs. Genome instability and telomere shortening alter the signals and form mutant clones resistant to apoptosis and consequently AML develops (Lensch et al., 1999; Tischkowitz & Dokal, 2004).

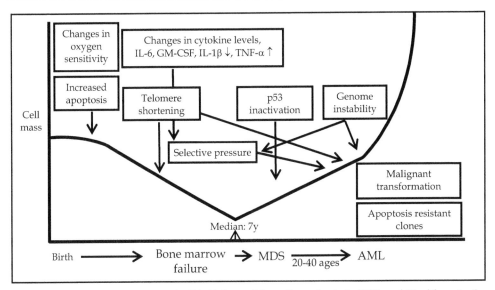

Fig. 6. Defective Hematopoiesis in FA (Adapted from Lensch et al., 1999 and Tischkowitz & Dokal, 2004).

The role of p53 in preventing DNA damage in FA cells was shown in a theoretical model (Kennedy & D'Andrea 2005). As revealed in Fig. 7, when severe DNA damage occurs in FA cells, p53 activates apoptosis and tumor progression is inhibited. If this process occurs in embryonic stem cells, it may cause anomalies. Stem cell loss in bone marrow leads to progressive anemia associated with FA.

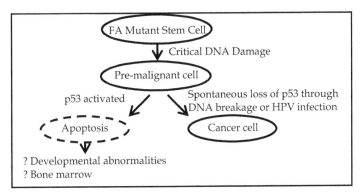

Fig. 7. p53-mediated apoptosis (From Kennedy, R.D. & D'Andrea, A.D., The Fanconi Anemia/BRCA Pathway: New Faces in the Crowd. Genes and Development, 2005; 19:2925-2940).

Loss of p53 or other genes related to apoptosis due to DNA breakage by viral infection or cross-link agents, might inhibit the cell apoptosis. Cells with severe DNA damage continue dividing and this, in turn, may result in malignant transformation. Also a tumor may develop with human papilloma virus (HPV) infections. Since HPV E6 protein decreases the p53 protein level, the apoptotic pathway activation is inhibited. Loss of p53 function may lead to cancer by allowing premalignant cells to survive (Kennedy & D'Andrea 2005).

2.4 Complementation groups, genes and DNA repair

Fifteen complementation groups have been identified in patients with FA (Table 3) and new complementation groups may be identified in the future.

Complementation group	gene	frequency* %	chromosome
FA – A	FANCA	60	16q 24.3
FA – B	FANCB	<1	Xp 22.3
FA – C	FANCC	15	9q 22.3
FA – DI	BRCA2	<5	13q 12.3
FA – D2	FANCD2	<5	3p 25.3
FA – E	FANCE	<1	6p 21.3
FA – F	FANCF	<1	11p 15
FA – G	FANCG	10	9p 13
FA – I	FANCI	<1	15q 25 - q 26
FA – J	BRIP1	<1	17q 22
FA – L	FANCL	<1	2p 16.1
FA – M	FANC M	<1	14q 21.3
FA – N	PALB2	<1	16p 12
FA – O	RAD51C	<1	17q 22
FA – P	SLX4	<1	16p 13.3

Table 3. FA complementation groups and genes (Adapted from Alter & Kupfer, 2011; Kennedy & D'Andrea, 2005).

FA-A mutations are the most frequent ones observed in about 60% of the cases; FA-C and FA-G mutations are recognized in 15% and 10% of the cases, respectively. While the frequencies of FA-D1 (BRCA2) and FA-D2 are 5% each, the prevalence of other complementation groups is rare (Kennedy & D'Andrea, 2005). The first gene cloned is the FA-C complementation group gene composed of 1674 nucleotides and 14 exons (Fig. 8). Six mutations are recognized in the gene. More than 90% of FA-C mutations are in exon 1 and in exon 4. There is a mild form of FA in mutation related with "dG 322" deletion in exon 1. IV S4 + 4A > T mutations are distinguished for the majority of FA in Ashkenazi Jewish patients having severe phenotype of multiple congenital malformations and early onset of hematological disease (Joenje et al., 1995a, 1995b).

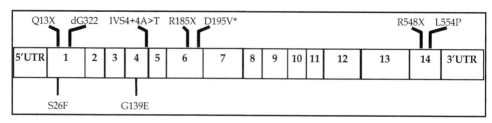

Fig. 8. Mutations in FA-C gene (From Joenje, H. et al., Fanconi Anemia Research: Current Status and Prospects, European Journal of Cancer 1995; 31:268-272).

Several types of, sometimes overlapping, DNA repair processes are identified based on the targeted types of damage. Three types of excision repair processes have been described: base excision repair (BER), nucleotide excision repair (NER) and mismatch repair (MMR). Two additional types of DNA repair, homologous recombination (HR) and nonhomologous end-joining (NHEJ) are employed in response to a double strand break, the most serious type of DNA damage. HR is considered to be an error-free pathway since it uses a copy of the damaged segment. NHEJ is accepted as an error-prone pathway since free ends are joined in the absence of a template which might cause an associated loss of nucleotides or translocation (Risinger & Groden, 2004). FA pathway has an important role in three classic DNA repair processes, namely homologous recombination, nucleotide excision repair andtranslesion synthesis which is DNA polymerization on damaged templates (Moldovan & D'Andrea, 2009).

FA proteins have a significant role in regulating DNA repair by homologous recombination. FA proteins cooperate in a common pathway known as the FA/BRCA pathway. Eight of the FA proteins (A, B, C, E, F, G, L, M and possibly I subunits) form a nuclear core complex required for the monoubiquitination of FANCD2 protein. In response to DNA damage, the FA complex (complex 1) is activated and initiates the monoubiquitination of FANCD2. Then FANCD2 – Ub interacts with BRCA2 in complex 2, leading to repair of the cross-link possibly through homologous recombination and translesion synthesis. The FANCD1 gene is identical to the breast and ovarian cancer susceptibility gene, BRCA2. FANCD2 is deubiquitinated by USP1, thereby inactivating the pathway (Fig. 9). The FA proteins are also important in the arrangement of an intra-S-phase checkpoint (D'Andrea, 2003; Kennedy & D'Andrea, 2005; Wang & D'Andrea, 2004). In the absence of BRCA2, DNA repair cannot be performed by homologous recombination. DNA damage is repaired by nonhomologous end-joining (Fig. 10).

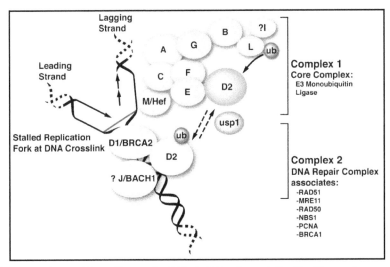

Fig. 9. The FA pathway (From Kennedy, R.D. & D'Andrea, A.D., The Fanconi Anemia/BRCA Pathway: New Faces in the Crowd. Genes and Development 2005; 19: 2925-2940).

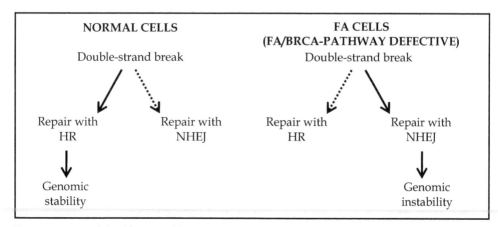

Fig. 10. Repair of double-strand break in normal and FA cells (Adapted from Venkitaraman, 2004). HR: Homologous recombination; NHEJ: Nonhomologous end-joining.

In the cytoplasm, only FANCA, FANCC, FANCF and FANCG proteins are present. Cytoplasmic functions and interactions of FANCC and FANCG are decoded. The FANCC protein binds to NADPH cytochrome P-450 reductase and regulates the major detoxification pathway. FANCC also interacts with glutathion-S-transpherase PI-I, and protects the cell from oxidative stress. FANCC interacts with HSP70 to prevent the apoptosis in hematopoietic cells exposed to IFN–γ and TNF-α. FANCC is required for optimal activation of STAT1 in the JAK/STAT pathway. FANCG protein directly interacts with CYP2E1 and prevents oxidative DNA damage (Thompson et al., 2005).

2.5 Fanconi anemia and cancer

Mutations in FA genes cause a disorder characterized by bone marrow failure, developmental defects and cancer proneness (Moldovan & D'Andrea, 2009). The FANCD2 knockout mice exhibit micropthalmia, perinatal lethality, and severe hypogonadism. Fancd2knockout mice also has increased incidences of epithelial cancers such as breast, ovarian and liver cancers (D'Andrea, 2003). FA is a rare cancer susceptibility syndrome that increases the predisposition of the patient to leukemia, squamous cell carcinomas of the head and neck or female genitelia as well as liver tumors. Predisposition to cancer in heterozygotes was also reported by Swift (Alter, 2003a). One thousand three hundred cases of FA were evaluated during the years between 1927 and 2001. Nine percent of these cases had leukemia, 7% had myelodysplastic syndrome, 5% had solid tumors and 3% liver tumors. In approximately 25% of patients with cancer, the malignancy preceded the diagnosis of FA. It is unclear which patients are prone to develop such tumors (Alter, 2003c). In another study, the cumulative incidence of malignancies among 145 patients with FA was 9 leukemias and 18 solid tumors in 14 patients. The ratio of observed to expected neoplasm (O/E) was 50 for all cancers, 48 for all solid tumors and 785 for leukemia. These increased risks were calculated to be statistically significant. The highest solid tumor O/E ratios were 4317 for vulvar cancer, 2362 for esophageal cancer, and 706 for head and neck cancer. The median age of onset of leukemia was 11.3 years, which is significantly lower compared to the median 28.9 years of onset for solid tumors (Rosenberg et al., 2003). Actuarial risk of developing MDS or AML by 40 years of age was 52% (Butturini et al., 1994).

The types of leukemia occurring in FA are primarily non-lymphocytic leukemia although a few lymphoblastic types have also been reported (Alter, 1993a; Yetgin et al., 1994). The incidence of AML in FA patients is 15.000 times more compared to children in the population (Auerbach & Allen, 1991). In these patients, all FAB sub-types occur; the myelomonocytic (M_4) and acute monocytic (M_5) types (Fig.11, Fig.12) are the most common (Alter, 2003c, Tischkowitz & Dokal, 2004).

Certain cytogenetic abnormalities are commonly seen in these patients with MDS/AML. In one study of the cytogenetic findings of 23 MDS and AML cases in FA homozygotes in high incidence of monosomy 7, 7q-, rearrangement of 1p36, 1q24-34 and 11q22-25, abnormalities was reported (Butturini et al., 1994). The most frequently observed chromosomal abnormalities in FA-associated leukemia are monosomy 7, duplication of 1 q and chromosome 3q abnormalities. Gain of 3q is associated with poor prognosis (Taniguchi & D'Andrea, 2006). As suggested, all FA patients may be considered as preleukemic state and this disorder represents a model for study of the etiology of AML (Auerbach & Allen, 1991). Leukemia may be the first hematologic manifestation of FA (Auerbach et al., 1982). Five out of the 52 patients with FA developing 3 AML, 1 squamous cell carcinoma of the gingiva, 1 hepatocellular carcinoma were mentioned in another clinical research (Altay et al., 1997).

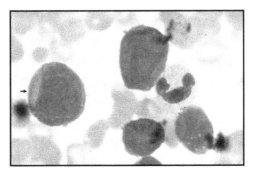

Fig. 11. Auer rods positivity in myeloblast.

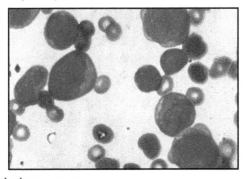

Fig. 12. Monoblasts in the bone marrow.

In our series, four out of 39 cases developed AML and one had two malignancies.There were no other cancers among family members in these four patients whereas the sister of a boy with FA developed acute leukemia in another hospital. (Gözdaşoğlu et al., 1980, Gözdaşoğlu et al., 2009). The majority of solid tumors occurs after the first or second decade of life (Alter, 2011).

FA-D1 complementation group is different from other complementation groups in its severity. In this group, leukemia and solid tumors develop as early as before 5 years of age. A cell line (termed FA-AML1) was obtained from blast cells after a second relapse following the bone marrow transplantation in a 2 years old boy with FA and AML. FA-AML1 is the first AML cell line obtained from a FA patient. FA-AML1 cells have failed to reveal FA phenotype such as hypersensitivity to growth inhibition and chromosomal breakage by the cross-linking agent mitomycin C. Genomic DNA showed biallelic mutations in FANCD1/BRCA2. Genetic reversion has been observed resulting in the loss of the FA cellular phenotype (Ikeda et al., 2003). In another report, a cross-linker-sensitive AML cell line also was derived from a 2 years old boy who had biallelic FANCD1/BRCA2 (Meyer et al., 2005). FA-D1 subgroup, however, can be associated with a high incidence of leukemia and specific solid tumors such as Wilms tumor and medulloblastoma in very early childhood (Hirsch et al., 2004). BRCA2 mutations predisposes to cancers like the familial breast, ovary, prostate and pancreas (Shivji & Venkitaraman, 2004). From several studies on the issue, it is possible to conclude that the diagnosis of leukemia and solid tumors at early age and worse prognosis are the most important features of FA-D1 complementation group. FA is found as the most common form of inherited bone marrow failure syndrome associated with worst prognosis. A high percentage of patients developed severe bone marrow failure and cancer in a study based on 127 patients whose 66 cases (52%) are with FA. One of the striking findings of this study is the high rate of consanguinity, 68 % of patients with FA. Leukemia in 7 patients (11%), MDS in 11 patients (16%) and solid tumors in 6 patients (9%) out of these 66 cases were diagnosed (Tamary et al., 2010). In another study of 181 patients, however, bone marrow failure in 66 patients, acute myeloid leukemia in 14 patients and solid tumors in 10 patients were determined. The ratio of O/E was 44 for all cancers, 26 for all solid tumors and 868 for acute myeloid leukemia. These increased risks were statistically significant. In this study, absent or abnormal radii and a five-item congenital abnormality score were significant risk factors for bone marrow failure. In three of the 48 patients who received a transplant, the three malignancies, namely tongue, liver and esophagus, occurred after 2, 16 and 17 years following the transplants. The age-specific risk of solid tumors was 3.8-fold higher in cases with transplants compared to the cases without (Rosenberg, Alter & Ebell, 2008). Hematopoietic stem cell transplant (HSCT) is presently the only therapy that can restore normal hematopoiesis in patients with FA. The risk of squamous cell cancers increased for FA patients irrespective of receiving and not receiving the transplants. HSCT conditioning regimes may also increase the occurrence of squamous cell cancers in cases with transplants. Rosenberg et al., compared two groups of patients; 117 receiving transplants and 145 not receiving. It was found that the age-specific risk of squamous cell cancer was 4.4 fold higher in patients who received transplants than who did not. Squamous cell cancers developed at significantly younger ages in the transplanted group. Acute and chronic graft-versus-host diseases were significant squamous cell cancer risk factors, and this cancer was also an adverse risk factor for death in both groups. Survival rate following squamous cell cancer was not significantly different between the two groups (Rosenberg et al., 2005). Liver tumors associated with androgens were reported in the patients with FA (Velazquez& Alter, 2004) and the cumulative probability of liver tumors has been estimated to be 46 % by age 50 (Alter, 2003c).

The patients with FA should be followed in the form of hematologic monitoring and cancer surveillance. Complete blood counts should be taken every 4 months. Annual bone marrow aspirates and biopsies should be performed on all patients. Dental and oropharyngeal(

including naso-laryngoscopy) exams should start at age 10 or within the first year after transplant. Gynecologic examination and Pap semears beginning at age 16, and if necessary, annual esophageal endoscopy should be done as part of cancer surveillance. The patients are advised to avoid toxic agents, smoking and alcohol. Radiographic studies should be minimally utilised. Vaccination of female patients with the human papillomavirus vaccine should be considered starting at nine years of age (Alter,2011).

3. Conclusion

FA is a rare autosomal recessive or x-linked inherited chromosomal instability syndrome. Affected individuals have a highly increased risk of developing bone marrow failure, hematologic malignancies and solid tumors. FA-pathway has an important role in repairing DNA damage namely homologous recombination, nucleotide excision repair and translesion synthesis. Fifteen complementation groups and genes that cause FA have been identified. FA-D1 subgroup can be associated with high incidence of leukemia and solid tumors such as Wilms tumor, medulloblastoma, neuroblastoma at early ages.   BRCA2 mutations predispose to cancers such as familial breast, ovary, prostate and pancreas. Leukemia in FA is generally very difficult to treat and survival is rare. The deficiency in DNA repair leads to increased sensitivity to the side effects of chemotherapy and the patients are either vulnerable to treatment toxicity or may receive inadequate treatment. The effective treatment modalities have to be further developed. Patients with FA should be followed with regard to AML and solid tumors which should be considered as first manifestations of FA. It is also important to note that the family members of the patients with FA must be scanned for cancer as well. Genetic counseling and psychosocial support should be employed as soon as possible.

4. Acknowledgements

This work is dedicated to the loving memory of my late husband Prof. Dr. Rıfat Gözdaşoğlu for his unwavering support throughout my career and his unrelenting dedication to the ethical and respectful treatment of his patients.

5. References

Akar, N. & Gözdaşoğlu, S. (1984). Spectrum of Anomalies in Fanconi Anemia, *Human Genetics,* Vol.21, No.1, pp. 75-76, ISSN 0340-6717

Altay, C.; Alikaşifoğlu, M.; Kara, A.; Tunçbilek, E.; Özbek, N.; Schroeder-Kurth, T.M. (1997). Analysis of 65 Turkish Patients with Congenital Aplastic Anemia (Fanconi Anemia and Non-Fanconi Anemia): Hacettepe Experience, *Clinical Genetics,* Vol.51, No.5, pp. 296-302, ISSN 0009-9163

Alter, B.P. & Kupfer, G. (2011). Fanconi Anemia, In: *Gene Reviews-(internet) NCBI Bookshelf, ID: NBK 1401, PMID: 20301575,* R.A. Pagon, T.D. Bird, C.R. Dolan, et al., (Eds.), pp. 1-42

Alter, B.P. (1992). Fanconi's Anemia. Current Concepts, *American Journal of Pediatric Hematology/Oncology,* Vol.14, No.2, pp. 170-176, ISSN 0192-8562

Alter, B.P. (1993a). Annotation. Fanconi's Anemia and its Variability, *British Journal of Haematology,* Vol.85, No.1, pp. 9-14, ISSN 0007-1048

Alter, B.P. (2003b). Cancer in Fanconi Anemia 1927-2001, *Cancer,* Vol.97, No.2, pp. 425-440, ISSN 0008-543X

Alter, B.P. (2003c). Inherited bone marrow failure syndrome, In: *Nathan and Oski's Hematology of Infancy and Childhood,* D.G. Nathan, S.H. Orkin, D. Ginsburg, A.T. Look, (Eds.), pp. 280-299, W.B. Saunders Company, ISBN 0-7216-9317-1, Philadelphia

Alter, B.P. (2005). Fanconi's Anemia, Transplantation and Cancer, *Pediatric Transplantation,* Vol.9, (Suppl.7), pp. 81-86, ISSN 1397-3142

Auerbach, A.D. & Allen, R.G. (1991). Leukemia and Preleukemia in Fanconi Anemia Patients. *Cancer Genetics and Cytogenetics,* Vol.51, No.1, pp. 1-12, ISSN 0165-4608

Auerbach, A.D.; Adler, B. & Chaganti, S.K. (1981). Prenatal and Postnatal Diagnosis and Carrier Detection of Fanconi Anemia by a Cytogenetic Method, *Pediatrics,* Vol.67, No.1, pp. 128-135, ISSN 0031-4005

Auerbach, A.D.; Weiner, M.A.; Warburton, D.; Yeboa, K.; Lu, L. & Broxmeyer, H.E. (1982). Acute Myeloid Leukemia as the First Hematologic Manifestation of Fanconi Anemia, *American Journal of Hematology,* Vol.12, No.3, pp. 289-300, ISSN 0361-8609

Butturini, A.; Gale, R.P.; Verlander, P.C.; Adler-Brecher, B.; Gillio, P. & Auerbach, A.D. (1994). Hematologic Abnormalities in Fanconi Anemia Registry Study, *Blood,* Vol.84, No.5, pp. 1650-1655, ISSN 0006-4971

D'Andrea, A.D. (2003). The Fanconi Road to Cancer, *Genes & Development,* Vol.17, No.16, pp. 1933-1936, ISSN 0890-9369

Ebell, W.; Friedrich, W. & Kohne, E. (1989). Therapeutic Aspects of Fanconi Anemia, In: *Fanconi Anemia Clinical, Cytogenetic and Experimental Aspects,* T.M. Schroeder-Kurth, A.D. Auerbach, G. Obe, (Eds.), pp. 47-60, Springer-Verlog, ISBN 3-540-50401-X, New York, Berlin, Heidelberg

Gözdaşoğlu, S.; Çavdar, A.O.; Arcasoy, A.; Babacan, E.; Sanal, Ö. (1980). Fanconi's Aplastic Anemia, Analysis of 18 Cases, *Acta Haematologica,* Vol.64, No.3, pp. 131-135, ISSN 0001-5792

Gözdaşoğlu, S.; Ertem, M.; Uysal, Z.; Babacan, E.; Yüksel, M.; Bökesoy, I.; Sunguroğlu, A.; Arcasoy, A. & Çavdar, A.O. (2009). Acute Myeloid Leukemia in Turkish Children with Fanconi Anemia. One Center Experience in the Period Between 1964-1995, *Turkish Journal of Hematology,* Vol.26, No.3, pp. 118-122, ISSN 1300-7777

Hanson, H.; Mathew, C.G.; Docherty, Z.; Ogilvie, M. & Mackie, M. (2001). Telomere Shortening in Fanconi Anaemia Demonstrated by a Direct FISH Approach, *Cytogenetic and Genome Research,* Special issue, Vol.93, No.3-4, p.203-206, ISSN 1424-8581

Hirsch, B.; Shimamura, A.; Moreau, L.; Baldinger, S.; Hag-alshiek, M.; Bostrom, B.; Sencer, S.; D'Andrea, A.D. (2004) Association of Biallelic BRCA2/FANCD1 Mutations with Spontaneous Chromosomal Instability and Solid Tumors of Childhood, *Blood,* Vol. 103, No. 7, p. 2554-2559 ISSN 0006-4971

Ikeda, H.; Matsushita, M.; Waisfisz, W.; Kinoshita, A.; Oostra, A.B.; Nieuwint, A.W., deWinder, J.P., Hoatlin, M.E., Kawai, Y., Sasaki, M.S., D'Andrea, A.D., Kawakami, Y., Joenjo, H., (2003). Genetic Reversion in an Acute Myelogenous Leukemia Cell Line from a Fanconi Anemia Patient with Biallelic Mutations in BRCA2, *Cancer Research,* Vol.63, No.10, pp. 2688-2694, ISSN 0008-5472

Joenje, H.; Lo Ten Foe, J.R.; Oostra, A.B. & et al. (1995a). Classification of Fanconi Anemia Patients by Complementation Analysis: Evidence for a Fifth Genetic Subtype, *Blood,* Vol.86, No.6, pp. 2156-2160, ISSN 0006-4971

Joenje, H.; Mathew, C. & Gluckman, E. (1995b). Fanconi Anemia Research: Current Status and Prospects, *European Journal of Cancer*, Vol.31, No.2, pp. 268-272, ISSN 0959-8049

Kennedy, R.D. & D'Andrea, A.D. (2005). The Fanconi Anemia/BRCA Pathway: New Faces in the Crowd, *Genes & Development*, Vol.19, No.24, pp. 2925-2940, ISSN 0890-9369

Koç, A.; Pronk, J.C.; Alikaşifoğlu, M.; Joenje, H. & Altay, Ç. (1999). Variable Pathogenicity of Exon 43del (FAA) in Four Fanconi Anaemia Patients within a Consanguineous Family, *British Jornal of Haematology*, Vol.104, No.1, pp. 127-130, ISSN 007-1048

Kwee, M.L. & Kuyt, L.P. (1989). Fanconi Anemia in the Netherlands, In: *Fanconi Anemia Clinical, Cytogenetic and Experimental Aspects*, T.M. Schroeder-Kurth, A.D. Auerbach, G. Obe, (Eds.), pp. 18-33, Springer-Verlog, ISBN 3-540-50401-X, New York, Berlin, Heidelberg

Lanzkowsky, P. (1999). *Manual of Pediatric Hematology and Oncology*, (third ed.), Academic Pres, ISBN 0-12-436635-x, San Diego, San Francisco, New York, Boston, London, Sydney, Tokyo

Lensch, MW., Rathbun, PK., Olson, SB., Jones, GR &Bagby Jr, GC. (1999). Selective Pressure as an Essential Force in Molecular Evolution of Myeloid Leukemic Clones: A View from the Window of Fanconi Anemia, *Leukemia*, Vol.13, No.11, pp. 1784-1789, ISSN 0887-6924

Li, X.; Leteurtre, F.; Rocha, V.; Guardiola, P.; Berger, R.; Daniel, M.T.; Noguera, M.H.; Maarek, O.; Roux, G.L.; de la Salmoniere, P.; Richard, P. & Glueckman, E. (2003). Abnormal Telomere Metabolism in Fanconi's Anemia Correlates with Genomic Instability and the Probability of Developing Severe Aplastic Anemia, *British Journal of Hematology*, Vol.120, No.5, pp. 836-845, ISSN 0007-1048

Lo Ten Foe, J.R.; Kwee, M.L.; Rooimans, M.A.; Oostra, A.B.; Veerman, A.J.P.; van Well, M.; Pauli, R.M.; Shahidi, N.T.; Dokal, I.; Roberts, I.; Altay, Ç.; Gluckman, E.; Gibson, R.A.; Mathew, C.G.; Arwert, F. & Joenje, H. (1997). Somatic Mosaicism in Fanconi Anemia: Molecular Basis and Clinical Significance, *European Journal of Human Genetics*, Vol.5, No.3, pp. 137-148, ISSN 1018-4813

Meetei, A.R.; Levitus, M.; Xue, Y.; Medhurst, A.L.; Zwann, M.; Ling, C.; Rooimans, M.A.; Bier, P.; Hoatlin, M.; Pals, G.; de Winter, J.P.; Wang, W. & Joenje, H. (2004). X-Linked Inheritance of Fanconi Anemia Complementation Group B, *National Genetics*, Vol.36, No.11, pp. 1219-1224, ISSN 1061-4036

Meyer, S.; Fergusson, W.D; Oostra, A.B. & et al. (2005). A Cross-linker. Sensitive Myeloid Leukemia Cell Line from a 2-year-old Boy with Severe Fanconi Anemia and Biallelic FANCDI/BRCA2 Mutations, *Genes Chromosomes Cancer*, Vol.42, No.4, pp. 404-415, ISSN 1045-2257

Moldovan, G.L. & D'Andrea, A.D. (2009). How the Fanconi Anemia Pathway Guards the Genome, *Annual Review Genetics*, Vol.43, pp. 223-249, ISSN 0066-4197

Risinger, M.A. & Groden, J. (2004). Crosslinks and Crosstalk: Human Cancer Syndromes and DNA Repair Defects, *Cancer Cell*, Vol.6, No.6, pp. 539-545, ISSN 1535-6108

Rosenberg, P.S.; Alter, B.P. & Ebell, W. (2008). Cancer Risks in Fanconi Anemia: Finding from the German Fanconi Anemi Registry, *Haematologica*, Vol.93, No.4, pp. 511-517, ISSN 0390-6078

Rosenberg, P.S.; Greene, M.H. & Alter, B.P. (2003). Cancer Incidence in Person with Fanconi Anemia, *Blood*, Vol.101, No.3, pp. 822-826, ISSN 0006-4971

Rosenberg, P.S.; Huang, Y. & Alter, B.P. (2004). Individualized Risks of First Adverse Events in Patients with Fanconi Anemia, *Blood*, Vol.104, No.2, pp. 350-355, ISSN 0006-4971

Rosenberg, P.S.; Socié, G.; Alter, B.P. & Gluckman, E. (2005). Risk of Head and Neck Squamous Cell Cancer and Death in Patients with Fanconi Anemia Who Did and Did Not Receive Transplants, *Blood*, Vol.105, No.1, pp. 67-73, ISSN 0006-4971

Schultz, J.C. & Shahidi, N.T. (1993). Tumor Necrosis Factor-alpha Overproduction in Fanconi's Anemia, *American Journal of Hematology*, Vol.42, No.2, pp. 196-201, ISSN 0361-8609

Shimamure, A. (2003). Treatment of Hematologic Abnormalities in FA, In: *Fanconi Anemia, Standards for Clinical Care*, pp. 17-37, Fanconi Anemia Research Fund, Inc., Second Edition, Eugene, Oregon

Shivji, M.K.K. & Venkitaraman, A.R. (2004). DNA Recombination, Chromosomal Stability and Carcinogenesis: Insights into the Role of BRCA2, *DNA Repair*, Vol.3, No.8-9, pp. 835-843, ISSN 1568-7864

Smith, S.; Marx, M.P.; Jordaan, C.J. & van Niekerk, C.H. (1989). Clinical Aspects of a Cluster of 42 Patients in South Africa with Fanconi Anemia, In: *Fanconi Anemia Clinical Cytogenetic and Experimental Aspects*, T.M. Schroeder-Kurth, A.D. Auerbach, G. Obe, (Eds.), pp. 18-33, Springer-Verlag, ISBN 3-540-50401-X, Newyork, Berlin, Heidelberg

Stark, R.; Andre, C.; Thierry, D.; Cherel, M.; Galibert, F. & Gluckman, E. (1993). The Expression of Cytokine and Cytokine Receptor Genes in Long-term Bone Marrow Culture in Congenital and Acquired Bone Marrow Hypoplasias, *British Journal of Haematology*, Vol.83, No.4, pp. 560-566, ISSN 0007-1048

Tamary, H.; Nishri, D.; Yacobovich, J.; Zilber, R.; Dgany, D.; Krasnow, T.; Aviner, S.; Stepensky, P.; Ravel-Vilk, S.; Bitan, M.; Kaplinsky, C.; Barak, A.B.; Elhasid, R.; Kapelusnik, J.; Koren, A.; Levin, C.; Attias, D.; Laor, R.; Yaniv, I.; Rosenberg, P.S. & Alter, B.P. (2010). Frequency and Natural History of Inherited Bone Marrow Failure Syndromes: The Israeli Inherited Bone Marrow Failure Registry, *Haematologica*, Vol.95, No.8, pp. 1300-1307, ISSN 0390-6078

Taniguchi, T. & D'Andrea, A.D. (2006). The Molecular Pathogenesis of Fanconi Anemia: Recent Progress, *Blood*, Vol.107, No.11, pp. 4223-4233, ISSN 0006-4971

Thompson, L.H.; Hinz, J.M.; Yamada, N.A. & Jones, N.J. (2005). How Fanconi Anemia Proteins Promote the Four Rs: Replication, Recombination, Repair, and Recovery, *Environmental and Molecular Mutagenesis*, Vol.45, No.2-3, pp. 128-142, ISSN 0893-6692

Tischkowitz, M. & Dokal, I. (2004). Fanconi Anaemia and Leukemia – Clinical and Molecular Aspects, *British Journal of Haematology*, Vol.126, No.2, pp. 176-191, ISSN 0007-1048

Velazquez, I. & Alter, B.P. (2004). Androgens and Liver Tumors: Fanconi's Anemia and Non-Fanconi's Conditions, *American Journal of Hematology*, Vol.77, No.3, pp. 257-267, ISSN 0361-8609

Venkitaraman, A.R. (2004). Tracing the Network Connecting BRCA and Fanconi Anaemia Proteins. *Nature Reviews Cancer*, Vol.4, No.4, pp. 266-276, ISSN 1474-175X

Wang, X.Z. & D'Andrea, A.D. (2004). The Interplay of Fanconi Anemia Proteins in the DNA Damage Response, *DNA Repair*, Vol.3, No.8-9, pp. 1063-1069, ISSN 1568-7864

Yetgin, S.; Tuncer, M.; Güler, E.; Duru, F. & Kaşifoğlu, M.A. (1994). Acute Lymphoblastic Leukemia in Fanconi's Anemia, *American Journal of Hematology*, Vol.45, No.1, p. 101, ISSN 0361-8609

10

Anemia in Chronic Obstructive Pulmonary Disease

Karina Portillo Carroz and Josep Morera
Department of Pneumology Hospital Germans
Trias i Pujol. Universitat Autónoma de Barcelona
Spain

1. Introduction

Chronic obstructive pulmonary disease (COPD) is the fourth leading cause of death worldwide, and it is projected to be the third by 2020 or earlier. Patients with COPD frequently have other chronic diseases and systemic effects that worsen their clinical status and prognosis. The best recognized manifestations include the presence of concomitant cardiovascular disease, skeletal muscle wasting, osteoporosis and lung cancer. Although COPD is "traditionally" associated with polycythemia there is a growing body of literature on the relationship between anemia and COPD. Recent studies described that anemia in patients with COPD is more frequent than expected, with a prevalence ranging from 8 to 33%. Systemic inflammation may be an important pathogenic factor, but anemia in COPD can also be the result of a number of factors, such as nutritional and endocrine disorders, treatment with certain drugs (theophylline or angiotensin-converting enzyme inhibitors), acute exacerbations and oxygen therapy.

The level of hemoglobin in COPD patients is strongly associated with increased functional dyspnea, decreased exercise capacity as well as a poor quality of life. Moreover, some studies have showed that anemia is an independent predictor of mortality. Despite the possible clinical benefit of successfully treating anemia in these patients, evidence supporting the importance of its effect on the prognosis of COPD is limited.

2. Prevalence of anemia in COPD

The prevalence of anemia in COPD remains unclear and varies widely. This variability depends on the population under study (stable COPD or patients hospitalized for acute exacerbation), the tools to identifying anemic subjects, and the definitions used for anemia. Contrary to common thinking, recent studies have shown that anemia is a frequent comorbid associated disease in COPD, ranging from nearly 10 to 30% of patients, particularly in patients with severe disease, whereas polycythemia (erythrocytosis) is relatively rare (Barnes & Celli, 2009).The World Health Organization defines anemia in the general population as hemoglobin concentration of less than 13.0 g/dL in men and less than 12.0 g/dL in women (WHO 1968). However, when determining anemia using hemoglobin, it is important to account for the following aspects: firstly, the prevalence of anemia in the general population increases with age and COPD is a chronic disease that affects an aging population; secondly, appropriate hemoglobin threshold for anemia definition in older post-menopausal females remains controversial (Cote et al, 2007) and finally, COPD patients could have a "relative anemia" — a term used to describe cases in which apparently normal hemoglobin values do not correlate with level of hypoxemia.

John et al., reported for first time anemia prevalence in a stable COPD population. They found that among 101 severe COPD patients (forced expiratory volume in one second [FEV$_1$]37 ±2% predicted) 13 were anemic, which means a prevalence of 13%. (John et al, 2005) The data extracted from large national database in France maintained by the Association Nationale pour le Traitement à Domicile de l'Insuffisance Respiratoire (ANTADIR study) showed a similar prevalence in a cohort of 2524 COPD individuals under long-term oxygen therapy (LTOT) (12.6% in males and 8.2% in females) (Chambellan et al, 2005). Cote and colleagues estimated a prevalence of anemia of 17% in contrast with 6% of polycythemia among 683 COPD outpatients. (Cote et al, 2007). In hospitalized patients, described prevalence in anemia rises up to 33%.John and colleagues compared the prevalence of anemia between hospital-admitted COPD and other chronic diseases (asthma, chronic heart failure, chronic renal insufficiency, and cancer).They found in a sample of 7,337 patients an overall prevalence of anemia in COPD of 23%. This was comparable to that in patients with heart failure, higher than in asthmatic individuals, but lower than that in the groups with cancer or chronic renal insufficiency (John et al, 2006). In another study, based on 177 COPD admitted patients due to acute exacerbation (AECOPD) the prevalence reported was 31%. The normocytic normochromic anemia was the most common morphological pattern in 32 cases (58%) and anemia of chronic disease (ACD)or anemia of inflammation was also the more frequent etiology founded. Ultimately, only 8 (4.5%) had polycytemia. (Portillo et al, 2007).

It is worthwhile saying that studying the prevalence of anemia in patients with acute syndromes may overestimate the real number of cases, however, the frequency of anemia during AECOPD is also a relevant issue, since it represents a state of augmented systemic inflammation which also could affect hemoglobin levels in COPD, as described later.

Two recent reports have provided data in large series of patients, obtained from ICD-9/10 code of the discharge diagnoses in order to analyze mortality and healthcare resource variables. In a study performed on US Medicare population, anemia was diagnosed in 21% of COPD patients (Halpern et al, 2006); whereas Shorr and co-workers identified 788 cases in a population of 2404 COPD patients (33%). Anemic patients were older, more likely to be male and non-caucasian, and had a greater co-morbidity burden than non-anemic individuals. (Shorr et al, 2008)

In summary, anemia seems to be common entity among COPD patients, but current available data about its frequency are provided from retrospective analysis or single-center studies, therefore, are subject to the general biases inherent in such designs. Efforts to determine the true prevalence of anemia as comorbid disease in COPD are needed.

3. Mechanisms of anemia in COPD

Increasing evidence indicates that COPD is a complex disease involving more than airflow obstruction (Barnes & Celli 2009).In many patients the disease is associated with several extra pulmonary manifestations that could be the expression of systemic inflammatory state of COPD. In the light of this and together with presence of normocytic anemia in some reported series, it has considered that COPD is another disease likely to be associated with anemia of chronic disease or anemia of inflammation (ACD) (Similowski et al, 2006). In any case, besides the possible role that inflammation may play in the etiology of anemia in COPD, it should not forget that the aging process itself increases the prevalence of anemia as mentioned above and the hemoglobin concentration in COPD can also be influenced by intervention of other mechanisms (Fig. 1). There is a growing interest in the literature about this issue, but the evidence is still scarce. We briefly review the most cited pathophysiologic aspects of this association.

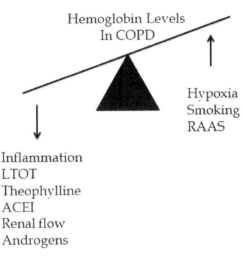

Fig. 1. Possible factors related to hemoglobin levels in COPD. ACEI indicates angiotensin-converting enzyme inhibitors; LTOT, long-term oxygen therapy; and RAAS, renin-angiotensin-aldosterone system.

3.1 Anemia of chronic disease

ACD is an immune disorder that has been reported in numerous diseases with an inflammatory component. Inflammatory cytokines exert various effects on pathogenesis of this form of anemia and ultimately interfere with the normal process of erythropoiesis. The underlying mechanisms are complex, including dysregulation in iron homeostasis and erythropoietin production, impaired proliferation of erythroid progenitor cells and reduced life span of red blood cells. (Weiss 2005). In addition, activation of these inflammatory mediators may stimulate the production of hepcidin, a polypeptide that is the principal regulator of extracellular iron homeostasis and is thought to play a key role of development of ACD.

ACD is usually normocytic, normochromic anemia, but it can become microcytic and hypochromic as the disease progresses. Characteristic changes in systemic iron distribution develop such that the serum iron concentration and transferrin saturation are low, while macrophage iron stores remain replete (Roy, 2010).

COPD is a disorder that could be related with ACD, due the existence of systemic inflammation documented in some patients with COPD. A wide variety of inflamatory markers are isolated in both peripheral blood and sputum in these patients and are higher than controls (Gan et al, 2004). The most important mediators that have been identified are: C-reactive protein (CRP), fibrinogen, circulating leukocytes, and several interleukines (IL) such as IL- 6, IL-8 and tumor necrosis factor alfa (TNF-α) (Fig. 2). Increased of oxidative stress also have been demonstrated in COPD, especially during exacerbations. (McNee 2005).

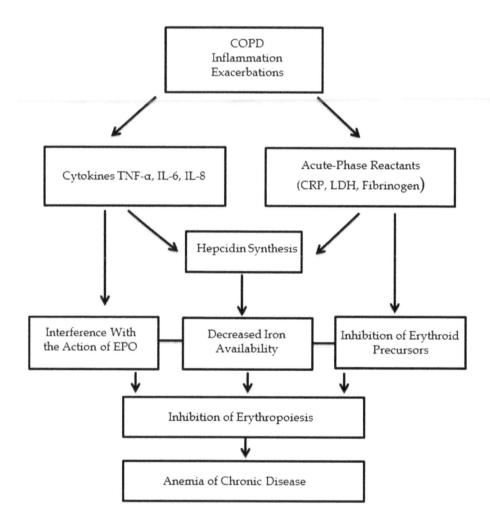

Fig. 2. Possible mechanisms of anemia of inflammation, or anemia of chronic disease, in chronic obstructive pulmonary disease (COPD). EPO indicates erythropoietin; IL, interleukin; LDH, lactate dehydrogenase; CRP, C-reactive protein; and TNF-α, tumor necrosis factor α. (Taken from Portillo, 2007)

One of the first studies that linked the ACD in patients with COPD was made by Tassiopoulos and co-workers, in 2001. Their initial objective was to evaluate the characteristics of anemia and compare the compensatory erythropoietic response in clinically stable patients with idiopathic pulmonary fibrosis and COPD individuals in respiratory failure. The assumption was that the hematologic mechanism would function differently in these two diseases and that the phenomenon of secondary erythrocytosis would be retained in COPD hypoxemic patients. However, they found that the expected response (an increase in red cell mass) was inconsistent in a subgroup of patients with COPD. These individuals had normal or below normal hemoglobin values in spite of higher than normal concentrations of erythropoietin (EPO) in plasma, a suggestion that inflammation was probably the cause of the inconsistent response (Tassiopoulus et al, 2001). These observations were confirmed later by the previously mentioned study performed by John and colleagues. In these patients, the serum levels of CRP and IL-6 were significantly higher than in a group of control subjects. CRP was significantly higher in the anemic subgroup than in non anemic patients as well the level of serum EPO. Moreover, an inverse correlation was showed between hemoglobin and EPO levels, an indication of the existence of a certain resistance to the action of this hormone. These results, together with the lack of any correlation between anemia with nutritional abnormalities present in these patients (weight loss and cachexia), led to the conclusion that the development of anemia in some patients with COPD may fulfilled the criteria for ACD. (John et al, 2005).

3.2 Exacerbations

One of the inherent characteristics of COPD is the occurrence of exacerbations, (AECOPD) which succeed in the curse of the natural history of disease. During AECOPD typically occurs an amplification inflammatory response, both locally and systemically. It has been postulated that the existence of this increased systemic inflammation may worsen some of extrapulmonary manifestations of COPD including anemia. (Portillo 2007; Soler- Cataluña et al, 2010)

Two recent reports assessed the role of inflammatory mechanisms over hemoglobin levels during AEPOC with dissimilar results regarding EPO response. Sala et al., compared the plasma levels of EPO and CRP in patients hospitalized because of AECOPD (n = 26; FEV_1: 48 ±15% predicted), patients with clinically stable COPD (n = 31; FEV_1 :49 ± 17% predicted), smokers with normal lung function (n = 9), and healthy never smokers (n = 9). The main findings were: 1) EPO plasma levels were significantly lower during AECOPD and 2) in COPD group EPO was significantly related to CRP (r = -0.55, p < 0.0001) and with circulating neutrophils (r = -0.48, p <0.0001). Finally, in a subset of 8 COPD patients who could be studied both during AECOPD and clinical stability, EPO levels were significantly higher in stability compared to those recorded during the AECOPD (p < 0.0001). These observations suggest that EPO is downregulated during AECOPD related to the burst of systemic inflammation. (Sala et al, 2010)

In the other study, hemoglobin, EPO and serum biomarkers of systemic inflammation (CRP, TNF-α, fibrinogen and IL-6]) were measured at three time points (admission, resolution and stable phases) in a selected cohort of 93 COPD patients. Hemoglobin levels were significantly lower on admission compared to resolution and stable phases (p=0.002), whereas EPO was significantly higher on admission compared to resolution and stable phases. EPO and hemoglobin were negatively associated during AECOPD. This association was related to increased IL-6 levels, indicating a possible EPO resistance through the mechanism of increased systemic inflammatory process (Markoulaki et al, 2011).

3.3 Macrocytosis

An increase in mean corpuscular volume (MCV) has been reported in patients with COPD, although the cause is still poorly understood. Tsantes et al., investigated this phenomenon among 32 hypoxemic COPD patients and 34 healthy volunteers. They evaluated the following parameters: complete blood count, percentage of F-cells (erythrocytes containing fetal hemoglobin), arterial blood gases, and EPO levels. Red cell macrocytosis (defined as MCV>94 fL) was found in almost half of the patients with COPD (43.75%), and 37% of this group had erythrocytosis. The EPO response was not associated with the degree of hypoxemia, erythrocytosis, or macrocytosis, and in some cases the phenomenon occurred independently. The F-cell percentage was significantly higher in the patients with COPD, and this parameter correlated with MCV values. Based on their findings, the authors hypothesized that erythropoietic stress occurs repeatedly in COPD as a result of exacerbations and nocturnal or exercise-related desaturation. This may triggers a compensatory mechanism, as the release of immature cell forms in the bone marrow to optimize oxygen carrying capacity. Even when they are within the normal range, hemoglobin concentrations can be suboptimal in these patients given the severity of their baseline hypoxemia (Tsantes et al, 2004). Garcia-Pachón et al., also reported macrocytosis in COPD patients but without respiratory insufficiency. It was present in 17 of the 58 stable COPD patients (29%). The most interesting finding, was a significant correlation between macrocytosis, dyspnea, and FEV_1 in a subgroup of 9 COPD (36%), that presumably reflects a correlation between macrocytosis and a deterioration in the clinical situation (García-Pachón & Padilla-Navas 2007).

3.4 Renin-angiotensin-aldosterone system

There are some clinical and experimental studies demonstrating that COPD causes neurohumoral activation, which presumably contributes to a self- maintaining pathogenic cycle that may be related to the systemic effects of the disease (Andreas et al, 2005). An increase in EPO secretion has been observed in experimental animals after administration of renin or angiotensin II. Thus, administration of angiotensin converting enzyme inhibitors is accompanied by a reduction in EPO and hematocrit values. Vlahakos et al., analyzed the degree to which activation of renin-angiotensin system (RAS) was associated with the development of compensatory erythrocytosis in hypoxemic COPD individuals. Renin and aldosterone levels were 3 times higher in the patients with erythrocytosis than in the control group of hypoxemic COPD patients who did not have erythrocytosis. Therefore, it has been contemplated that the alteration in the activation could, partially, help to explain the differences found in the values of hemoglobin in patients with COPD with the same degree of hypoxemia (Vlahakos et al, 1999).

3.5 Renal flow

As EPO is synthesized primarily in the kidney, any impairment of renal hemodynamics — a comorbidity also reported in COPD as a consequence of decreased renal blood flow — causes an imbalance in the supply and demand of oxygen that affects the production of this hormone possibly as a result of an effect on the oxygen sensor (Pham et al, 2001).

3.6 Androgens

Androgens can also stimulate erythropoiesis directly by stimulation of erythroid progenitors or indirectly by activating the renin-angiotensin-aldosterone system; in fact, anemia is a common finding in men who have hypogonadism or are receiving antiandrogenic treatment. Furthermore, testosterone levels decline with age. There is evidence that testosterone concentrations are low in men with COPD (Casaburi et al, 2004).Various predisposing factors for these low values have been proposed, including hypoxia, corticosteroid treatment, and the chronic nature of the disease. A published study of a sample of 905 patients over 65 years of age concluded that low testosterone levels are associated with a higher risk of developing anemia (Ferrucci et al, 2003).

3.7 Other factors

It has been observed that, like the angiotensin-converting enzyme inhibitors, which reduce hematocrit values, theophylline also gives rise to a reduction in the production of red blood cells. The suppression mechanism is complex and in principle may be the result of direct inhibition of erythropoiesis through apoptosis induced by this drug rather than any effect on EPO (Tsantes et al, 2003).

Oxygen therapy can theoretically blunt hypoxia-driven erythropoyiesis, (Similowski et al, 2005) while smoking habit might exert negative effect on folate status and oxygen carrying capacity through tendency to increase red blood cell mass.

4. The effects of anemia in COPD

The relationship between anemia and adverse clinical outcomes is wide recognized in other chronic disease states. The hemoglobin is the principal oxygen transport molecule. Any decrease in hemoglobin levels results in a corresponding reduction in the oxygen-carrying capacity of the blood. Thus, while arterial oxygen pressure may remain normal, the absolute amount of oxygen transported per unit blood volume declines. Impairment of this mechanism exerts a negative impact on clinical status. Although there are few related studies, those published so far it appears that anemia plays an important role in various domains and outcomes of disease including mortality.

4.1 Symptoms, exercise tolerance

It is well known that anemia is a cause per se of dyspnea and that it contributes to functional limitation in the anemic individual. Fatigue is also a common finding among COPD and is the primary symptom of anemia. In fact, anemia is one of the most treatable causes of fatigue in general. Cote and colleagues demonstrated that anemia was independently associated with increased dyspnea, by means modified Medical Research Council dyspnea scale (MRC) and reduced exercise capacity measured by 6- min walk distance in a cohort of stable COPD patients (Cote et al, 2007). Recently, another study was aimed to investigated specifically the impact of ACD on dyspnea and exercise capacity utilizing cardiopulmonary exercise testing (CPET) in a group of 283 COPD patients. The results of these report also showed a negative effect of low hemoglobin on breathlessness. COPD patients whom fulfilled criteria of ACD had higher MRC dyspnea score compared to controls and lower exercise capacity (lower peak oxygen uptake[VO2], peak work rate, peak VO2/heart rate, as well a trend for lower anaerobic threshold) (Boutou et al, 2010).

There is only restrospective study that analyzed the relationship between anemia in COPD and health related quality of life (HRQL) based on general population (n=2704). Among patients with COPD (n = 495) physical functioning (PF) and physical component summary (PCS) scores from Short Form-36 questionnaire were significantly lower in individuals with anemia compared to those without. In conclusion, anemia associated with COPD was an important contributor to poor quality of life. (Krishnan et al, 2006)

4.2 Health resources

COPD generates a large consumption of resources that involves a significant economic burden worldwide due to its high prevalence and morbidity. Moreover, presences of comorbidities in COPD appear to be a cost multiplier. (Shorr et al, 2008)

The ANTADIR study founded that a reduced hematocrit level was associated with more frequent hospitalizations and a longer mean hospital stay (Chambellan et al, 2005).Two studies mentioned above have been measured the economic impact of anemia in COPD based on large sample of patients. Both documented that anemia significantly and independently contributes to the cost of care for COPD. (Halpern et al, 2006; Shorr et al, 2008).

4.3 Mortality

There is some evidence available to suggest that anemia is associated with a reduced survival in COPD. In cohort of stable COPD used to described the BODE index (body mass index, airflow obstruction, dyspnea and exercise capacity) Celli and colleagues showed that patients who died were found to have significantly lower hematocrit levels than those who survived (Celli et al, 2004).

In survival data derived from the ANTADIR study, multivariate analysis proved that hematocrit was important independent predictor of survival in COPD patients receiving LTOT and showed that the survival rate at three years was 24% in patients with hematocrit <35%, and 70% in patients with hematocrit > 55%(Chambellan et al, 2005).These findings are consistent with a recent report also conducted on patients under LTOT in which 67% had a diagnosis of COPD. Hemoglobin and hematocrit were significantly lower in the nonsurvivor group. Multiple regression analysis demonstrated that the main risk factors for mortality after three years of follow-up were male gender, lower values of hemoglobin, hematocrit and carbon dioxide pressure more intense hypoxemia and dyspnea sensation. The cut-off point associated with higher mortality in this study was hemoglobin ≤ 11 g/dl (sensitivity 95% specificity 85%) or hematocrit ≤33%(sensitivity 97% specificity 89%)(Lima et al, 2010).

In the National Emphysema Treatment Trial, in which randomized patients to be treated medically or surgically, also found that the decrease in hemoglobin acted as an independent predictor of mortality (Martinez et al, 2006).

Lastly, Rasmussen and co-workers analyzed the effects of anemia in critically ill patients with COPD admitted to the intensive care unit (ICU) requiring invasive mechanical ventilation. With a cutoff point of hemoglobin to define anemia of 12g/dL, it found that low hemoglobin levels were associated with substantially increased mortality within the first 90 days following admission (Rasmussen et al, 2011).

5. Should anemia be treated in COPD?

Throughout this review we have discussed some clinical and pathophysiological aspects that would justify therapeutics efforts to correct anemia in COPD. However, the degree of uncertainty in fundamental aspects, as well limited available evidence do not establish whether the treatment of this condition will result in improvement in COPD outcomes.

Schonhofer et al., published the only two studies in the literature on this subject. After treating anemia by blood transfusion in 20 patients with severe COPD in an ICU, it documented a statistically significant reduction in minute-ventilation and work of breathing, with unloading of the respiratory muscles (Schonhofer et al, 1999) The earlier study involved 5 COPD patients in whom weaning from invasive mechanical ventilation had proved difficult. By increasing hemoglobin levels to over 12 g/dL by blood transfusion, the physicians were able to extubate satisfactorily (Schonhofer et al, 1998)

Another treatment options to correct anemia as used in other chronic disease such congestive heart failure, cancer or chronic kidney disease have not been explored in COPD (i.e. erythropoietic agents, iron supplements or combined therapy). Is not known whether treating the underlying inflammation could improve the hematological values. Future prospective trials are needed to establish the appropriate threshold for initiation treatment and effect of improvement of hemoglobin on clinical outcomes in COPD population.

6. Conclusions

Anemia seems to be a common feature in COPD, although its real prevalence remains to be determined. While the mechanisms involved in the genesis of anemia in COPD are poorly studied and the evidence is scarce, we can talk about an imbalance in hemoglobin levels because there are factors that stimulate erythropoiesis as well as others that blunt this process.

Recent data support that low hemoglobin and hematocrit concentrations can have a detrimental impact on certain respiratory variables in COPD, including mortality. Whether the treatment of anemia will result in improvement in functional outcome measures remains uncertain. However, before a treatment strategy can be devised, the influence of anemia on the natural history of COPD should be properly evaluated in further prospective studies.

7. References

Andreas S, Anker SD, Scanlon PD, Somers VK. Neurohumoral activation as a link to systemic manifestations of chronic lung disease. *Chest*. 2005; 128:3618-25.

Barnes PJ, Celli BR. Systemic manifestations and comorbidities of COPD. *Eur Respir J*. 2009; 33:1165-85.

Boutou AK, Stanopoulos I, Pitsiou GG, Kontakiotis T, Kyriazis G, Sichletidis L, Argyropoulou P. Anemia of Chronic Disease in Chronic Obstructive Pulmonary Disease: A Case-Control Study of Cardiopulmonary Exercise Responses. *Respiration*. 2011 [Epub ahead of print]

Casaburi R, Bhasin S, Cosentino L, Porszasz J, Somfay A, Lewis MI, et al. Effects of testosterone and resistance training in men with chronic obstructive pulmonary disease. *Am J Respir Crit Care Med*. 2004;170:870-8.

Celli BR, Cote CG, Marin JM, Casanova C, Montes de Oca M, Méndez RA, et al. The body-mass index, airflow obstruction, dyspnea, and exercise capacity index in chronic obstructive pulmonary disease. *N Engl J Med*. 2004; 350: 1005-1012.

Chambellan A, Chailleux E, Similowski T, ANTADIR Observatory Group. Prognostic value of hematocrit in patients with severe COPD receiving long-term oxygen therapy. *Chest*. 2005; 128: 1201-1208.

Cote C, Zilberberg MD, Mody SH, Dordelly LJ, Celli B. Haemoglobin level and its clinical impact in a cohort of patients with COPD. *Eur Respir J*. 2007;29: 923-9.

Ferrucci L, Maggio M, Bandinelli S, Basaria S, Lauretani F, Ble A, et al. Low testosterone levels and the risk of anemia in older men and women. *Arch Intern Med*. 2006; 166:1380-8.

Gan WQ, Man SF, Senthilselvan A, Sin DD. Association between chronic obstructive pulmonary disease and systemic infl ammation: a systematic review and a meta-analysis. *Thorax*. 2004;59:574-80.

García-Pachón E, Padilla-Navas I. Red cell macrocytosis in COPD patients without respiratory insufficiency: a brief report. *Respir Med*. 2007;101:349-52.

Halpern MT, Zilberberg MD, Schmier JK, Lau EC, Shorr AF. Anemia, costs and mortality in chronic obstructive pulmonary disease. *Cost Eff Resour Alloc*. 2006 16;4:17.

John M, Hoernig S, Doehner W, Okonko DD, Witt C, Anker SD. Anemia and inflammation in COPD. *Chest*. 2005; 127: 825-829.

John M, Lange A, Hoernig S, Witt C, Anker SD. Prevalence of anemia in chronic obstructive pulmonary disease: comparison to other chronic diseases. *Int J Cardiol*. 2006;111:365-70.

Krishnan G, Grant BJ, Muti PC, et al. Association between anemia and quality of life in a population sample of individuals with chronic obstructive pulmonary disease. *BMC Pulm Med*. 2006; 6: 23.

Lima DF, Dela Coleta K, Tanni SE, Silveira LV, Godoy I, Godoy I. Potentially modifiable predictors of mortality in patients treated with long-term oxygen therapy. *Respir Med*. 2011;105:470-6.

MacNee W. Pulmonary and systemic oxidant/antioxidant imbalance in chronic obstructive pulmonary disease. *Proc Am Thorac Soc*. 2005;2:50-60.

Markoulaki D, Kostikas K, Papatheodorou G, Koutsokera A, Alchanatis M, Bakakos P, et al. Eur J Hemoglobin, erythropoietin and systemic inflammation in exacerbations of chronic obstructive pulmonary disease. *Intern Med*. 2011 ;22:103-7.

Martínez FJ, Foster G, Curtis JL, Criner G, Weinmann G, Fishman A, et al; NETT Research Group. Predictors of mortality in patients with emphysema and severe airflow obstruction. *Am J Respir Crit Care Med.* 2006;173:1326-34.

Pham I, Andrivet P, Sediame S, Defouilloy C, Moutereau S, et al. Increased erythropoietin synthesis in patients with COLD or left heart failure is related to alterations in renal haemodynamics. *Eur J Clin Invest.* 2001;31:103-9.

Portillo K, Belda J, Antón P, Casan P. High frequency of anemia in COPD patients admitted in a tertiary hospital. *Rev Clin Esp.* 2007; 207:383-7.

Portillo K. Anemia in COPD: should it be taken into consideration?.Arch Bronconeumol. 2007;43:392-8.

Rasmussen L, Christensen S, Lenler-Petersen P, Johnsen SP. Anemia and 90-day mortality in COPD patients requiring invasive mechanical ventilation. *Clin Epidemiol.* 2011;3:1-5.

Roy CN. Anemia of inflammation. *Hematology Am Soc Hematol Educ Program.* 2010;2010: 276-80.

Sala E, Balaguer C, Villena C, Ríos A, Noguera A, Núñez B,et al. Low erythropoietin plasma levels during exacerbations of COPD. *Respiration.* 2010;80:190-7.

Schonhofer B, Bohrer H, Kohler D. Importance of blood transfusion in anemic patients with COPD and unsuccessful weaning from respirator. *Med Klin.* 1999;Suppl 1:108-10.

Schonhofer B, Wenzel M, Geibel M, Kohler D. Blood transfusion and lung function in chronically anemic patients with severe chronic obstructive pulmonary disease. *Crit Care Med.* 1998;26:1824-8.

Shorr AF, Doyle J, Stern L, Dolgitser M, Zilberberg MD. Anemia in chronic obstructive pulmonary disease: epidemiology and economic implications. *Curr Med Res Opin.* 2008;24:1123-30.923

Similowski T, Agusti A, MacNee W, Schonhofer B. The potential impact of anaemia of chronic disease in COPD. *Eur Respir J.* 2006; 27:390–6.

Soler-Cataluña JJ,Martínez-García MA, Catalán Serra P. Impacto multidimensional de las exacerbaciones de la EPOC. *Arch Bronconeumol.*2010; 46(Supl.11) :12-9.

Tassiopoulos S, Kontos A, Konstantopoulos K, Hadzistavrou C, Vaiopoulos G, Aessopos A, et al. Erythropoietic response to hypoxaemia in diffuse idiopathic pulmonary fibrosis, as opposed to chronic obstructive pulmonary disease. *Respir Med.* 2001;95: 471-5.

Tsantes AE, Papadhimitriou SI, Tassiopoulos ST, Bonovas S, Paterakis G, Meletis I, et al. Red cell macrocytosis in hypoxemic patients with chronic obstructive pulmonary disease. *Respir Med.* 2004;98:1117-23.

Tsantes AE, Tassiopoulos ST, Papadhimitriou SI, Bonovas S, Poulakis N, Vlachou A, et al. Theophylline treatment may adversely affect the anoxia-induced erythropoietic response without suppressing erythropoietin production. *Eur J Clin Pharmacol.* 2003;59:379-83.

Vlahakos D, Kosmas E, Dimopoulou I, Ikonomou E, Jullien G, Vassilakos P, et al. Association between activation of the reninangiotensin system and secondary

erythrocytosis in patients with chronic obstructive pulmonary disease. *Am J Med.*
   1999;106:158- 64.

Weiss G, Goodnough LT. Anemia of chronic disease. *N Engl J Med.* 2005;352:1011-23.

World Health Organization. Nutritional anemias: report of a WHO scientific group. WHO
   Technical Report Series 405. Geneva, World Health Organization, 1968; pp. 1–37

11

The Molecular Connection Between Aluminum Toxicity, Anemia, Inflammation and Obesity: Therapeutic Cues

Adam Bignucolo, Joseph Lemire, Christopher Auger, Zachary Castonguay,
Varun Appanna and Vasu D. Appanna
Laurentian University
Canada

1. Introduction

Anemia is reported to be the most common blood disorder. A variety of anemic conditions affecting various groups of people exist and each of the types of anemia has different underlying causes. Iron (Fe) deficiency, a potent instigator of anemia, is the most common mineral deficiency and its effects have been linked to slow physical development and impaired cognitive function along with behavioral and learning disturbances (De Giudice *et al*, 2009). Exacerbating the iron deficiency epidemic is obesity, a disease defined by an excess accumulation of body fat leading to adverse health effects. It has been demonstrated that there is an association between poor iron status and obesity. The relationship between the two conditions has been shown in children, adolescents and adults including post-menopausal women.

Obesity is now considered an independent factor contributing to iron deficiency (McClung *et al*, 2009). Gaining incredible importance as a global health issue, obesity rates are increasing worldwide. The World Health Organization estimated that in 2005, 1.6 billion adults were overweight (body mass index (BMI) =25), and over 400 million adults were obese (BMI =30). Notably, there is an increase in the incidence of childhood and adolescent obesity in industrialized countries where the number of affected population has more than doubled over the past few decades. A similar trend has been observed in developing countries such as Egypt, Brazil and Mexico. What used to be considered a "rich" country issue has now become a worldwide epidemic and the situation is continuously worsening (Hintze *et al*, 2010).

2. Hepcidin: Function and regulation

A significant proportion of the world's population is iron-deficient, obese, or both. This makes an understanding of the mechanisms underlying obesity-induced iron deficiency and anemia crucial. Recently, the discovery of the peptide hormone hepcidin, a regulator of organismal iron metabolism has shed light on the relationship between anemia and obesity. Hepcidin is a 25 amino acid long peptide secreted by the liver and adipose tissue that was initially studied for its modulation of iron-homeostasis during infection. Increases in hepcidin levels cause the depletion of serum iron levels and prevent the efflux of iron through the cellular iron exporter ferroportin from hepatocytes, enterocytes and macrophages (**Figure 1**). Therefore, hepcidin is the iron/inflammation/oxygen sensor that can act as a signal for numerous physiological responses including i) the decreased dietary iron uptake during an overload situation, ii) the anemia seen during infection to prevent free iron from promoting pathogen proliferation and iii) an increase of iron uptake during hypoxia (Atkinson *et al*, 2011; Choi *et al*, 2007; Vecchi *et al*, 2009).

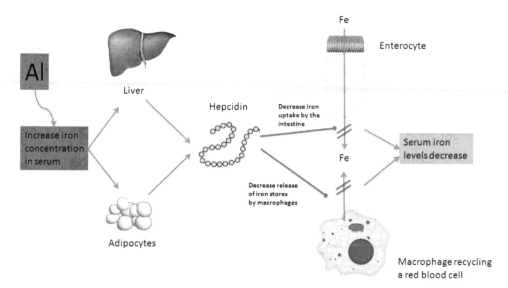

Fig. 1. Al toxicity leads to an increased Fe concentration in the serum of the body. High blood Fe levels cause the liver and adipose tissue to secrete hepcidin, a Fe homeostasis regulator, which signals the decrease in Fe absorption by enterocytes as well as a decrease in Fe release from cellular stores such as red blood cells.

Interestingly, chronic inflammation is one of the hallmarks of obesity (Ausk *et al*, 2008, Yanoff *et al*, 2007). Adipose tissue in obese mice has been shown to be considerably more hypoxic than adipose tissue from lean mice. As a result of the difference in O_2 tension there is an important shift in gene expression, not only for expected genes induced by hypoxia but also the increased levels of inflammatory cytokines including interleukin-6 (IL-6) (Lee *et al*, 2005). The latter appears to be the mediator of the induction of hepatic hepcidin secretion during inflammation. IL-6 and other hepcidin-inducing factors such as the adipokine leptin may explain the increased hepcidin levels in obese individuals compared to healthy patients (Barisani *et al*, 2008; Choi *et al*, 2007; Hintze *et al*, 2010).

3. The link between Fe-deficiency, anemia, inflammation and obesity

When studied separately, the development of anemia, inflammation and obesity have all been associated with aluminum (Al) toxicity. It is well established that Al disrupts iron homeostasis leading to the dysfunction of essential biochemical processes dependent on this redox-active ion. Al negatively influences the absorption of iron via the intestine, hinders its transport in the serum, and displaces iron by binding to transferrin (**Figure 2**) (Turgut *et al,* 2007).

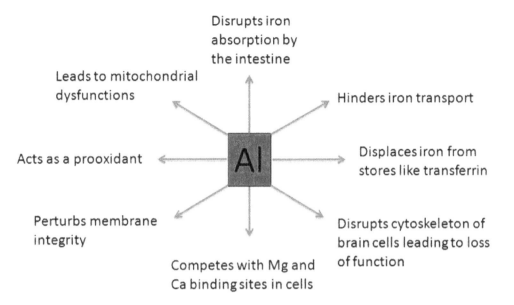

Fig. 2. Al has various toxic effects on cellular processes, notably on Fe homeostasis.

Al plays an important role in the immune response by being a trigger of the inflammatory cascade. For this reason, Al salts are administered with vaccines and act as adjuvants. Al stimulates an inflammatory response which promotes the effectiveness of the immune system to respond to the vaccine and acquire immunity. The effect of Al toxicity on fatty acid metabolism is just starting to emerge. The modulation of energy metabolism at the mitochondrial level caused by this metal leads to an accumulation of triglycerides and an increase in fat deposits. In addition, there is a marked increase in very low density lipoprotein (VLDL) secretion caused by Al toxicity. This phenomenon is directly related to the accumulation of fatty tissue observed during obesity. The information presented in this chapter delineates the molecular mechanism of Al toxicity and thus affords insights into the implication of this metal in dysfunctional Fe homeostasis, inflammation, obesity and anemia.

4. Aluminum and the environment

Aluminum is an environmentally abundant element that has a wide variety of uses and industrial applications. Industrialization and anthropogenic activities have led to a further increase in bioavailable Al. Exposure to this non-redox active metal occurs in daily life where the major sources of exposure for the average individual are diet and drinking water. Additional aluminum exposure can be brought upon by certain medications such as antacids, while individuals can also be subjected to high Al levels due to occupational exposure from breathing in contaminated air. Although drinking water was first thought to be the main delivery method of Al to the body, it was shown that 95% of the exposure to the element occurs through diet whereas the soluble water form of Al only accounts for 1-2%. The average human Al intake ranges between a total of 4 to 9 mg/day. Although small, these values are easily influenced by factors such as the type of food consumed in one's diet, the country/place of residence, one's age and sex. Alternate sources contribute to the amount of Al an individual is subjected to (**Table 1**), with antacids representing a significant dose, as they are generally composed of aluminum hydroxide salts (Lopez *et al*, 2002; *et al*, 2006; Yokel *et al*, 2008b).

Source	Al exposure contribution
Antacids	5000000 µg/day
Environmental air inhalation	4-20 µg/day
Industrial air inhalation	25000 µg/day
Antiperspirants	70000 µg/day
Cigarettes	500-2000 µg/cigarette
Vaccines	1-8 µg/day
Allergy immunotherapy	7-40 µg/day

Table 1. Various sources of Al and their average Al exposure contribution (Yokel *et al*, 2008b).

The use of aluminum salts is not restricted to stomach acidity neutralizing agents, but are rather quite frequently used in the food industry. Sodium aluminum phosphates (SALPs) are generally recognized as safe (GRAS) FDA-approved food additives that contribute the most important source of Al to the diet. Basic SALP ($Na_8Al_2(OH_2)((PO)_4)_4$) is one of the many emulsifying salts added to processed cheese, cheese food and cheese spread. This salt is added to cheese since it reacts with proteins resulting in modifications that produce a smooth, uniform film around each fat droplet, preventing separation and bleeding of fat from cheese. Ultimately this allows for a soft texture, easy melting characteristics and desirable slicing properties. The FDA approves up to 3% concentrations of basic SALP. Unprocessed cheese has been shown to have an Al concentration of < 10 mg Al/kg. In contrast the aluminum levels in processed cheese can range from 320-1440 mg Al/kg. Cheese is not the only processed food containing higher levels of aluminum. Both fruit juices and soft drinks contain aluminum levels ranging from 49.3 to 1144.6 µg/l in fruit juices and from 44.6 to 1053.3 µg/l in soft drinks respectively (Lopez *et al*, 2002). The benefits of processed foods include a longer shelf life, change in taste and texture, minimal meal preparation and lower cost. The increased consumption of processed food has been shown to be related to the rise in obesity rates in industrialized nations for many reasons including the high simple sugar levels. Perhaps the high levels of Al found in processed food are amplifying the risk of obesity that is associated with food processing (**Figure 3**) (Yokel *et al*, 2008a; 2008b; 2006).

The food processing industry is responsible for an increase in bioavailable Al, however it is not working alone. Industrialization has led to a higher frequency of acid rain which in turn lowers the pH in soil. Consequently, Al is leaching into groundwater thus causing the bioaccumulation of this toxic metal in various non-processed food such as vegetation and livestock. Once consumed, these sources increase the accumulation of aluminum in the body. Various fresh food sources contain relatively high levels of Al, as shown in **Table 2.**

Food Group	Mean Al concentration (mg/kg of fresh weight)	Food Group	Mean Al concentration (mg/kg of fresh weight)
Bread	6.6	Potatoes	0.9
Poultry	0.3	Canned vegetables	0.97
Fish	6.1	Fresh fruit	0.29
Oils & fats	1.1	Fruit products	0.82
Eggs	0.14	Milk	0.07
Green vegetables	3.1	Nuts	4.0

Table 2. Occurrence of Al in food according to the Food Standards Agency, United Kingdom.

Aluminum toxicity has been extensively studied for its implication in neurodegenerative diseases such as Alzheimer's disease (AD) and multiple sclerosis (MS). The brain is an important Al accumulating organ, yet Al can also concentrate more severely in other tissues of the human body (**Figure 4**) (Gomez *et al*, 2008; Rondeau *et al*, *2008*). Nonetheless, aluminum salts such as aluminum hydroxides and aluminum phosphates are routinely used in medical practices as the only licensed adjuvants in vaccines. Aluminum adjuvants, referred to as "alum", are proven effective in stimulating an immune response towards the vaccine being administered. However, the mode of action remains unclear. It is generally accepted that the alum particles adhere to the surface of the antigen (Ag), forming an Ag deposit at the injection site. This process maximizes the interaction time between the Ag and the immune system's antigen presenting cells (APCs) which initiate a response cascade (**Figure 4**). Alum have also been shown to act on the immune system's compliment system of the immune machinery, along with causing the formation of granulomas containing antibody (Ab)-producing cells and other immune response mediators. Recent studies have illustrated the ability of alum to stimulate the release of pro-inflammatory cytokines such as IL-1β and IL-18 that have pleiotropic functions, including adjuvant capacity. Although several mechanisms are proposed (**Figure 5**), the exact way by which aluminum promotes inflammation has yet to be solved (Aimanianda *et al*, 2009; HogenEsch, 2002; Li *et al*, 2008). Nonetheless, Al is an active instigator of inflammation (Campbell *et al*, 2002). Regardless of the source of Al the reality remains that the element is bioavailable and at significant concentrations. For this reason, the toxic effects of Al are of interest to the human population and the study of these effects could help explain Al-associated dysfunctions such as neurodegenerative diseases, obesity and chronic inflammation. More importantly, the link between these disease states, aluminum toxicity and anemia is beginning to be understood.

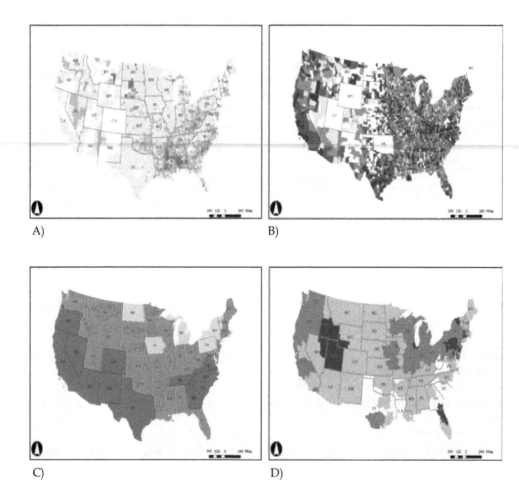

Fig. 3. These maps illustrate the link between processed food (commonly served in the fast food industry or found in prepared meals) and the obesity epidemic in the United-States. **A) Adult obesity rate in 2007**. Grey (12.5% - 25%). Light blue (25.1% - 30%). Blue (30.1% - 35%). Dark blue (35.1% - 43.5%); **B) Low-income preschool obesity rate in 2008.** Light pink (2.1% - 10%). Pink (10.1% - 14%). Red (14.1% - 18%). Dark red (18.1% - 39.7%); **C) Fast food expenditure per capita in 2007**. Light pink ($402.10 - $500.00). Pink ($500.01 - $700.00). Red ($700.01 - $1,043.86). **D) Prepared food (lbs) per capita in 2006**. Grey (229 - 280lbs). Light green (281 - 300lbs). Green (301 - 320lbs). Dark green (321-374lbs). (Centers for Disease Control and Prevention).

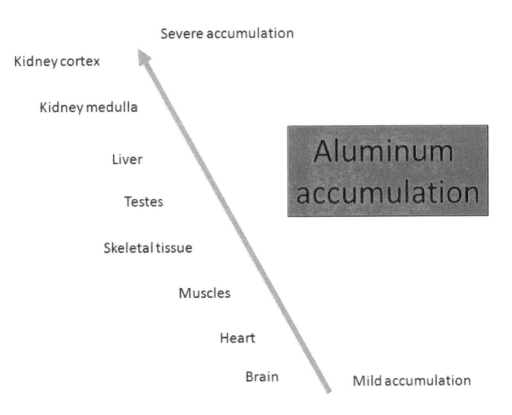

Fig. 4. The hierarchy of Al accumulation in the various tissues of the human body. Although the brain is an important location for Al accumulation, there are many other organs that accumulate much greater concentrations of Al (Ward *et al*, 2001).

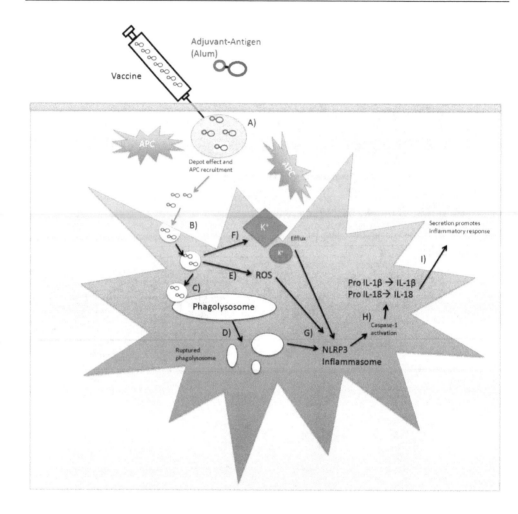

Fig. 5. Proposed mechanism of action for Al being used as an adjuvant A) As a vaccine is injected into the skin, the alum adjuvant bound to the Ag form a deposit at the injection site. This promotes APC recruitment and maximizes the interaction between the Ag and the immune system's cells. B) The innate immune system cells intake the Alum salts. C) The engulfed adjuvants interact with the phagolysosome of the APCs. D) Intereaction with the Alum salts leads to rupture of the phagolysosomes and the release of activators of NLRP3 inflammasome (not shown in image). E) Al within the cell promotes the formation of ROS which also activates the NLRP3 inflammasome. F) The Alum salts also lead to potassium (K+) efflux, thus further activating the NLRP3 inflammasome. G) The NLRP3 inflammasome, an intracellular innate immune response system, senses the K+ efflux, the ROS formation and the lysosomal damage and activates caspase-1. H) Caspase-1 processes pro-IL-1β and pro-IL-18 into IL-1β and IL-18, respectively, resulting in the release of these mature cytokines (Modified from Aimanianda *et al*, 2009; HogenEsch, 2002; Li, 2008).

5. Aluminum and dyslipidemia: A metabolic perspective

Metal toxicity has been linked to cancers, neurological disorders, nephrological complications and pulmonary diseases. Environmental pollution is a growing concern in today's society causing the increased bioavailability of metals that pose a serious threat to living organisms. Toxic elements like mercury (Hg) and lead (Pb) have been extensively studied. While Hg has been shown to react with critical thiol moieties and impede normal immunological responses and mental cognition, Pb dislocates the essential zinc (Zn) found in enzymes responsible for heme production. Ultimately these toxic metals lead to various diseases (Mailloux et al, 2007b). The molecular aspects of Al toxicity have begun to emerge. It has been reported that a variety of ion channels are inactivated by micromolar quantities of Al, subsequently disrupting biological membranes. In addition, Al has an ionic radius that resembles that of magnesium (Mg), which leads to its interaction with naturally-occurring Mg-dependent enzymes. Al has also been shown to perturb cytoskeletal structure of astrocytoma cells causing a disruption of their shape and hence their biological function. Exposure to Al, however, is primarily characterized by the disruption of Fe homeostasis which in turn interferes with essential biochemical processes that are dependent on this metal (Lemire et al, 2009; Mailloux et al, 2011).

Fe is an important cofactor of many enzymes and a structural component of proteins. It is redox-active and therefore can act as an electron acceptor and donor, a critical attribute for its involvement in metabolic processes. Notably, Fe is required for protein components such as iron-sulfur clusters (Fe-S clusters) and hemes. When Al interacts with these constituents, it mimics the Fe atoms forcing the liberation of the transition metal and its subsequent intracellular accumulation. Free Fe poses a threat to cells as it leads to the formation of reactive oxygen species (ROS) through Fenton chemistry (figure 6). The Al-triggered oxidative environment enhances the toxic effect of the trivalent metal. Together, Al and its concomitant ROS greatly affect cellular metabolism. Metabolism is the foundation of any biological system and metabolic processes allow organisms to react and adapt to intracellular and extracellular fluctuations. It enables the maintenance of an environment suitable for the production and storage of energy and for cellular growth (Kim et al, 2007; Mailloux et al, 2011; Vergara et al, 2008).

The importance of Fe as a cofactor in metabolic processes is made evident in energy metabolism. The redox active metal is essential for the ATP-producing machinery in the mitochondria of eukaryotes. The central metabolic pathway known as the tricarboxylic acid cycle (TCA cycle), along with the electron transport chain (ETC) which is responsible for oxidative phosphorylation, are composed of enzymes that depend on Fe for proper functioning. For example, the Fe-containing enzyme aconitase (ACN) is considered the "gatekeeper" to the TCA cycle. ACN are Fe-S cluster proteins that catalyze the reversible isomerization of citrate to isocitrate. The enzymatically active form of the ACN Fe-S clusters are predominantly [4Fe-4S]. In mammalian systems, ACN with [3Fe-4S] clusters play an alternate role, acting as an oxygen sensor therefore aiding in energy homeostasis. This form of the enzyme serves as a regulatory protein that controls the stability and translation of messenger RNAs (mRNAs) encoding proteins involved in iron and energy homeostasis. The regulatory ACN is referred to as iron-responsive protein, which binds to iron-responsible elements localized in the RNA-stem loop (figure 7). This action leads to the modulation of gene expression (Middaugh et al, 2005).

It has been demonstrated that cells exposed to Al have severely impeded mitochondrial functions. Most importantly, these cells appear to have limited ATP production due to diminished TCA cycle and oxidative phosphorylation activity. As the trivalent metal Al displaces Fe in key enzymes of the TCA cycle such as ACN, fumarase (FUM) along with the Fe found in enzymes of the ETC (notably succinate dehydrogenase (SDH) and cytochrome C oxidase (Cyt c ox)), an evident shift in metabolism occurs as these enzymes become inactive. Impairment of ACN by Al triggers a decrease in NADH production by the TCA cycle. NADH is a reducing equivalent essential for oxidative phosphorylation, thus as the levels of NADH diminish and Al displaces Fe from ETC enzymes, mitochondrial production of ATP is hindered (figure 8). This perturbation in oxidative phosphorylation is advantageous during Al exposure since the ETC is a known endogenous ROS generator. Inefficient electron transport through the chain leads to the univalent reduction of oxygen, a process that creates free radical species that exacerbates the toxic effect of Al. It is in a cell's favor to maintain redox homeostasis by limiting its own production of oxidative species during Al-stressed conditions. In order to meet its energy demands, Al-stressed cells evoke the anaerobic respiratory machinery to produce ATP, notably substrate level phosphorylation (SLP) (Mailloux et al, 2011; 2007a; 2007b; Middaugh et al, 2005; Lemire et al, 2011a).

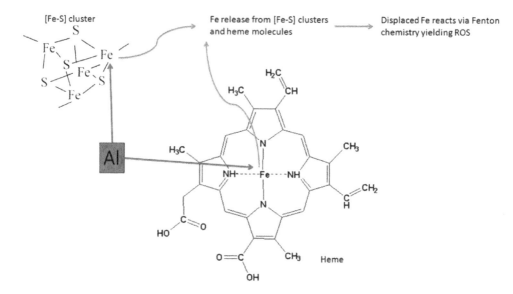

Fig. 6. Al displaces the Fe in biological molecules such as heme and [Fe-S] clusters. The presence of free Fe leads to the formation of ROS.

Al can severely impede mitochondrial function, however the consequences of its effects are not limited to a decrease in energy production. The disruption of oxidative phosphorylation by the trivalent metal evokes not only a limited supply of ATP but also an increased lipid production. This phenomenon is common in obese individuals who tend to experience diminished levels of ATP and an accumulation of fatty tissue. In human liver cells, it has been demonstrated that dyslipidemia is due to the ability of Al to perturb iron metabolism and promote oxidative stress. By displacing Fe in metabolically active enzymes, Al favors a hypoxic environment and stimulates lipogenesis. Lipogenesis is the series of chemical reactions leading to the carboxylation and subsequent polymerization of acetyl CoA through the use of the anabolic nucleotide NADPH. Under Al toxicity, pivotal enzymes in the lipid production pathway of hepatocytes show an increase in activity. First, acetyl-CoA carboxylase (ACC) is up-regulated under ROS and Al-stress conditions. This enzyme is responsible for the production of malonyl-CoA, an inhibitor of the transport of lipids into the mitochondria and an activator of lipogenesis. Second, glycerol-3-phosphate dehydrogenase (G3PDH) diverts trioses from glycolysis into the lipid generating machinery by producing glycerol, the backbone of triglycerides. Finally, the much-needed supply of NADPH for lipogenesis during Al toxicity is ensured by an ensemble of enzymes including glucose-6-phosphate dehydrogenase (G6PDH), 6-phosphogluconate dehydrogenase (6PGDH), malic enzyme (ME), NADP$^+$-dependent glutamate dehydrogenase (GDH), NAD kinase (NADK) and NADP$^+$-dependent isocitrate dehydrogenase (IDH) (**Figure 9**). Since Al disrupts Fe homeostasis, rendering the TCA cycle and oxidative phosphorylation inactive, carbon sources coming from upstream metabolism are funneled towards the production of fatty acids. Al toxicity instigates the metabolic shift from NADH production to the synthesis of the anabolic reducing agent and antioxidant, NADPH (**Figure 10**) (Mailloux *et al*, 2011; 2007b; Lemire *et al*, 2008).

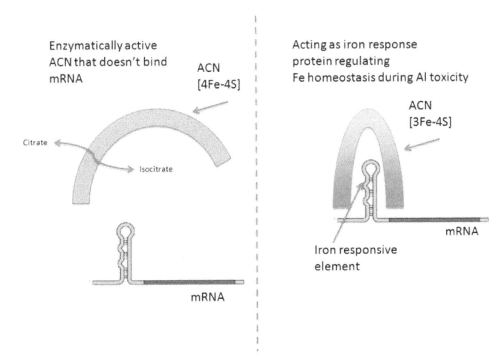

Fig. 7. ACN is recognized as the "gatekeeper" to the TCA cycle. When the [4Fe-4S] cluster is intact, the protein is enzymatically active. However under conditions that favor the [3Fe-4S] form of the enzyme, such as Fe starvation, Al toxicity and oxidative stress, the protein is no longer metabolically active. ACN [3Fe-4S] acts as the Fe response protein which regulates Fe homeostasis at the gene expression level by binding to the Fe responsive element in mRNA coding for various genes involved in Fe metabolism.

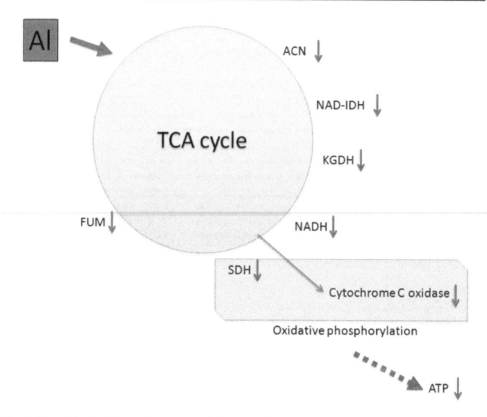

Fig. 8. Al toxicity leads to a disruption of the central metabolic pathways known as the TCA cycle. ACN, IDH (NAD-dependent), KGDH and FUM are all hindered under Al stress. This limits the production of NADH and therefore oxidative phosphorylation lacks the substrate for ATP production. Furthermore, the activity of the ETC enzymes SDH and Cyt C oxidase is perturbed under Al toxicity.

The Al-triggered increase in lipogenesis in liver cells has been recently demonstrated. When cultured hepatocytes are stressed with Al, there is a marked increase in lipoproteins and cholesterol levels in comparison to non-stressed cultures. ApoB-100 is a glycoprotein that plays a critical role in the formation of very low density lipoproteins (VLDL) and low density lipoproteins (LDL). As apoB-100 accumulates, insoluble intracellular aggregates form leading to their co-translational or post-translational degradation. However, nascent apoB-100 is stabilized by the presence of lipids, a process mediated by the microsomal triglyceride transfer protein (MTP), ultimately leading to the formation of VLDL and LDL. Al leads to the increased lipid production needed to stabilize apoB-100, allowing the maturation of VLDL molecules which are subsequently excreted out of the cell. Once out of the cells VLDL molecules can be transported to different organs via a receptor-mediated process. The concentration of the apoB-100 glycoprotein in the spent media of cultured liver cells is directly proportional to the concentration of Al utilized, thus showing direct evidence of the link between Al toxicity, lipogenesis and fatty acid accumulation. What is of further interest is the fact that the carbon source used to grow the cultured cells has an effect on the concentration of lipids accumulated and the monosaccharide D-fructose, a common product in processed food and a compound chemically linked to cancer development and obesity, lead to enhanced VLDL secretion in the Al-stressed hepatocytes (figure 9) (Mailloux et al, 2007b).

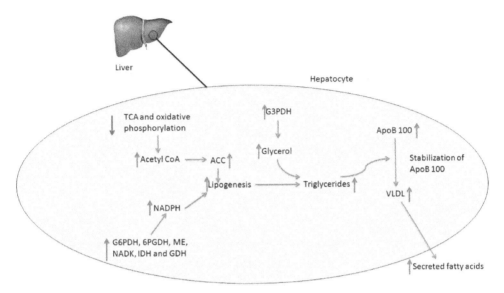

Fig. 9. Al toxicity leads to an increase in lipogenesis which can be observed by the increased levels of VLDL excreted by Al-stressed hepatocytes. As Al disables the TCA cycle and oxidative phosphorylation, there is an accumulation of acetyl-CoA, an important cofactor for lipogensis. Al also induces an increase in NADPH production through IDH and G6PDH along with an increase in glycerol synthesis, two essential substrates for triglyceride synthesis. The elevated levels of lipids in the cell stabilized the glycoprotein ApoB-100, leading to the formation and secretion of VLDL (Mailloux et al, 2007b).

The accumulation of lipids during Al exposure is partially due to the increased lipogenesis brought upon by a hindered mitochondrial TCA cycle and ETC. However, the Al stressed cells are also unable to degrade lipids, a phenomenon which also contributes to the accumulation of fatty acids. L-Carnitine is a non-essential amino acid involved in the transport of fatty acid-derived acyl groups into the mitochondria, a key step in the lipid degradation process known as β-oxidation. During Al-stressed conditions, L-carnitine levels have been shown to decrease in both liver and brain cells. The synthesis of L-carnitine is a multistep enzymatic process that requires the participation of lysine, methionine and α-ketoglutarate (KG). The decrease in L-carnitine levels appear to be triggered by the diminished activity and expression of two key enzymes involved in its synthesis, namely γ-butyrobetainealdehyde dehydrogenase (BADH) and butyrobetaine dioxygenase (BBDOX) (Lemire et al, 2011b). Along with the downregulated enzymes, the impeded TCA cycle blocks the steady supply of KG needed for L-carnitine synthesis. Al-toxicity is associated with the formation of ROS and under oxidative stress cells undergo metabolic reconfigurations. As previously mentioned the TCA cycle is modulated during Al exposure and therefore also during oxidative stress. An important aspect of this metabolic adaptation is the downregulation of KG dehydrogenase (KGDH). This enzyme is particularly sensitive to ROS due to the reactivity of its covalently bound lipoic acid cofactor with oxidizing species. It has been shown that oxidation products in the lipid membranes can go on to react with membrane bound proteins. For example the aldehydic product of lipid peroxidation, 4-hydroxy-2-nonenal (HNE), reacts with the lipoic acid of KGDH, leading to the disruption of enzyme activity. The advantage of KGDH downregulation is the accumulation of the potent antioxidant KG. Like other ketoacids such as pyruvate and oxaloacetate, KG reacts with and nullifies ROS releasing succinate (KG's respective product) and CO_2, by a process referred to as non-enzymatic decarboxylation. As KG is being syphoned towards ROS sequestration, L-carnitine synthesis decreases due to a lack of this pivotal cofactor (**Figure 11**) (Lemire *et al*, 2011b).

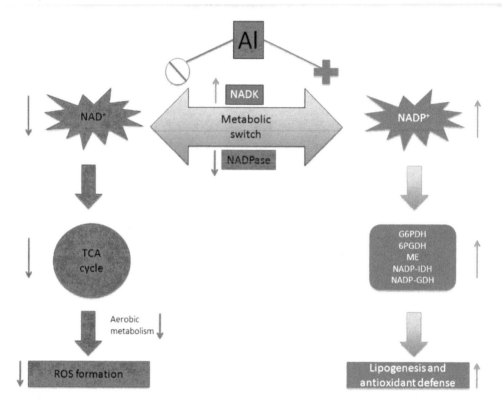

Fig. 10. Al leads to decreased levels of NAD+ through the inhibition of the TCA cycle. Under Al toxicity, aerobic metabolism comes to a halt in order to prevent further ROS formation by endogenous sources such as the electron transport chain in the mitochondria. Al triggers the metabolic shift gated by NADK towards NADP+ production. This substrate is subsequently reduced by various enzymes to produce NADPH. This last compound is essential in antioxidant defense and just as importantly, for lipogenesis (Mailloux *et al*, 2007b).

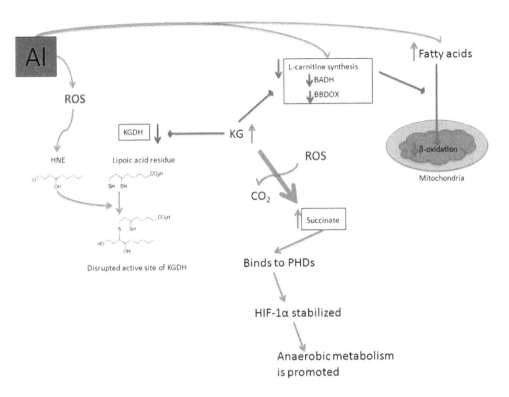

Fig. 11. Al leads to the formation of ROS, which ultimately disrupts KGDH activity (through interactions with the lipoic acid residue in the enzyme's active site). The resulting KG is accumulated in the cell and funneled towards ROS scavenging yielding an accumulation of succinate. Elevated levels of succinate leads to the stabilization of the transcription factor HIF-1α leading to the promotion of anaerobic metabolism. The supply of KG is utilized for sequestration of ROS and L-carnitine synthesis is hindered. Hence, there is decreased expression of key enzymes in the synthesis pathway. This amino acid is responsible for fatty acid transport into the mitochondria for degradation (β-oxidation) and so accumulation of lipids caused by Al is further enabled by a decrease in fatty acid catabolism (Lemire *et al*, 2011b).

The concomitant production of succinate during ROS scavenging by KG is a key contributor to the switch to anaerobic respiration. This adaptive response is initiated by the heterodimeric transcription factor HIF-1. HIF-1 consists of HIF-1α, HIF-2α and HIF-1β subunits. HIF-1α is extremely sensitive to oxygen tension and, under normoxic conditions (when the ETC can function properly), HIF-1α is quickly degraded by prolyl hydroxylases (PHDs) and the ubiquitin-proteosomal degradation pathway. When the proline residues undergo hydroxylation (via PHD), HIF-1α is targeted for degradation by the proteosome. Succinate is known to perturb substrate binding sites in PHD thus interfering with the degradation of HIF-1α. As Al and ROS lead to an accumulation of succinate due to an altered TCA cycle, HIF-1α is stabilized and anaerobic metabolism is promoted (Mailloux *et al*, 2009; 2007a; 2006; Peyssonnaux *et al*, 2007).

6. Aluminum: The missing link between obesity, chronic inflammation and anemia

It is well established that Al disrupts Fe homeostasis. As exposure to this toxin leads to decreased absorption of Fe in the intestine, hinders its transport in the serum, and displaces Fe by binding to transferrin, the involvement of Al in anemia is evident. In a similar fashion to insulin resistance in diabetic individuals, which leads to high levels of glucose in the serum and low intracellular glucose concentrations, Al toxicity causes a disproportionate ratio of serum and cellular Fe levels. When the body experiences Al toxicity, Fe is displaced and released into the bloodstream. This increase in serum Fe tricks the body into thinking there is an excess of Fe, which would lead to limited Fe uptake and release (regulated by hepcidin), when in fact the Al exposed cells are in an anemic state (Del Giudice *et al*, 2009). However, the effects of Al-altered Fe metabolism extend beyond these aforementioned phenomena. As described in the previous section, Al displaces Fe from important enzymatically active proteins leading to a disruption of metabolic processes. This event results in a dysfunctional mitochondria geared towards lipogenesis rather than energy production. An excess fat accumulation and an increase in adipose tissue evoked by Al toxicity can lead to obesity (Mailloux *et al*, 2011). Obese individuals are faced with many obstacles including being at greater risk for cardiovascular diseases, diabetes, obstructive sleep apnea, certain cancers and osteoarthritis (Ausk *et al*, 2008). One of the hallmarks of obesity is chronic inflammation. Inflammation associated with obesity may be linked to Al exposure, a well known and readily used adjuvant. There exists a correlation between unhealthy eating habits and obesity and so an increased intake of processed and "fast" foods by an individual would suggest an increased exposure to Al. This Al could be responsible for the chronic inflammatory response observed in obese patients.

Fe release from various proteins including the [Fe-S] clusters and hemes of enzymes is facilitated by Al. This would cause an increase in free Fe in the body, an event which is hazardous to an organism due to potential ROS formation and promotion of pathogen infection. The body's response to increase Fe levels is the secretion of the hormonal peptide hepcidin. Secreted by the liver and adipose tissues, this peptide limits absorption of Fe by the intestine and release from stores. When gene deletions for hepcidin were performed in mice, unregulated hyperabsorption of Fe in the intestine and unregulated discharge of Fe from spleen macrophages was observed. Overexpression of the hepcidin gene in the mice led to Fe deficiencies and death. It is therefore obvious that this peptide is the regulator of Fe homeostasis.

As an organism is exposed to Al, multiple effects can be observed. The dysfunctional mitochondria leads to increased intracellular lipid accumulation. Obesity sets in and chronic inflammation occurs. Fe homeostasis is disrupted. Together, these events may favor an increase in hepcidin levels in the serum which would limit further absorption of Fe, ultimately causing Al-induced anemia (figure 12) (Ganz, 2003). As Al is associated with ROS toxicity and metabolic shifts leading to the accumulation of the ketoacid antioxidants, such as KG and pyruvate, perhaps dietary supplementation with these potent scavengers might offset the effects of the metal toxin.

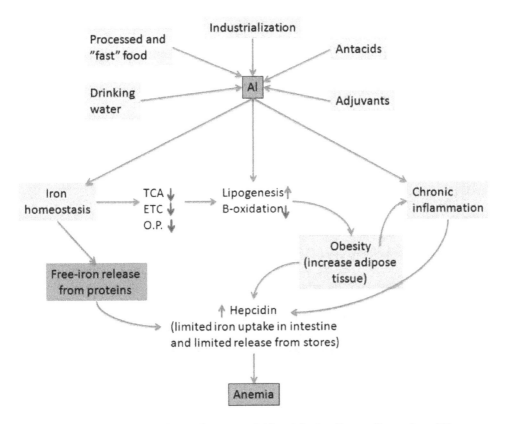

Fig. 12. A global outlook on the implications of Al toxicity leading to disruption of Fe homeostasis, increased lipogenesis and induction of chronic inflammation. Ultimately Al causes the release of Fe into the bloodstream which can signal the secretion of hepcidin by the liver and adipose tissue leading to the limited Fe uptake in the intestine and limited release from cellular stores. Al, by mimicking Fe, tricks the body into thinking it has an overload of the redox active metal and the body response leads to an Al induced anemic state.

7. The therapeutic potential of α-ketoacids

An important factor contributing to Al toxicity is its ability to generate an oxidative environment within the cell. As Al displaces Fe, this redox-active element can participate in ROS-generating reactions leading to the formation of toxic moieties such as hydrogen peroxide (H_2O_2), superoxide ($O_2 \cdot^-$) and the hydroxyl radical ($\cdot OH$). Due to the nature of our oxygen-rich environment, cells are constantly challenged with the burden of oxidative stress. Situations such as Al toxicity worsen the oxidative load that aerobic organisms are exposed to. Hence, organisms possess a battery of antioxidant systems that maintain the redox balance of their cells. With the classical antioxidants molecules such as glutathione

(GSH), ascorbic acid (AA) and vitamin E being extensively studied, the importance of α-ketoacids as ROS scavengers has begun to emerge.

α-Ketoacids are organic compounds that contain a carboxylic acid group adjacent to a ketone group. They play an essential role in cellular metabolism as intermediates in many pathways including the TCA cycle and glycolysis. Examples of biologically relevant α-ketoacids include pyruvate, α-ketoglutarate, oxaloacetate and glyoxylate. The antioxidant potential of these substrates has been demonstrated in a variety of ways. For example, in the soil microbe *Pseudomonas fluorescens* the α-ketoacids KG and pyruvate are readily accumulated for ROS scavenging in conditions of oxidative stress induced by exogenous H_2O_2, menadione (a $O_2\cdot-$ generator), and Al (Mailloux *et al,* 2008). Similarly, metabolic adaptations occur in cultured human hepatocytes and astrocytes leading to the accumulation of these α-ketoacids when the cells are exposed to Al and other oxidizing agents (Lemire *et al,* 2011, Mailloux *et al,* 2011).

In a clinical setting, numerous studies have shown the benefits of α-ketoacid supplementation in an effort to prevent or rectify oxidative damage. An area of this research includes the prevention of cataract formation by pyruvate. Cataracts cause the clouding that develops in the crystalline lens of the eye, which can vary from a slight or complete degree of opacity and obstruction of the passage of light. Cataract formation has been linked to diabetes, hypertension and the over-exposure to UV-radiation. Although treatment with surgery and replacement with synthetic implants are options, there is a push for the development of pharmacological means of cataract prevention, which would reduce invasiveness and cause less secondary effects. The UV-radiation hypothesis of cataract formation states that photons penetrate through to the cornea and subsequently cause the generation of photochemically derived ROS in the aqueous humour and lens of the eye. Fittingly, cataract formation is accompanied by many signs of oxidative stress such as excessive protein glycation and lipid peroxidation, depletion of GSH and a decrease in ATP levels. *In vitro* incubation of mice and rat eye lens with pyruvate demonstrated the beneficial effect of this α-ketoacid in preventing cataract formation by scavenging ROS. These studies demonstrate the therapeutic potential of pyruvate in offsetting the cataractogenesis effects of solar radiation and other factors that act via ROS toxicity (Hegde, 2007, Hegde, 2005).

The use of α-ketoacids in the detoxification of ROS has been shown in many other cases. In numerous brain pathologies such as neurodegenerative diseases or in acute injuries such as ischemia or trauma, H_2O_2 is a suspected culprit in the development of neuropathogenesis. A study by Desagher *et al.* examined the ability of pyruvate to improve the survival of cultured striatal neurons exposed to oxidative agents. Pyruvate protected neurons against both H_2O_2 added to the external medium and $O_2\cdot-$ endogenously produced through the redox cycling agent menadione. The neuroprotective effect of pyruvate appeared to result from the ability of the α-ketoacid to undergo non-enzymatic decarboxylation in the presence of ROS. In addition, several other α-ketoacids including α-ketobutyrate, which is not an energy substrate, also provided the neuroprotective effect of pyruvate. This study also showed that optimal neuroprotection was achieved with relatively low concentrations of pyruvate (>1mM) and that due to its low toxicity and its capacity to cross the blood-brain barrier, this α-ketoacid opens a new therapeutic perspective in ROS associated-brain pathologies (Desagher, 1997).

The advantages of α-ketoacid supplementation for the cardiovascular system have been demonstrated in numerous settings including cardiopulmonary bypass surgery, cardiopulmonary resuscitation, myocardial stunning, and cardiac failure. An important factor in these situations includes the trauma brought upon by myocardial ischemia. As the muscles of the heart are re-oxygenated after a prolonged anaerobic period, the tissue is faced with a depleted energy supply and a massive burst of ROS formation. Therapy with pyruvate has been shown to decrease the damage caused to the ischemic myocardium after reperfusion (Mallet *et al.*, 2005).

The clinical use of α-ketoacids along with their natural occurrence as an antioxidant shows promise of a new line of therapeutic drugs against a wide variety of diseases and dysfunctions. Since Al toxicity is linked to disease states such as obesity, chronic inflammation and anemia, α-ketoacids supplementation may perhaps offer a treatment for the effects of this ROS-forming metal toxin.

8. Acknowledgments

Research in our laboratory is funded by Laurentian University, Industry Canada and NATO. Adam Bignucolo is a recipient of the OGSST TEMBEC Scholarship. Joseph Lemire is a recipient of the Alexander Graham Bell Doctoral Canada Graduate Scholarship. Christopher Auger is a recipient of the Ontario Graduate Scholarship.

9. References

Aimanianda, V., Haensler, J., Lacroix-Desmazes, S., Kaveri, S.V., & Baryr, J. (2009) Novel cellular and molecular mechanisms of induction of immune responses by aluminum adjuvants. *Trends in Pharmacological Sciences*. Vol. 30(6): 287-295

Atkinson, M.A., & White, C.T. (2011) Hepcidin in anemia of chronic kidney disease: review for the pediatric nephrologist. *Pediatric Nephrology*. (in press)

Ausk, K.J., & Ioannou, G.N. (2008) Is obesity associated with anemia of chronic disease? A population-based study. *Obesity*. Vol. 16: 2356-2361

Barisani, D., Pelucchi, S., Mariani, R., Galimberti, S., Trombini, P., Fumagalli, D., Meneveri, R., Nemeth, E., Ganz, T., & Piperno, A. (2008) Hepcidin and iron-related gene expression in subjects with dysmetabolic hepatic iron overload. *Journal of Hepatology*. Vol. 49: 123-133

Campbell, A., Yang, E., Tsai-turton, M., & Bondy, S. (2002) Pro-inflammatory effects of aluminum in human glioblastoma cells. *Brain Research*. Vol. 933: 60-65

Choi, S-O., Cho, Y-S., Kim, H-L., & Park, J-W. (2007) ROS mediate the hypoxic repression of the *hepcidin* gene by inhibition C/EBPα and STAT-3. *Biochemical and Biophysical Research Communications*. Vol. 356: 312-317

Del Giudice, E.M., Santoro, N., Amato, A., Brienza, C., Calabro, P., Wiegerinck, E.T., Cirillo, G., Tartaglione, N., Grandone, A., Swinkels, D.W., & Perrone, L. (2009) Hepcidin in obese children as a potential mediator of the association between obesity and iron deficiency. *Journal of Clinical Endocrinology and Metabolism*. Vol. 94: 5102-5107

Desagher, S., Glowinski, J., & Prémont, J. (1997) Pyruvate protects neurons against hydrogen peroxide- induced toxicity. *Journal of Neuroscience*. Vol. 17(23): 9060–9067

Ganz, T. (2003) Hepcidin, a key regulator of iron metabolism and mediator of anemia of inflammation. *Blood*. Vol. 102(3): 783-788

Gomez, M., Esparza, J.L., Cabre, M., Garcia, M., & Domingo, J.L. (2008) Aluminum exposure through diet: metal levels in AβPP transgenis mice, a model for Alzheimer's disease. *Toxicology*. Vol. 249: 214-219

Hegde, K.R., Kovtun, S., & Varma, S.D. (2007) Induction of ultraviolet cataracts in vitro: prevention by pyruvate. *Journal of Ocular Pharmacology and Therapeutics*. Vol 23(5): 492-502

Hegde, K.R. & Varma, S.D. (2005) Prevention of cataract by pyruvate in experimentally diabetic mice. *Molecular and Cellular Biochemistry*. Vol. 269: 115–120

Hintze, K.J., Snow, D., Nabor, D., & Timbimboo, H. (2010) Adipocyte hypoxia increases hepatocyte hepcidin expression. *Biological Trace Element Research*. (in press)

HogenEsch, H. (2002) Mechanisms of stimulation of the immune response by aluminum adjuvants. *Vaccine*. Vol. 20: 534-539

Kim, Y., Olivi, L., Cheong, J.H., Maertens, A., & Bressler, J.P. (2007) Aluminum stimulate uptake of non- transferrin bound iron and transferrin bound iron in human glial cells. *Toxicology and Applied Pharmacology*. Vol 220: 349-356

Lee, P., Peng, H., Gelbart, T., Wang, L., & Beutler, E. (2005) Regulation of hepcidin transcription by interleukin-1 and interleukin-6. *PNAS*. Vol. 102(6): 1906-1910

Lemire, J., & Appanna, V. (2011a) Aluminum toxicity and astrocyte dysfunction: a metabolic link to neurological disorders. *Journal of Inorganic Biochemistry*. (in press)

Lemire, J., Mailloux, R.J., Darwich, R., Auger, C., & Appanna, V. (2011b) The disruption of L-carnitine metabolism by aluminum toxicity and oxidative stress promotes dyslipidemia in human astrocytic and hepatic cells. *Toxicology letters*. Vol. 203: 219-226

Lemire, J., Mailloux, R.J., Puiseux-Dao, S., & Appanna, V. (2009) Aluminum-induced defective mitochondrial metabolism perturbs cytoskeletal dynamics in human astrocytoma cells. *Journal of Neuroscience research*. Vol. 87: 1474-1483

Lemire, J., Kumar, P., Mailloux, R.J., Cossar, K., & Appanna, V. (2008) Metabolic adaptation and oxaloacetate homeostasis in *P.fluorescens* exposed to aluminum toxicity.

Li, H., Willingham, S.B., Ting, J., & Re, F. (2008) Cutting edge: inflammasome activation by alum and alum's adjuvant effect are mediated by NLRP3. *The Journal of Immunology*. Vol. 181: 17-21

Lopez, F.F., Cabrera, C., Lorenzo, M.L., & Lopez, M.C. (2002) Aluminum content of drinking waters, fruit juices and soft drinks: contribution on dietary intake. *The Science of the Total Environment*. Vol. 292: 205-213

Mailloux, R.J., Lemire, J., & Appanna, V. (2011) Hepatic response to aluminum toxicity: dyslipidemia and liver diseases. *Experimental Cell Research*. (in press)

Mailloux, R.J., Puiseux-Dao, S., & Appanna, V. (2009) α-ketoglutarate abrogates the nuclear localization of HIF-1α in aluminum-exposed hepatocytes. *Biochimie*. Vol. 91: 408-415

Mailloux, R.J., Lemire, J., Kalyuzhnyi, S., & Appanna, V. (2008) A novel metabolic network leads to enhanced citrate biogenesis in *Pseudomonas fluorescens* exposed to aluminum toxicity. *Extremophiles*. Vol. 12: 451-459

Mailloux, R.J. & Appanna, V. (2007a) Aluminum toxicity triggers the nuclear translocation of HIF-1α and promotes anaerobiosis in hepatocytes. *Toxicology in Vitro.* Vol. 21: 16-24

Mailloux, R.J., Lemire, J., & Appanna, V. (2007b) Aluminum-induced mitochondrial dysfunction leads to lipid accumulation in human hepatocytes: a link to obesity. *Cellular Physiology and Biochemistry.* Vol. 20: 627-638

Mailloux, R.J., Hamel, R., & Appanna, V. (2006) Aluminum toxicity elicits a dysfunctional TCA cycle and succinate accumulation in hepatocytes. *Journal of Biochemical and Molecular Toxicology.* Vol. 20(4): 198-208

Mallet, R.T., Sun, J., Knott., E.M., Sharma, A.B., & Olivencia-Yurvati, A.H. (2005) Metabolic cardioprotection by pyruvate: recent progress. *Experimental and Biological Medicine.* Vol. 230(7): 435-443

McClung, J.P., & Karl, J.P. (2009) Iron deficiency and obesity: the contribution of inflammation and diminished iron absorption. *Nutrition Reviews.* Vol. 67(2): 100-104

Middaugh, J., Hamel, R., Hean-Baptiste, G., Beriault, R., Chenier, D., & Appanna, V. (2005) Aluminum triggers decreased aconitase activity via Fe-S cluster disruption and the overexpression of isocitrate dehydrogenase and isocitrate lyase: a metabolic network mediating cellular survival. *The Journal of Biological Chemistry.* Vol. 280(5): 3159-3165

Peyssonnaux, C., Zinkermagel, A., Schuepbach, R., Rankin, E., Vaulont, S., Haase, V., Nizet, V., & Johnson, R. (2007) Regulation of iron homeostasis by the hypoxi-inducible transcription factors (HIFs). *The Journal of Clinical Investigation.* Vol. 117(7): 1926-1932

Rondeau, V., Jacqumin-Gadda, H., Commenges, D., Helmer, C., & Dartigues, J-F. (2008) Aluminum and silica in drinking water and the risk of Alzeihmer's disease or cognitive decline: findings from 15- year follow-up of the PAQUID cohort. *American Journal of Epidemiology.* Vol. 169(4): 489-496

Turgut, S., Bor-Kucukaty, M., Emmungil, G., Atsak, P., & Turgut, G. (2007) The effect of low dose aluminum on hemorheological and hematological parameters in rats. *Archives of Toxicology.* Vol. 81: 11-17

Vecchi, C., Montosi, G., Zhang, K., Lamberti, I., Duncan, S., Kaufman, R., & Pietrangelo, A. (2009) ER stress controls iron metabolism through induction of hepcidin. *Science.* Vol 325: 877-880

Vergara, S.V., & Thiele, D.J. (2008) Post-transcriptional regulation of gene expression in response to iron deficiency: coordinated metabolic reprogramming by yeast mRNA-binding proteins. *Biochemical Society Transactions.* Vol. 36(5): 1088-1090

Ward, R.J., Zhang, Y, & Critchon, R.R. (2001) Aluminum toxicity and iron homeostasis. *Journal of Inorganic Biochemistry.* Vol. 87: 9-14

Yanoff, I.B., Menzie, C.M., Denkinger, B., Sebring., N.G., McHugh, T., Remaley, A.T., & Yanovski, J.A. (2007) Inflammation and iron deficiency in the hypoferremia of obesity. *International Journal of Obesity.* Vol. 31: 1412-1419

Yokel, R.A., & Florence, R.L. (2008a) Aluminum bioavailability from tea infusion. *Food and Chemical Toxicology.* Vol. 46: 3659-3663

Yokel, R.A., Hicks, C.L., & Florence, R.L. (2008b) Aluminum bioavailability from basic sodium aluminum phosphate, an approved food additive emulsifying agent, incorporated in cheese. *Food and Chemical Toxicology*. Vol. 46: 2261-2266

Yokel, R.A., & Florence, R.L. (2006) Aluminum bioavailability from the approved food additive leavening agent acidic sodium aluminum phosphate, incorportated into a baked is lower than from water. *Toxicology*. Vol. 227: 86-93

12

Hemolysis and Anemia
Induced by Dapsone Hydroxylamine

Gabriella Donà[1], Eugenio Ragazzi[2], Giulio Clari[1] and Luciana Bordin[1,*]

[1]Department of Biological Chemistry, University of Padova,
[2]Department of Pharmacology and Anesthesiology, University of Padova
Italy

1. Introduction

Dapsone (4,4'-diaminodiphenylsulfone, DDS) has been used for over half a century in the treatment of leprosy, for anti-inflammatory conditions and, in the chlorproguanil-dapsone and artesunate–dapsone–proguanil combinations, for treating malaria. It is also a second-line treatment for AIDS-related Pneumocystis pneumonia (Sangiolo et al., 2005), and is increasingly applied to a variety of immuno-related conditions (Bahadir et al., 2004; Ujiie et al., 2006), despite its well-documented toxicity, which is closely related to its routes of biotransformation.

Dapsone is mono and diacetylated and the monoacetylated derivative and the parent drug can be oxidised by cytochrome P (CYP) family to hydroxylamines, both of which are methaemoglobin formers. However, both dapsone and mono-N-acetyl dapsone are 97% to 100% bound to plasma proteins. Both hydroxylamines are auto-oxidisable to nitroso arenes, which can covalently bind proteins. In erythrocytes, hydroxylamines react with hemoglobin to form methemoglobin and nitrosoarenes and produce reactive oxygen species (ROS). In turn, ROS reacts with glutathione (GSH) and with hemoglobin thiols to generate thiyl radicals (RS· where R is residue from glutathione or hemoglobin cysteine residue). The thiyl free radicals are responsible for glutathione-protein mixed disulfide and skeletal protein-hemoglobin disulfide formation, which causes alterations in cell morphology (McMillan et al., 2005; Bradshaw et al., 1997) (Fig. 1).

Mono- and diacetylated metabolites of dapsone (MADDS and DADDS) are not associated with toxicity (Coleman et al., 1991), although N-hydroxylation of the parent drug and MADDS lead to the formation of the toxic hydroxylamines DDS-NHOH and MADDS-NHOH (Israili et al., 1973; Coleman et al., 1989) (Fig. 1). These species, formed either by CYP2C9 (Winter et al., 2000), one isoform of the cytochrome P450 (CYP) family, or other oxidative enzyme systems, are linked with several immune-mediated hypersensitivity reactions (Vyas et al., 2006). The hydroxylamines are also responsible for the clinical methaemoglobinaemia associated with dapsone therapy (DT) (Israili et al., 1973; Schiff et al., 2006).

DDS-NHOH cannot be directly detected in human plasma as it is rapidly taken up by erythrocytes prior to its redox cycling with haemoglobin, forming methaemoglobin (Coleman & Jacobus, 1993). In any case, the metabolic elimination of dapsone is N-hydroxylation, which accounts for between 30% and 40% of an oral dapsone dose, and the efficiency of N-hydroxylation is related to dapsone clearance (May et al., 1990; May et al., 1992; Bluhm et al., 1999). Dapsone therapy includes a daily administration of 50-100 mg for leprosy and 100-300 mg for dermatitis herpetiformis (Leonard and Fry, 1991), leading to serum concentrations of 0.5-5 mg/L (equivalent to 2-20 microM); therapeutical doses up to 400 mg have been reported in literature (Elonen et al., 1979; Zuidema et al., 1986), as well as some cases of intoxication with DDS, such as after an overdose with 10 g of DDS, leading to serum concentrations of 120 mg/L (about 0.5 mM, comparable to those used in our in vitro experiments). Another case of intoxication produced methaemoglobinemia at serum concentrations of 18.8 mg/L (76 μM) (Woodhouse et al., 1983). The acetylation ratio (MADDS:DDS) shows a genetically determined bimodal distribution, allowing the definition of 'slow' and 'rapid' acetylators (Zuidema et al., 1986).

2. DDS-NHOH toxicity

Adverse effects of dapsone therapy are the cause of an idiosyncratic reaction, called dapsone hypersensitivity syndrome (DHS) (Orion et al., 2005; Sener et al., 2006), and, more frequently, dose-related methaemoglobinaemia and haemolytic anemia (Cream, 1970).

DHS includes a number of adverse effects including fever, rash, and internal organ involvement, all related to the bioactivation of DDS into DDS-NHOH (Prussick R & Shear NH, 1996). Bioactivated drug represent the first step in the formation of toxic intermediates, which bind covalently to or modify various molecules through the process defined haptenation, where a small molecule can elicit an immune response by attaching to a large carrier, such as a protein. Once the body has generated antibodies to a hapten-carrier adduct, it will usually initiate an immune response.

It has been recently demonstrated that skin (Roychowdhury et al., 2007) and human keratinocytes are able to convert DDS to hydroxylamine by the action of myeloperoxidase (MPO). Once formed, these highly reactive metabolites can bind to cellular proteins and act as haptens, promoting autoimmunity in susceptible individuals (Vyas et al., 2006).

DDS mediated haemolytic anemia is closely related to erythrocyte membrane alterations leading to premature cell removal, which can occur both extravascularly, by spleen-mediated subtraction of damaged erythrocytes, or intravascularly, by DDS induced cell fragility. All haematological side effects reported for DDS therapy are due to the N-hydroxy metabolites of the drug, dapsone hydroxylamine (DDS-NHOH).

3. Erythrocytes and DDS-NHOH toxicity

3.1 In vitro alterations of normal erythrocyte membranes

DDS-NHOH undergoes a coupled oxidation-reduction reaction with haemoglobin and molecular oxygen yielding methaemoglobin and ROS formation (ferryl haem and hydroxyl radicals) (Fig. 1), respectively (Bradshaw et al., 1997).

To date, no direct evidence of the mechanism whereby DDS-NHOH shortens the erythrocyte lifespan has ever been reported. Only the fact that DDS-NHOH affects the integrity of the erythrocyte lipid bilayer has been excluded, since neither lipid peroxidation nor phosphatidylserine (PS) externalisation have ever been detected (McMillan et al., 1998; McMillan et al., 2005).

Erythrocyte

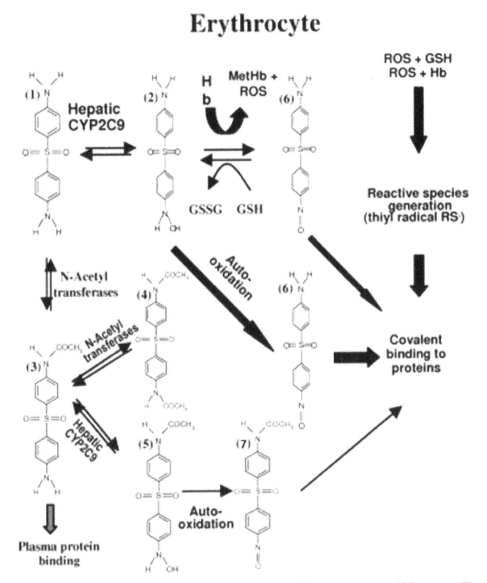

Fig. 1. Scheme showing main features of metabolic fate of dapsone in man. (1) Dapsone; (2) dapsone hydroxylamine; (3) monoacetyl dapsone (MADDS), (4) diacetyl dapsone (DADDS); (5) monoacetyl dapsone hydroxylamine; (6) dapsone nitrosoarene derivatives (7). monoacetyl dapsone nitrosoarene derivative.

In a recent report (Bordin et al., 2010a) we proposed tyrosine phosphorylation (Tyr-P) level of erythrocyte membrane as diagnostic method to evaluate erythrocyte membrane status. In human erythrocytes, Tyr-P of membrane proteins is the result of the antithetic actions of protein tyrosine kinases (TPKs) and protein tyrosine phosphatases (PTPs) and involves mainly band 3 protein. This is the most abundant membrane protein of red blood cells and is divided into three regions: an external domain, enriched in glycosyl chains that probably allow band 3 protein to be recognised as a specific antigens (Bratosin et al., 1998); a transmembrane domain, representing the anionic exchanger of cells; and a cytosol portion (Wang, 1994), containing all phosphorylatable residues. Although serine/threonine (Ser/Thr)-phosphorylation of the band 3 cytosol domain has been demonstrated to regulate the anion flux rate (Baggio et al., 1993a,; Baggio et al., 1993b), Tyr-P is involved in multiple functions, including regulation of glycolysis (Low et al., 1993), alteration of erythrocyte morphology (Bordin et al., 1995) and volume (Musch et al., 1999), and senescence (Bordin et al., 2009; Pantaleo et al., 2009).

When triggered by oxidative (diamide) or hyperosmotic stress, the band 3 Tyr-P level can predict both pathological and particular physiological conditions. In glucose-6-phosphate dehydrogenase (G6PD) deficiency, the higher band 3 Tyr-P level, compared with normal control cells, correlates well with chronic impairment of cell anti-oxidative defences (Bordin et al., 2005b); conversely, the lower band 3 Tyr-P level observed in pregnancy is synonymous of characteristically increased anti-oxidative defences (Bordin et al., 2006).

Methemoglobinemia occurs to some extent in all patients receiving DDS and becomes less pronounced as treatment is continued because of an adaptative increase in the activity of NADH-dependent reductase in erythrocytes (Orion et al., 2005). Methemoglobin (MetHb) production is due to oxidation of hemoglobin by nitroso species which react with NADPH (Kiese et al., 1966) or glutathione (GSH) (Coleman et al., 1994) to regenerate hydroxylamines. Reilly and co-workers (Reilly et al., 1999) showed that GSH, rather than NADPH, is the key reducing specie responsible for regenerating hydroxylamine metabolites and that any GSH consumed must be rapidly regenerated.

We observed that DDS-NHOH, when added to intact erythrocytes in in vitro experiments, triggered the formation of both MetHb and Tyr-P level of band 3 (Bordin et al., 2010b). This last process was time and dose-dependent by DDS-NHOH but only for the early 30 minutes of incubation and to 0.3 mM concentration. Increasing incubation time (50 min) and effector dose (0.6 mM), band 3 Tyr-P decreased to negligible level.

We compared these effects with those induced by diamide (Bordin et al., 2005a), which increased protein phosphorylation level by inhibiting tyrosine phosphatase activities by directly oxidising cysteine located in the catalytic domain of the enzyme (Hecht & Zick, 1992), and by inducing immediate band 3 clustering (Bordin et al., 2006; Fiore et al., 2008).

Our findings showed that both Tyr-kinase and phosphatase activities were promptly inhibited by DDS-NHOH in both dose- and time-dependent manners, and total inactivation was reached in both after 60 min incubation with 0.15 and 0.3 mM. At 0.6 mM, DDS-NHOH treatment was almost completely inhibitory after only 15 minutes of incubation. This suggests that the triggering of band 3 Tyr-P is not due to an imbalance between enzymatic activities but, more probably, by a favoured substrate-kinase interaction, at least up to 0.3 mM within 30 min. Longer incubation times or higher compound concentrations resulted in the total disappearance of band 3 Tyr-P, as well as total enzyme inhibition. This time-dependent increasing effect of DDS-NHOH indicated that there is progression in the action mechanism of the compound.

In addition, it has been previously demonstrated that band 3 structural alterations can be useful to further reveal the status of membranes (Bordin et al., 2006). DDS-NHOH treatment induced band 3 aggregation in high molecular weight aggregates (HMWA) mainly located in the Triton-soluble part of the membrane. This effector differentiated greatly from diamide: its time-dependent effect increased in a sort of amplifying system, leading to further increases in band 3 HMWA, but, more interestingly, also to their total relocation within the membrane, accompanied by reorganization of both PTKs (Brunati et al., 2000) and PTPs (Bordin et al., 2002), independently from band 3 Tyr-P level. This new membrane set up was easily recognized and marked by autologous IgG, representative of damaged cells (Bordin et al., 2010b).

This raises the hypothesis that the gradual band 3 Tyr-P tailing off within the first 45 min may represent the time threshold between the formation of two differently located band 3 aggregates - Triton-soluble, and, successively, cytoskeleton bound. Accordingly, the Tyr-phosphorylative process may be considered a cellular defence against the incoming oxidative modifications induced by DDS-NHOH. In this process, introduction of negative charges, represented by phosphate groups, to band 3 protein would slow down its aggregation, at least up to the total arrest of the phosphorylative process. Subsequently, modifications would continue more profoundly, inducing not only more marked clustering of band 3 but also totally redistributing HMWA from soluble to insoluble (cytoskeleton) membrane fractions. This is further suggested by total rearrangement of band 3 HMWA at 0.6 mM DDS-NHOH: in these conditions, band 3 Tyr-P is very slight, and band 3 HMWA were located in the cytoskeleton even after 30 min incubation (Bordin et al., 2010b).

This may fit the hypothesis that reactive radicals also generate a second species of radicals, probably a thiyl radical (McMillan et al., 2005), more reactive and efficacious in generating so many and drastic alterations in membrane structure and composition.

Taken together, the direct evidence of the mechanism whereby DDS-NHOH shortens the erythrocyte lifespan is consistent with progressive oxidative alteration starting from cytosol, where it induces methaemoglobin formation (Israili et al., 1973; Schiff et al., 2006), glutathione oxidation, and initial impairment of Tyr-protein kinase and phosphatase activities. Later, the effect of DDS-NHOH advances, with progressive reorganisation of membrane/proteins, as evidenced by enzyme recruitment and the formation of band 3 aggregates (HMWA) (Bordin et al., 2010b). Lastly, general membrane reorganisation is achieved, with protein relocation from the Triton-soluble compartment to the cytoskeleton and with autologous antibody recognition (Bordin et al., 2010b). The fact that DDS-NHOH affects the integrity of the erythrocyte lipid bilayer has been excluded, since neither lipid peroxidation nor phosphatidylserine externalisation have ever been detected (McMillan et al., 1998; McMillan et al., 2005).

3.2 Erythrocyte membrane alterations in Glucose-6-Phosphate Dehydrogenase (G6PD) deficient patients in dapsone therapy

In order to verify whether the above mechanism of DDS-NHOH-induced membrane reorganisation was the mechanism effectively leading to erythrocyte denaturation/removal in vivo, we analysed membranes from two patients in dapsone treatment (DT) for dermatitis herpetiformis (Bordin et al., 2010b). The two patients were diagnosed as suffering from dermatitis herpetiformis (DH) according to skin biopsies and cell surface deposition of IgA, and were given oral dapsone. At admission, both had normal blood and urine samples. Their treatment started with 100 mg/day DT, as usual dose (Leonard & Fry 1991).

Patient 1 remained successfully in treatment for the length of the study; blood was withdrawn before and during dapsone administration (after 14 days' treatment).

Patient 2, was hospitalised for a haemolytic episode following 3 days of 100 mg/day DT (P2$_{100}$). His laboratory tests revealed that he had Glucose-6-Phosphate Dehydrogenase (G6PD) deficiency, class II, according to the WHO directive (Betke et al., 1967). G6PD residual activity in red cells was < 10%, measured spectrophotometrically at 340 nm on a

Sigma diagnostic kit (Sigma-Aldrich, Italy). Dapsone was discontinued for a month, after which laboratory test results had returned to normal range. Dapsone treatment (DT) was later re-administered, starting with two days with 30 mg/day, and then 50 mg/day, with partial relief but not total remission of symptoms.

Blood samples from both patients were taken before and during treatments. Samples from patient 1 were called P1 and $P1_{100}$ to indicate samples before administration and during 100 mg/day DT; erythrocytes from patient 2 were called P2, $P2_{30}$, and $P2_{50}$ to indicate samples withdrawn before and after 2 days at 30 mg/day, or after 3 days at 50 mg/day DT, respectively. Erythrocytes were analysed for their band 3 HMWA and IgG bound contents. DT in patient 1 (P1) induced a slight increase in band 3 HMWA, which was correlated with an increase in bound IgG (Fig. 2, panel A). Erythrocyte membranes from patient 2 showed a higher level of basal band 3 HMWA (P2), which increased (+18%) during the 30 mg/day DT, but reached a dramatic level at 50 mg/day (+215%). The effect was correlated with a 30% increase in bound IgG in $P2_{30}$ and with more than 120% in $P2_{50}$.

$P1_{100}$ was chosen as arbitrary unit to indicate erythrocyte membrane alterations (band 3 HMWA and IgG binding) induced by DT (A) or band 3 Tyr-P induced by diamide (B) in normal patients.

In addition, when analysed for Tyr-P level extent, membranes from erythrocytes of both patients showed that the basal level of band 3 Tyr-P was negligible. Successive analysis of glutathione content evidenced that DT induced a decrease in total GSH content in both patients (Bordin et al., 2010b). However, $P1_{100}$ maintained about 85% of total glutathione in reduced form (GSH), but P2 showed progressive depletion of glutathione, with an alarming rise in oxidised glutathione (GS-SG) which, at $P2_{50}$, reached almost 60% of total glutathione. To induce weak oxidative stress, addition of 0.3 mM diamide to isolated erythrocytes from both patients was performed. $P1_{100}$ showed a reduction in total glutathione content and a rise of GS-SG. P2 and $P2_{30}$ highlighted a net reduction in the amount of total glutathione which, at $P2_{50}$, was only 50%, compared with the glutathione content of P2. Diamide induced net increase in the GS-SG form, which reached almost 100% glutathione at $P2_{50}$.

When analysed also for their Tyr-P content after 0.3 mM diamide treatment (inconsistent with Tyr-P triggering in normal subjects), patients presented clear differences (Bordin et al., 2006) (Fig. 2, panel B). The first patient showed a slight trace of band 3 Tyr-P only after DT ($P1_{100}$). Instead, P2 evidenced net band 3 Tyr-P (as expected, due to his G6PDdeficiency), which dramatically escalated on increasing DT (Fig. 2 panel B). Syk and SHP-2 content in membranes from P2 also rose after DT, in both the absence and presence of diamide incubation (Bordin et al., 2010b).

This is in line with what evidenced in vitro from normal erythrocytes: in normal subjects, therapy leads to weakening of anti-oxidant defences (as indicated by decreased GSH content) and triggers membrane reorganisation, as indicated by increased band 3 HMWA formation (Fig. 2, panel A) and higher sensitivity towards diamide-induced oxidative stress. When dapsone was administered to G6PDd patient (P2), drops in both haemoglobin content and haematocrit were observed at $P2_{50}$, suggesting the onset of the haemolytic process. This cannot be explained by the simple fall in GSH content since, even at 50 mg/day dapsone ($P2_{50}$), almost one-third of total glutathione is in reduced form, but incapable of preventing DT-induced erythrocyte modification. In other words, glutathione is not sufficient to counteract membrane oxidisation induced by dapsone, because its metabolite, DDS-NHOH, acts on different substrates in a time-dependent progressive ROS formation. That hydroxylamine is the responsible of the alterations is confirmed by the fact that DT induces the same membrane alterations than those previously shown in *in vitro* experiments with DDS-NHOH, such as band 3 HMWA formation and IgG binding increase. Instead, band 3 Tyr-P was not detected, even in $P2_{50}$ erythrocytes, although Tyr-protein kinases and/or phosphatases were not inhibited in these conditions, as indicated by the following diamide-induced band 3 Tyr-P of patients' erythrocytes (especially in P2). This was probably because the concentration of this effector is insufficient to have immediate effects on the enzymes, like those evidenced in in vitro experiments, which would be representative of high toxicity. Band 3 Tyr-P level, therefore, is to be dependent on the net alteration of erythrocyte membrane following DT.

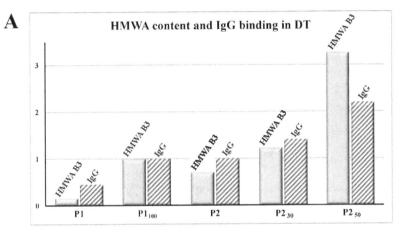

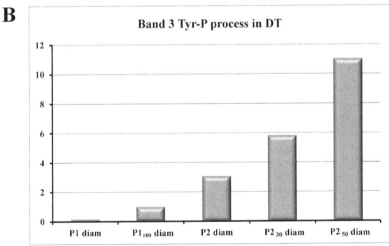

Fig. 2. Effect of dapsone treatment (DT) on erythrocyte membrane rearrangement. Erythrocytes from patients 1 and 2 before (P1 and P2) and after DT ($P1_{100}$ and $P2_{30}$ and $P2_{50}$) were directly analysed for high molecular weight aggregate (HMWA) of band 3 and IgG binding (panel A), or incubated with 0.3 mM diamide to trigger band 3 Tyr-P level (panel B).

3.3 DDS-NHOH-induced alterations in erythrocyte from endometriotic patients: Potential toxicity in inflammatory disease

In the above paragraph, it has been reported that band 3 Tyr-P levels were negligible in erythrocytes from patients during DT, and diamide addition was useful to investigate membrane status, mainly cell capacity of counteracting additional oxidative stress.

To evidence the direct effect of pre-existing inflammatory status on DDS-NHOH treatment, we compared band 3 Tyr-P levels induced by increasing concentrations of DDS-NHOH on erythrocytes from endometriotic patients with that obtained in normal erythrocytes (Figures 3 and 4).

Figure 3 shows band 3 Tyr-P obtained with 0.15, 0.3 and 0.6 mM DDS-NHOH in erythrocytes from endometriotic patients (panel A, lanes b-d), which result much higher than that obtained in the control (lane a) with 0.3 mM (concentration able to induce maximum Tyr-P level in normal erythrocytes (Bordin et al., 2010b).

DDS-NHOH and endometriosis

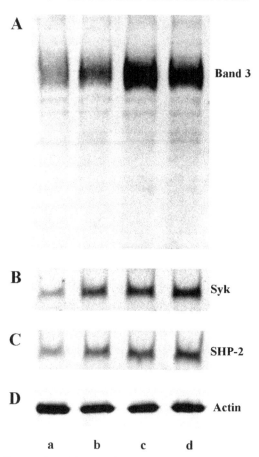

Fig. 3. DDS-NHOH effect on band 3 Tyr-P level (panel A), Syk (panel B) and SHP-2 (panel C) recruitments.

This higher sensitivity of endometriotic erythrocytes towards hydroxylamine was further confirmed by the increased amounts of enzymes, Syk PTK (panel B) and SHP-2 PTP (panel C) bound to membranes following DDS-NHOH treatment. In addition, band 3 HMWA, synonymous of a predisposition of the cell to be recognized by IgG and removed from circulation (Bordin et al., 2010b, Arese et al., 2005; Ciccoli et al., 2004; Kay, 2005; Lutz et al., 1987), were markedly higher in endometriotic cells (Fig. 4) following DDS-NHOH treatment (lanes b-d, compared with lane a, control erythrocytes incubated with 0.3 mM DDS-NHOH).

In order to verify if the patterns of figures 3 and 4 obtained in vitro would mirror potential toxicity for endometriotic patients in DT, we compared them with those obtained by incubating erythrocytes from G6PDd patients in the same above conditions (Fig. 5). Diamide-induced band 3 Tyr-P level and Syk and SHP-2 recruitments were very similar between G6PDd and endometriotic patients, the former reaching the highest values for all parameters, especially when compared with healthy controls.

The high similarity present in in vitro DDS-NHOH treatment between G6PDd and endometriosis erythrocytes strengthens the idea that inflammation status-related alteration would predispose cell to be highly sensitive to the presence of arylamine derivatives, which would lead to potential toxicity to DT.

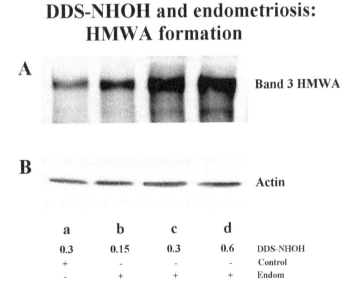

Fig. 4. Effect of increasing DDS-NHOH on band 3 HMWA formation in normal (lane a) and endometriotic patients (lanes b-d).

A

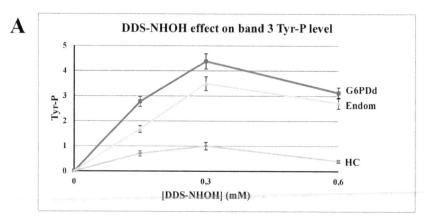

B

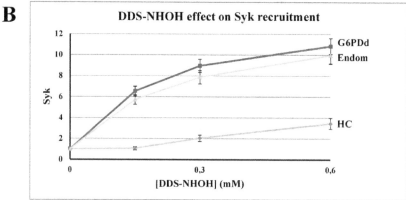

C

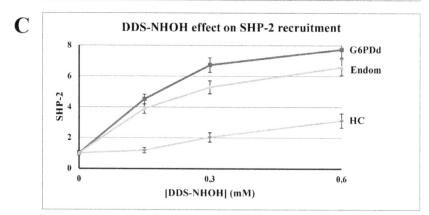

Fig. 5. DDS-NHOH effect on erythrocytes: membrane band 3 Tyr-P level (Panel A), Syk (Panel B) and SHP-2 (Panel C) recruitments, in in vitro experiments: comparison among Healthy Controls (HC), G6PDd and Endometriotic (Endom) patients.

4. Conclusions

G6PD in the hexose (HMP) shunt regulates the production of NADPH, an obligatory substrate for several redox systems, in particular for glutathione, which protects the cell from oxidative stress. It has been previously shown that conditions of oxidative stress lowering NADPH content immediately raise the HMP shunt rate up to 30-fold. Red blood cells with G6PD deficiency cannot increase their shunt sufficiently during an oxidative load, and thus show a weakened cellular redox defence (Jacobasch & Rapoport 1996). In several antimalarial, antipyretics or analgesic drugs' treatments, G6PD deficient patients can not provide an adequate antioxidant defence and their erythrocytes present degenerative parameters, revealing the formation of anomalies in cell morphology and deformability (Jacobasch & Rapoport 1996). Oxidative stress induces haemoglobin (Hb) denaturation and membrane binding of hemichromes, Heinz body precursors, and provokes aggregation of band 3 and deposition of antibodies and complement C3c fragments. In fact, it has been described that membrane clustering of band 3 can allow immune recognition by naturally occurring antibodies, inducing antibody-dependent phagocytosis of senescent/alterate erythrocytes (Arese et al., 2005; Kay, 1984; Low et al. 1985; Schluter & Drenekhanh 1986; Lutz et al. 1988; Arese & De Flora 1990; Hebbel, 1990). Also, band 3 Tyr-P level induced by pathological conditions, could make structural alterations, which probably lead cell into apoptosis, by exposing new band 3 epitopes and favouring cell removal from circulation. Both can induce membrane alterations as well as binding of multivalent ligands, leading to hemolysis (Bottini et al., 1997).

All these facts, together with the G6PDd cell inability to response powerfully to oxidants, indicates that the physiological status of band 3 is essential for erythrocytes survival/apoptosis.

In G6PDd anti-oxidative defences are much lower than those present in endometriosis, which has been demonstrated to correlate with chronic oxidative assault induced by inflammation, rather than impairment in glutathione (GSH) restoring. In addition, pre-existing membrane alterations have been postulated even for endometriotic erythrocytes, as indicated by their higher sensitivity to diamide (Bordin et al., 2010a). In fact, diamide-triggered band 3 Tyr-P level was two or three times higher than those of controls, owed to an altered redox system, predisposing membrane proteins to be more markedly oxidized. This was confirmed by the observation that total cell glutathione does not differ from that of healthy controls (data not shown) but, once the erythrocytes are incubated with diamide, patients' GSH contents are far lower, probably due to membrane oxidative status alterations which retained glutathione under the form of protein glutathionylation (Bordin et al., 2010a).

Our study confirms previous reports, stressing that sensitiveness to the compound is clearly idiosyncratic and dependent on the patho/physiological patients' status (May et al., 1990; May et al., 1992; Wertheim et al., 2006).

From these considerations, the assessment of the pre-existent oxidative status of erythrocytes should be carefully evaluated prior to the choice of the appropriate therapy.

5. References

Arese, P. & De Flora, A. (1990). Pathophysiology of hemolysis in glucose-6-phosphate dehydrogenase deficiency. *Seminars in Hematolology*, Vol.27, No.1, pp. 1-40.

Arese, P.; Turrini, F. & Schwarzer, E. (2005). Band 3/complement-mediated recognition and removal of normally senescent and pathological human erythrocytes. *Cellular Physiology and Biochemistry*, Vol.16, No.4-6, pp. 133-146.

Baggio, B.; Bordin, L.; Clari, G.; Gambero, G. & Moret, V. (1993a). Functional correlation between the Ser/Thr-phosphorylation of band 3 and band 3-mediated transmembrane anion transport in human erythrocytes. *Biochimica and Biophysica Acta*, Vol.1148, No.1, pp. 157-160.

Baggio, B.; Bordin, L.; Gambaro, G.; Piccoli, A.; Marzaro, G. & Clari, G. (1993b). Evidence of a link between band 3 phosphorylation and anion transport in patients with "idiopathic" calcium oxalate nephrolithiasis. *Mineral and Electrolyte Metabolism*, Vol.19, No.1, pp. 17-20.

Bahadir, S.; Cobanoglu, U.; Cimsit, G.; Yayli, S. & Alpay, K. (2004). Erythema dyschromicum perstans: response to dapsone therapy. *International Journal of Dermatolology*, Vol.43, No.3, pp. 220-222.

Betke, K.; Beutler, E.; Brewer, G.J.; Kirkman. H.N.; Luzzato, L.; Motulsky, A.G.; Ramot, B. & Siniscalco, M. (1967). Standardization of procedures for the study of glucose-6-phosphate dehydrogenase. *Report of a WHO scientific group-WHO*, Technical Report-Serial 366.

Bluhm, R.E.; Adedoyin, A.; McCarver, D.G. & Branch R.A. (1999). Development of dapsone toxicity in patients with inflammatory dermatoses: activity of acetylation and hydroxylation of dapsone as risk factors. *Clinical Pharmacology & Therapeutics*, Vol.65, No.6, pp. 598-605.

Bordin, L.; Brunati, A.M.; Donella-Deana, A.; Baggio, B.; Toninello, A. & Clari, G. (2002). Band 3 is a anchor protein and a target for SHP-2 tyrosine phosphatases in human erythrocytes. *Blood*, Vol.100, No.1, pp. 276-282.

Bordin, L.; Clari, G.; Moro, I.; Dalla Vecchia, F. & Moret, V. (1995). Functional link between phosphorylation state of membrane proteins and morphological changes of human erythrocytes. *Biochemical and Biophysical Research Communications*, Vol.213, No.1, pp. 249-257.

Bordin, L.; Fiore, C.; Bragadin, M.; Brunati, A.M. & Clari, G. (2009). Regulation of membrane band 3 Tyr-phosphorylation by proteolysis of p72(Syk) and possible involvement in senescence process. *Acta Biochimica et Biophysica Sinica*, Vol.41, No.10, pp. 846-851.

Bordin, L.; Fiore, C.; Donà, G.; Andrisani, A.; Ambrosini, G.; Faggian, D.; Plebani, M.; Clari, G. & Armanini, D. (2010a). Evaluation of erythrocyte band 3 phosphotyrosine level, glutathione content, CA-125, and human epididymal secretory protein E4 as combined parameters in endometriosis. *Fertility and Sterility*, Vol.94, No.5, pp. 1616-1621.

Bordin, L.; Fiore, C.; Zen, F.; Coleman, M.D.; Ragazzi, E. & Clari, G. (2010b) Dapsone hydroxylamine induces premature removal of human erythrocytes by membrane reorganization and antibody binding. *British Journal of Pharmacology*, Vol.161, No.5, pp. 1186-1199.

Bordin, L.; Ion-Popa, F.; Brunati, A.M.; Clari, G. & Low, P.S. (2005a). Effector-induced Syk-mediated phosphorylation in human erythrocytes. *Biochimica et Biophysica Acta*, Vol.1745, No.1, pp. 20-28.

Bordin, L.; Quartesan, S.; Zen, F.; Vianello, F. & Clari, G. (2006). Band 3 Tyr-phosphorylation in human erythrocytes from non-pregnant and pregnant women. *Biochimica et Biophysica Acta,* Vol.1758, No.5, pp. 611-619.

Bordin, L.; Zen, F.; Ion-Popa, F.; Barbetta, M.; Baggio, B. & Clari, G. (2005b). Band 3 Tyr-phosphorylation in normal and glucose-6-phospate dehydrogenase-deficient human erythrocytes. *Molecular Membrane Biology,* Vol.22, No.5, pp. 411-420.

Bottini, E.; Bottini, F.G.; Borgiani, P. & Businco, L. (1997). Association between ACP1 and favism: a possible biochemical mechanism. *Blood,* Vol.89, No.7, pp. 2613-2615.

Bradshaw, T.P.; McMillan, D.C.; Crouch, R.K, & Jollow, D.J. (1997). Formation of free radicals and protein mixed disulfides in rat red cells exposed to dapsone hydroxylamine. *Free Radical Biology and Medicine,* Vol.22, No.7, pp. 1183-1193.

Bratosin, D.; Mazurier, J.; Tissier, J.P.; Estaquier, J.; Huart, J.J.; Ameisen J.C.; Aminoff, D. & Montreuil, J. (1998). Cellular and molecular mechanisms of senescent erythrocyte phagocytosis by macrophages. A review. *Biochimie,* Vol.80, No.2, pp. 173-195.

Brunati, A.M.; Bordin, L.; Clari, G.; James, P.; Quadroni, M.; Baritono, E.; Pinna, L.A. & Donella-Deana, A. (2000). Sequential phosphorylation of protein band 3 by Syk and Lyn tyrosine kinases in intact human erythrocytes: identification of primary and secondary phosphorylation sites. *Blood,* Vol.96, No.4, pp. 1550-1557.

Ciccoli, L.; Rossi, V.; Leoncini, S.; Signorini, C.; Blanco-Garcia, J.; Aldinucci, C.; Buonocore, G. & Comporti, M. (2004). Iron release, superoxide production and binding of autologous IgG to band 3 dimers in newborn and adult erythrocytes exposed to hypoxia and hypoxia-reoxygenation. *Biochimica et Biophysica Acta,* Vol.1672, No.3, pp. 203-213.

Coleman, M.D.; Breckenridge, A.M. & Park, B.K. (1989). Bioactivation of dapsone to a cytotoxic metabolite by human hepatic microsomal enzymes. *British Journal of Clinical Pharmacology,* Vol.28, No.4, pp. 389-395.

Coleman, M.D. & Jacobus, D.P. (1993). Reduction of dapsone hydroxylamine to dapsone during methaemoglobin formation in human erythrocytes in vitro. *Biochemical Pharmacology,* Vol.45, No.5, pp. 1027-1033.

Coleman, M.D.; Simpson, J. & Jacobus, D.P. (1994). Reduction of dapsone hydroxylamine to dapsone during methaemoglobin formation in human erythrocytes in vitro. IV: Implications for the development of agranulocytosis. *Biochemical Pharmacology,* Vol.48, No.7, pp. 1349-1354.

Coleman, M.D.; Tingle, M.D.; Hussain, F.; Storr, R.C. & Park, B.K. (1991). An investigation into the haematological toxicity of structural analogues of dapsone in vivo and in vitro. *The Journal of Pharmacy and Pharmacology,* Vol.43, No.11, pp. 779-784.

Cream, J.J. & Scott, G.L. (1970). Anaemia in dermatitis herpetiformis. The role of dapsone-induced haemolysis and malabsorption. *The British Journal of Dermatology,* Vol.82, No.4, pp. 333-338.

Elonen, E.; Neuvonen, P.J.; Halmekoski, J. & Mattila, M.J. (1979). Acute dapsone intoxication: a case with prolonged symptoms. *Clinical Toxicology,* Vol.14, No.1, pp. 79-85.

Fiore, C.; Bordin, L.; Pellati, D.; Armanini, D. & Clari, G. (2008). Effect of glycyrrhetinic acid on membrane band 3 in human erythrocytes. *Archives of Biochemistry and Biophysics,* Vol.479, No.1, pp. 46-51.

Hebbel, R.P. (1990). The sickle erythrocyte in double jeopardy: autoxidation and iron decompartmentalization. *Seminars in Hematology*, Vol.27, No.1, pp. 51-69.

Hecht, D. & Zick, Y. (1992). Selective inhibition of protein tyrosine phosphatase activities by H2O2 and vanadate in vitro. *Biochemistry and Biophysic Research Communication*, Vol.188, No.2, pp. 773-779.

Israili, Z.H.; Cucinell, S.A.; Vaught, J.; Davis, E.; Lesser, J.M. & Dayton, P.G. (1973). Studies of the metabolism of dapsone in man and experimental animals: formation of N-hydroxy metabolites. *The Journal of Pharmacology and Experimental Therapeutics*, Vol.187, No.1, pp. 138-151.

Jacobasch, G. & Rapoport, S.M. (1996). Hemolytic anemias due to erythrocyte enzyme deficiencies. *Molecular Aspects of Medicine*, Vol.17, No.2, pp. 143-170.

Kay, M.M. (1984). Localization of senescent cell antigen on band 3. *Proceedings of the National Academy of Sciences of the United States of America*, Vol.81, No.18, pp. 5753-5757.

Kay, M. (2005). Immunoregulation of cellular life span. *Annals of the New York Academy of Sciences*, Vol.1057, pp. 85-111.

Kiese, M., Rauscher, E. & Weger, N. (1966). The role of N,N-dimethylaniline-N-oxide in the formation of hemiglobin following the absorption of N,N-dimethylaniline. *Naunyn-chmiedebergs Archive fur Pharmakologie und Experimentelle Pathologie*, Vol.254, No.3, pp. 253-260.

Leonard, J.N. & Fry, L. (1991). Treatment and management of dermatitis herpetiformis. *Clinics in Dermatology*, Vol. 9, No.3, pp. 403-408.

Low, P.S.; Rathinavelu, P. & Harrison, M.L. (1993). Regulation of glycolysis via reversible enzyme binding to the membrane protein band 3. *The Journal of Biological Chemistry*, Vol.268, No.20, pp. 14627-14631.

Low, P.S.; Waugh, S.M.; Zinke, K. & Drenckhahn, D. (1985). The role of hemoglobin denaturation and band 3 clustering in red blood cell aging. *Science*, Vol.227, No.4686, pp. 531-533.

Lutz, H.U.; Bussolino, F.; Flepp, R.; Fasler, S.; Stammler, P.; Kazatchkine, M.D. & Arese, P. (1987). Naturally occurring anti-band-3 antibodies and complement together mediate phagocytosis of oxidatively stressed human erythrocytes. *Proceedings of the National Academy of Sciences of the United States of America*, Vol. 84, No. 21, pp. 7368-7376.

Lutz, H.U.; Fasler, S.; Stammler, P.; Bussolino, F. & Arese, P. (1988). Naturally occurring anti-band 3 antibodies and complement in phagocytosis of oxidatively-stressed and in clearance of senescent red cells. *Blood Cells*, Vol. 14, No.1, pp. 175-195.

May, D.G.; Arns, P.A.; Richards, W.O.; Porter, J.; Ryder, D.; Fleming, C.M.; Wilkinson, G.R. & Branch, R.A. (1992). The disposition of dapsone in cirrhosis. *Clinical Pharmacology and Therapeutics*, Vol.51, No.6, pp. 689-700.

May, D.G.; Porter, J.A.; Uetrecht, J.P.; Wilkinson, G.R. & Branch, R.A. (1990). The contribution of N-hydroxylation and acetylation to dapsone pharmacokinetics in normal subjects. *Clinical Pharmacology and Therapeutics*, Vol. 48, No. 6, pp. 619-627.

McMillan, D.C.; Jensen, C.B. & Jollow, D.J. (1998). Role of lipid peroxidation in dapsone-induced hemolytic anemia. *The Journal of Pharmacology and Experimental Pharmaceutics*, Vol.287, No.3, pp. 868-876.

McMillan, D.C.; Powell, C.L.; Bowman, Z.S.; Morrow, J.D. & Jollow, D.J. (2005). Lipid versus proteins as major targets of pro-oxidant, direct-acting hemolytic agents. *Toxicological Sciences*, Vol. 88, No.1, pp. 274-283.

Musch, M.W.; Hubert, E.M. & Goldstein, L. (1999). Volume expansion stimulates p72(syk) and p56(lyn) in skate erythrocytes. *The Journal of Biological Chemistry*, Vol.274, No.2, pp. 7923-7928.

Orion, E.; Matz, H. & Wolf, R. (2005). The life-threatening complications of dermatologic therapies. *Clinics in Dermatology*, Vol.23, No.2, pp. 182-192.

Pantaleo, A.; Ferru E.; Giribaldi, G.; Mannu, F.; Carta, F.; Matte, A.; De Franceschi, L. & Turrini, F. (2009). Oxidized and poorly glycosylated band 3 is selectively phosphorylated by Syk kinase to form large membrane clusters in normal and G6PD-deficient red blood cells. *The Biochemical Journal*, Vol.418, No.2, pp. 359-367.

Prussick, R. & Shear, N.H. (1996) Dapsone hypersensitivity syndrome. *Journal of the American Academy of Dermatology*, Vol.35, No.2, pp. 346-349.

Reilly, T.P.; Woster, P.M. & Svensson, C.K. (1999). Methemoglobin formation by hydroxylamine metabolites of sulfamethoxazole and dapsone: implications for differences in adverse drug reactions. *The Journal of Pharmacology and Experimental Therapeutics*, Vol.288, No.3, pp. 951-959.

Roychowdhury, S.; Cram, A.E.; Aly, A. & Svensson, C.K. (2007). Detection of haptenated proteins in organotypic human skin explant cultures exposed to dapsone. *Drug Metabolism and Disposition*, Vol.35, No.9, pp. 1463-1465.

Sangiolo, D.; Storer, B.; Nash, R.; Corey, L.; Davis, C.; Flowers, M.; Hackman, R.C. & Boeckh, M. (2005). Toxicity and efficacy of daily dapsone as Pneumocystis jiroveci prophylaxis after hematopoietic stem cell transplantation: a case-control study. *Biology and Blood Marrow Transplantation*, Vol.11, No.7, pp. 521-529.

Schiff, D.E.; Roberts, W.D. & Sue YJ (2006). Methaemoglobinemia associated with dapsone therapy in a child with pneumonia and chronic immune thrombocytopenic purpura. *Journal of Pediatric Hematology/Oncology*, Vol.28, No.6, pp. 395-398.

Schluter, K. & Drenekhanh, D. (1986). Co-clustering of denatured hemoglobin with band 3: its role in binding of autoantibodies against band 3 to abnormal and aged erythrocytes, *Proceedings of the National Academy of Sciences of the United States of America*, Vol.83, No.16, pp. 6137-6141.

Sener, O.; Doganci, L.; Safali, M.; Besirbellioglu, B.; Bulucu, F. & Pahsa, A. (2006) Severe dapsone hypersensitivity syndrome. *Journal of Investigational Allergology and Clinical Immunology*, Vol.16, No.4, pp. 268-270.

Ujiie, H.; Shimizu, T.; Ito, M.; Arita, K. & Shimizu H (2006). Lupus erythematosus profundus successfully treated with dapsone: review of the literature. *Archives of Dermatology*, Vol.142, No.3, pp. 399-401.

Vyas, P.M.; Roychowdhury, S.; Koukouritaki, S.B.; Hines, R.N.; Krueger, S.K.; Williams, D.E.; Nauseef, W.M. & Svensson, C.K. (2006). Enzyme-mediated protein haptenation of dapsone and sulfamethoxazole in human keratinocytes: II. Expression and role of flavin-containing monooxygenases and peroxydases. *The Journal of Pharmacology and Experimental Therapeutics*, Vol.319, No.1, pp. 497–505.

Wang, D.N. (1994). Band 3 protein: structure, flexibility and function. *FEBS Letters*, Vol.346, No.1, pp. 26-31.

Wertheim, M.S.; Males, J.J.; Cook, S.D. & Tole, M.D. (2006). Dapsone induced haemolytic anaemia in patients treated for ocular cicatricial pemphigoid. *The British Journal of Ophthalmology*, Vol. 90, No.4, pp. 516.

Winter, H.R.; Wang, Y. & Unadkat, J.D. (2000). CYP2C8/9 mediate dapsone N-hydroxylation at clinical concentrations of dapsone. *Drug Metabolism and Disposition*, Vol.28, No.8, pp. 865-868.

Woodhouse, K.W.; Henderson, D.B.; Charlton, B.; Peaston, R.T. & Rawlins, M.D. (1983). Acute dapsone poisoning: clinical features and pharmacokinetic studies. *Human Toxicology*, Vol.2, No.3, pp. 507-510.

Zuidema, J.; Hilbers-Modderman, E.S. & Merkus, F.W. (1986). Clinical pharmacokinetics of dapsone. *Clinical Pharmacokinetics*, Vol.11, No.4, pp. 299-315.

13

Clinical Management of Hemolytic Disease of the Newborn and Fetus

Sebastian Illanes and Rafael Jensen
Fetal Medicine Unit, University of Los Andes, Santiago
Chile

1. Introduction

Hemolytic disease of the fetus and newborn (HDFN) is caused by maternal alloantibodies directed against antigens present in fetal red cells. Paternally inherited antigens of the Rh system, which differ to those from the mother, are present on fetal red cells and when the maternal immune system makes contact with a significant number of these cells create an immune response with antibodies against these antigens. This may happen because of fetomaternal transplacental bleeding (in traumatic events during pregnancy, obstetric procedures, labor, cesarean section) or by events unrelated with pregnancy, such as transfusion, contamination by needle use, etc. Maternal antibodies (IgG) can cross the placenta and activate macrophages in the fetal spleen which cause fetal red cell destruction with subsequent hemolytic anemia. This leads to jaundice and kernicterus in the newborn or hydrops and death in the fetus.

Before the 70's, HDFN was a major obstetric problem, that had a large impact on fetal and neonatal morbidity and mortality. Today, without an appropriate programme, up to 50% of untreated HDFN will result in death or severe brain damage. In developing countries, especially those lacking an efficient prophylactics progamme, this causes an important public health problem. In fact, it has been estimated that more than 50 thousand fetuses could be affected by this condition every year in India (Zipursky and Paul, 2010). With the established use of post-natal anti-D prophylaxis for rhesus (Rh) negative women, together with its increasing use for routine antenatal prophylaxis, the incidence of Rh-D sensitization has dramatically fallen (Hughes RG et al., 1994). Nevertheless, 15-17% of the Caucasian population in Europe and North America is D negative (Ubarkian S, 2002). With the sensitization against other red cell antigens such as Kell RhC/c, RhE/e, this pathology could still affect a large number of pregnancies every year, with significant health and financial implications (Abdel-Fattah SA et al., 2002; Illanes S and Soothill P, 2009). In England and Wales, about 520 fetuses develop HDFN each year, of which about 37 would die in the fetal or neonatal period and 28 would present developmental problems (Daniels G et al., 2004, NICE 2008).

On the other hand, in fetus affected by HDFN, survival rates can exceed 90 percent if anemia is diagnosed and treated with intrauterine blood transfusions in a timely manner (Van Kamp IL et al., 2001). Women with rising red cell antibody levels are usually referred to tertiary fetal medicine units for specialized management. The main challenge facing fetal medicine specialists today is not the skill required for invasive therapy, but rather the non-invasive monitoring of the disease so that its progress can be predicted to guide the need and timing of intrauterine transfusions to minimize unnecessary invasive testing (Ubarkian S, 2002).

2. Non-invasive management

2.1 Use of cell-free fetal DNA for the determination of fetal RhD genotype

The identification of blood group genes and subsequent detection of the molecular bases of blood group polymorphisms has made it possible to predict blood group phenotypes (Avent ND et al., 2000). The source of DNA used to predict fetal blood groups was initially done invasively by sampling amniotic fluid or chorionic villi (Finning KM et al., 2002). However, the related risk of the obstetric procedures (0.5–1% for fetal loss) (Nanal R et al., 2003) and risk of fetomaternal hemorrhage (amniocentesis 17%) (Tabor A et al., 1987) was associated with an unwanted increase in gestational maternal immunization (Murray JC et al., 1983).

The fact that cell-free fetal DNA (ffDNA) is present in the plasma of pregnant women in sufficient quantities for the determination of fetal RhD genotype (Lo YM, 1999), leads to the possibility of fetal D typing using a non-invasive approach. If the rhesus sequence is present in a D-negative women's blood it is indicative that the fetus is D-positive (Lo YM et al., 1997). Initially, cell-free DNA was studied as a tumor marker (Lo YM et al., 1998), but the presence of Y signals in pregnant women carrying a male fetus was the first evidence that this technique could be used to assess the fetus condition as well as for prenatal diagnosis (Lo YM et al., 1997). In a normal pregnancy, the placental tissue goes through a physiological remodeling via apoptosis and necrosis in the chorionic villus. As a consequence, ffDNA is released to the maternal plasma in increasing amounts as gestation progresses (Wataganara T and Bianchi DW, 2004; Alberry MS et al., 2009; Huppertz B et al., 2006; Fomigli L et al., 2000; Arnholdt H et al., 1991; Illanes S et al., 2009).

Non-invasive prenatal diagnosis using ffDNA is the focus of intense research nowadays because of its many potential uses. It's being evaluated for inherited diseases and genetic disorders such as trisomy 21 (Ehrich M et al., 2011; Deng YH et al., 2011; Sehnert AJ et al, 2011), trisomy 18 (Sehnert AJ et al, 2011), β-thalassaemia (Li Y et al, 2009; Hahn S et al., 2011), hemophilia (Tsui NB et al., 2011), X-linked genetic disorders (Miura K et al., 2011) and achondroplasia (Chitty LS et al., 2011). Genome-wide scanning may be implemented for fetal genetic prenatal non-invasive diagnosis (Lo YM el al., 2010) and quantitative changes in ffDNA blood levels have been proposed as a potential marker for preeclampsia (Hahn S et al., 2011). Finally, the combination of real-time PCR with improved rhesus D (RhD) typing enables a highly accurate prediction of fetal D status from maternal plasma (Finning KM et al., 2002). Moreover, this is now available as a world-wide service (Daniels G et al., 2004; Finning KM et al., 2002; Finning KM et al., 2004; Legler TJ et al., 2002; Rouillac-Le Sciellour C et al., 2004; Van der Schoot CE et al, 2006; Tynan JA et al., 2011; Tounta G et al., 2011)

A recent meta-analysis has been performed to evaluate the diagnostic sensitivity and specificity of fetal Rh genotyping using ffDNA (Geifman-Holtzman O et al., 2006). A total of 3261maternal plasma samples were analyzed in 37 publications and approximately 500 study protocols in order to assess fetal RhD status. Results showed total accuracy of 91.4% (94,8% if studies with small numbers of samples were excluded), with a wide variation, from 31.8 to 100 percent, depending on which protocol, gestational age at testing and study design was applied. Two recent studies have evaluated the feasibility of this testing in the first trimester of pregnancy. Akolekar et al tested patients at 11-13 weeks using a high-throughput robotic technique. They concluded that it was an accurate method with a positive predictive value of 100% and a negative predictive value of 96,5% (Akolekar R et al., 2011). The second study, reported a sensitivity of 100% and a specificity of 93%, with a 97% diagnostic accuracy for RhD genotyping in the first trimester of pregnancy using a quantitave PCR method (Cardo el al., 2010)

Non-invasive fetal RhD genotyping was compared to traditional postnatal serologic assay in a large scale validation study (Müller SP et al., 2008). The authors studied over one thousand samples of RH negative women who gave whole blood specimens at a gestational age of 25 weeks. Tests were drawn up using an innovative automated DNA extraction method using magnetic tips and spin columns that have been recently developed by members of Special Non-Invasive Advances in Fetal and Neonatal Evaluation Network of Excellence (SAFE NoE) (Chitty LS et al., 2008; Legler TJ et al., 2007). The sensitivity of fetal *RHD* genotyping was 99.7% for spin columns and 99.8% for magnetic tips, and these results were comparable to conventional serology (99.5%). In the case of specificity, the serology was slightly better (99.7% versus 99.2% for spin columns and 98.1% for magnetic tips). It has also been established that it is an accurate method in multi-ethnic populations such as Brazil, by using two or three exons for RHD gene (Amaral DR et al, 2011; Chinen PA et al., 2010). This new approach has significantly reduced the number of invasive procedures carried out in different fetal medicine units for fetal D grouping (Finning KM et al., 2004) and has proved that the automated DNA extraction method can be used in a clinical setting.

Non-invasive studies for other blood group antigens have also been flourishing, including Kell antigen, the second most important cause of hemolytic disease (Li Y et al., 2008), RhC/c and RhE/e (Li Y et al., 2008; Van der Schoot CE et al., 2003; Finning K et al., 2007). The International Blood Group Reference Laboratory, at Bristol (Finning K et al., 2007) has developed and tested allele-specific primers for detecting the K allele of KEL and alleles of RhC/c RhE/e (Van der Schoot CE et al., 2003), with great accuracy for each allele. The matrix assisted laser desorption/ionization time-of-flight mass spectrometry or MALDITOF MS (Li Y et al., 2008), is able to detect the fetal KEL1 allele in KEL negative mothers with an accuracy of 94%. In a recent meta-analysis, collective reported diagnostic accuracy of fetal RhCE genotyping, with a combined accuracy for fetal genotyping of 96.3% for RhC/c and 98.2% for RhE/e (Geifman-Holtzman O et al., 2009) was estimated. A recent Dutch report, after 7 years of non-invasive fetal blood group genotyping from maternal blood samples for D, K, c, and E groups, revealed that diagnosis could be achieved in 97% of cases in a medium gestational age of 17 weeks, with no false-positive or false-negative results, implying that it is an accurate and applicable diagnostic tool in clinic (Scheffer P et al., 2011). The use of cell-free fetal DNA in maternal plasma for fetal RhD genotype could eventually enable the screening of all D negative pregnant women, thereby confining the administration of prophylactic anti-D only to those pregnancies in which it is needed (Bianchi DW et al., 2005). Since the accuracy of the actual test is not 100%, there is an ongoing debate about the advantage of introducing such a policy. Some researchers propose that guided prophylaxis should have a lower cost than the routine prophylaxis to all RhD negative women (Daniels G et al., 2009). However, a recent cost benefits study evaluated the implementation of this strategy in England and Wales, and concluded that is unlikely to be sufficiently cost-effective for a large scale introduction. They estimated that only minor savings would be gained and that an increase in maternal sensitization may be unacceptably high due to test inaccuracies in different ethnic minority populations (Szczepura A et al., 2011). It is expected that new technologies should alter this picture. Nevertheless, any policy for the prevention of unnecessary administration of human-derived products, such as prophylactic anti-D, should be taken into account because of the potential contamination of blood products that at the present time cannot be tested, as unidentified viruses or prions (Avent ND. 2008, Avent ND. 2009).

3. Detection of fetal anemia non-invasively by ultrasonography

3.1 Ultrasound findings

Severe anemia causes tissue hypoxia (Soothill PW et al., 1987), with endothelial damage and increased capillary permeability. This may lead to protein loss into the interstitial space, hypoproteinaemia and consequently ascites (Nicolaides KH et al., 1985). Moreover, in response to red cell haemolysis and fetal anemia, extramedullary haematopoiesis occurs, increasing portal and umbilical venous pressures. This would impair hepatic function and protein synthesis, resulting in worsening hypoproteinaemia which would further deteriorate the hydrops process (Bowman JM, 1978; Socol ML et al., 1987). The ultrasonographic features of hydrops include ascites (the earliest sign), pleural effusions, pericardial effusions, scalp edema, subcutaneous edema and polyhydramnios. These findings are an indication of a hemoglobin deficit of more than 6 standard deviations below the normal mean for gestational age, and will need urgent intrauterine fetal transfusion (Nicolaides KH et al., 1988).

The many attempts to identify sonographic fetal anemia features which occur before the development of fetal hydrops have been unsuccessful (Queenan JT, 1982, De Vore GR et al., 1981,Nicolaides KH et al., 1988), because of their failure to quantify the real degree of the fetal anemia (Nicolaides KH et al., 1988). Moreover, these ultrasound findings, including the evaluation of the liver and spleen, have been abandoned, because when high quality Doppler measurements are used to predict fetal anemia, these anatomic evaluations add little useful independent information. In our practice, we don´t usually look for any structural measurement or appearance, save for the early signs of fetal ascites.

3.2 Fetal Doppler ultrasonography

Doppler ultrasonography is a non-invasive method used for studying fetal hemodynamic changes in vessels that supply fetal organs responding to pathological conditions. In anemic fetuses, the Doppler measurement that describes the hemodynamic changes occurring in response to this pathological condition has been attempted in several vessels. However, because of the rapid hemodynamic changes observed in the middle cerebral artery (MCA) (Mari G et al., 2000), have transformed the measurement of its peak systolic velocity (the maximum Doppler shift at the peak of the spectral curve) in the gold standard for anemia fetal prediction. (Campbell S et al., 1995). After Vyas et al in 1990 (Vyas et al., 1990) described an increase in the average MCA time for mean blood velocity in fetal anemia cases, Mari and colleagues reported that the degree of fetal anemia could be accurately detected by Doppler measurement of blood-flow velocity in the MCA, with an inverse relationship between the MCA peak velocity and the fetal hematocrit, with no false negative results for anemic fetuses (Mari G et al., 2000). The statistically significant increase in fetal hematocrit, following intrauterine transfusion, also resulted in a rapid reduction in the middle cerebral artery peak velocity. These results confirm that the traditional management of pregnancies complicated by Rh alloimmunization with serial invasive amniocentesis to determine bilirubin levels is no longer required. Even more, a recent study has shown that Doppler measurement of the peak velocity of systolic blood flow in the MCA can safely replace invasive testing in the management of Rh-alloimmunized pregnancies, avoiding all the complications related with the traditional invasive approach (Oepkes et al., 2006).

Several studies have used the MCA Dopplers in a clinical basis for the prediction of fetal anemia with at-risk cases, without ultrasound evidence of fetal hydrops. These have shown that there is a good correlation with fetal Hemoglobin (Abdel-Fattah SA et al., 2002). This non-invasive investigation can be reliable in predicting anemia in cases in which the need to sample fetal blood is not certain, therefore delaying invasive testing until treatment is likely to be required. The neonatal outcome where invasive testing has been avoided (based on reassuring MCA Doppler velocity results) did not result in life-threatening fetal or neonatal morbidities (Abdel-Fattah SA et al, 2005). Therefore, the routine use of MCA Doppler's can avoid unnecessary invasive procedures on at-risk fetuses. There are several normal reference ranges of fetal blood flow velocity in the middle cerebral artery. However, when compared in terms of discriminatory power, sensitivity and specificity, Mari's curve and its given cut-offs perform better when fetal anemia is predicted. (Mari G et al., 2000; Bartha JL et al., 2005).

4. Invasive approach

Intrauterine blood transfusion of anemic fetuses represents one of the great successes of fetal therapy. After the first approach with intraperitoneal blood transfusion introduced in 1963 by Liley (Liley AW, 1963), Rodeck (Rodeck CH et al., 1981) described intravascular fetal blood transfusion (IVT) by the needling of the chorionic plate or umbilical cord vessels via fetoscopy direct vision. In 1982, Bang in Denmark started IVT by umbilical cord puncture under ultrasound guidance. This is now the gold standart (Bang et al., 1982). IVT has produced a marked improvement in the survival rate of the anemic hydropic fetus. This in turn can also prevent complications from developing by treating anemic non-hydropic fetuses, where moderate or severe anemia is detected non-invasively by Doppler ultrasonography, by increased peak velocity of systolic blood flow or time-averaged mean velocity in the MCA in fetuses at risk (Abdel-Fattah SA et al., 2002; Mari G et al., 2000). It is estimated that between 10 and 12% of fetuses of sensitized RHD negative women will require IVT (NICE 2008) with the survival rate exceeding 95% in experienced centers, particularly when opportune IVT treatment is established in a timely manner (Van Kamp IL et al., 2001).

When possible the umbilical vein is sampled because artery puncture may pose a risk for bradycardia (Weiner CP et al., 1991). The hemoglobin concentration (Hb) is measured and interpreted according to gestational age, with the severity classified on the fetal hemoglobin deviation from the normal mean for gestation into mild (hemoglobin deficit less than 2 g/dl), moderate (deficit 2-7 g/dl), and severe (deficit greater than 7 g/dl) (Nicolaides KH et al., 1988). A blood transfusion will be attempted in cases were a moderate or severe anemia is detected. For IVT to be realized, the blood volume required to correct the fetal Hb needs to be calculated, using pre-transfusion fetal Hb, the donor blood Hb (adult blood usually packed to a hematocrit of about 70-80%) and the gestational age (Nicolaides KH et al., 1986). The volume required is given as fast as possible without causing changes to the fetal heart rate and it seems that the feto-placental unit is able to handle the blood volume expansion much more easily than when transfusing neonates without the benefit of a placenta. Infusion of packed blood through a 15-cm long, 20-gauge needle at rates of $1-10$ ml/min does not result in significant hemolysis (Nicolaides KH et al., 1986). After the volume calculated to correct the Hb deficit has been given a post-transfusion, Hb is measured to help time the subsequent transfusion. After two or three transfusions, fetal blood production is suppressed and instead adult blood cells become more dominant. The fall of Hb becomes very predictable at about 1% haematocrit point per day (Thein AT and Soothill P, 1998). We aim to complete the last transfusion at 35–36 weeks and then to induce labor at 37 weeks to allow maturation of both the pulmonary and hepatic enzyme systems. With this programme, we hope to avoid neonatal exchange transfusions.

As this management of anemic fetuses is increasing, and the number of cordocentesis and transfusions are decreasing, the problem of maintaining the skills needed is rising too. It has been suggested that operators should perform at least 10 procedures per year to keep competence. (Lindenburg IT et al., 2011). Complications associated with intrauterine procedures such as cord hematoma, hemorrhage, fetal bradycardia and intrauterine death could increase in the future (Illanes S and Soothill PW, 2006). A possible solution would be to introduce a health policy that gave transfusions, via some centers, to all those cases that needed one. This could potentially avoid any complications such as lack of operator training.

5. Neonatal outcome

For the neonate, the consequences of HDFN are anemia and hiperbilirrubinemia. Postnatal treatment options include top-up red blood cells transfusions for the former, and phototherapy and exchange transfusions for the latter. Top-up transfusions, even with a minimal risk, carry a theoretical possibility of anaphylactic reaction and transmission of viral disease. In contrast, exchange transfusion carries a high morbidity and mortality rate (5% and <0.3% respectively), but the number of neonates requiring exchange transfusions has reduced due to advances in phototherapy.

Few studies specifically investigate the short-term neonatal outcomes for pregnancies affected by hemolytic red cell alloimmunisation. Two recent retrospective studies have assessed this question. De Boer *et al.* (De Boer *et al* 2008) investigated the short-term morbidity for neonates treated for Rhesus disease with or without IVT. Those treated with IVTs were found to require a higher number of top-up red blood cell transfusions and had less need of phototherapy. However, both groups had a similar need for exchange transfusion. The second study, is a Scottish report of postnatal outcomes following intrauterine transfusion, and showed that 20% of newborn needed exchange transfusion, 50% had top-up transfusion, and most of them needed phototherapy (McGlone L et al., 2009). More studies are needed, to evaluate the neonatal outcomes and associated morbi mortality, related to the number of transfusions, the gestational age at first and last transfusion, and the hemoglobin level at first IVT.

6. Conclusion

The management of the HDFN represents one of the genuine successes of fetal therapy. The current aspects of this clinical management have shifted from a long-established invasive approach to a non-invasive one. This applies to the detection of fetuses at risk of HDFN with the use of cell-free fetal DNA in the plasma of pregnant women to determine fetal RhD genotype. If the fetus is D negative, then it is not at risk and no further procedures are required; if it is D positive the appropriate management of the pregnancy can be arranged. On the other hand, maternal plasma testing for fetal RhD genotype could eventually enable the screening of all D negative pregnant women, thereby confining the administration of prophylactic anti-D only to those pregnancies in which it is needed. In addition, when a fetus is antigen positive, the follow up of these fetuses is for the detection of moderate or severe anemia non-invasively by Doppler ultrasonography on the basis of an increase in the peak velocity of systolic blood in the middle cerebral artery. When anemia is suspected, an invasive approach is required in order to perform an intrauterine blood transfusion which should only be attempted when the fetus needs transfusion.

7. Summary

Hemolytic disease of the fetus and newborn (HDFN) is caused by maternal alloantibodies directed against paternally inherited antigens on fetal red blood cells. It was also a significant cause of fetal and neonatal morbidity and mortality until the introduction of anti-D immunoglobulin during pregnancy and shortly after delivery. However, it is still a major problem in affected pregnancies. The emphasis of current clinical management of HDFN is a non-invasive approach. This work is carried out on fetuses at risk with HDFN, with the use of cell-free fetal DNA in the plasma of pregnant women, in order to determine the fetal RhD genotype, or to see if the fetus is antigen positive. If the mother is sensitized, for the follow up and detection of moderate or severe anemia – this is done, primarily, non-invasively by Doppler ultrasonography of the middle cerebral artery. If anemia is suspected, an invasive approach is required in order to perform an intrauterine blood transfusion. This management represents one of the genuine successes of fetal therapy.

8. References

[1] Abdel-Fattah SA, Shefras J, Kyle PM, Cairns P, Hunter A, Soothill PW. Reassuring fetal middle cerebral artery doppler velocimetry in alloimmunised pregnancies: neonatal outcomes without invasive procedures. Fetal Diagn Ther. 2005 Sep-Oct;20(5):341-5

[2] Abdel-Fattah SA, Soothill PW, Carroll SG, Kyle PM. Middle cerebral artery Doppler for the prediction of fetal anaemia in cases without hydrops: a practical approach. Br J Radiol. 2002 Sep;75(897):726-30

[3] Akolekar R, Finning K, Kuppusamy R, Daniels G, Nicolaides KH. Fetal RHD Genotyping in Maternal Plasma at 11-13 Weeks of Gestation. Fetal Diagn Ther. 2011;29(4):301-6. Epub 2011 Jan 8.

[4] Alberry MS, Maddocks DG, Hadi MA, Metawi H, Hunt LP, Abdel-Fattah SA, Avent ND, Soothill PW. 2009. Quantification of cell free fetal DNA in maternal plasma in normal pregnancies and in pregnancies with placental dysfunction. Am J Obstet Gynecol. 200(1):98.e1-6.

[5] Amaral DR, Credidio DC, Pellegrino J Jr, Castilho L. Fetal RHD genotyping by analysis of maternal plasma in a mixed population. J Clin Lab Anal. 2011;25(2):100-4.

[6] Arnholdt H, Meisel F, Fandrey K, Lohrs U. 1991. Proliferation of villous trophoblast of the human placenta in normal and abnormal pregnancies. Virchows Arch B Cell Pathol Incl Mol Pathol.60: 365-72.

[7] Avent ND. 2008. RHD genotyping from maternal plasma: guidelines and technical challenges. Methods Mol Biol. 444:185-201.

[8] Avent ND. 2009. Large-scale blood group genotyping: clinical implications. Br J Haematol. 144(1):3-13.

[9] Avent ND, Finning KM, Martin PG, Soothill PW. Prenatal determination of fetal blood group status. Vox Sang. 2000;78 Suppl 2:155-62.

[10] Bang J, Bock JE, Trolle D Ultrasound guided fetal intravenous transfusion for severe rehus haemolytic disease. BMJ 1982; 284: 373–374.

[11] Bartha JL, Illanes S, Abdel-Fattah S, Hunter A, Denbow M, Soothill PW. Comparison of different reference values of fetal blood flow velocity in the middle cerebral artery for predicting fetal anemia. Ultrasound Obstet Gynecol. 2005 Apr;25(4):335-40

[12] Bianchi DW, Avent ND, Costa JM, van der Schoot CE.Noninvasive prenatal diagnosis of fetal Rhesus D: ready for Prime(r) Time. Obstet Gynecol. 2005 Oct;106(4):841-4. Review.

[13] Bowman JM. The management of Rh isoimmunization. Obstet Gynecol 1978; 52: 1-16

[14] Campbell S, Harrington K, Hecher K. The fetal arterial circulation. In: A colour atlas of Doppler ultrasonography in obstetrics, Eds Harrington K, Campbell S. Edward Arnold 1995; 59-69

[15] Cardo L, García BP, Alvarez FV. Non-invasive fetal RHD genotyping in the first trimester of pregnancy. Clin Chem Lab Med. 2010 Aug;48(8):1121-6.

[16] Chinen PA, Nardozza LM, Martinhago CD, Camano L, Daher S, Pares DB, Minett T, Araujo Júnior E, Moron AF. Noninvasive determination of fetal rh blood group, D antigen status by cell-free DNA analysis in maternal plasma: experience in a Brazilian population. Am J Perinatol. 2010 Nov;27(10):759-62.

[17] Chitty LS, Griffin DR, Meaney C, Barrett A, Khalil A, Pajkrt E, Cole TJ. New aids for the non-invasive prenatal diagnosis of achondroplasia: dysmorphic features, charts of fetal size and molecular confirmation using cell-free fetal DNA in maternal plasma. Ultrasound Obstet Gynecol. 2011 Mar;37(3):283-9. doi: 10.1002/uog.8893. Epub 2011 Feb 1.

[18] Chitty LS, van der Schoot CE, Hahn S, Avent ND. 2008. SAFE—the Special Non-invasive Advances in Fetal and Neonatal Evaluation Network: aims and achievements. Prenat Diagn.28: 83-8.

[19] Daniels G, Finning K, Martin P, Massey E. 2009. Noninvasive prenatal diagnosis of fetal blood group phenotypes: current practice and future prospects. Prenat Diagn. 29(2): 101-7.

[20] Daniels G, Finning K, Martin P, Soothill P. Fetal blood group genotyping from DNA from maternal plasma: an important advance in the management and prevention of haemolytic disease of the fetus and newborn. Vox Sang. 2004 Nov;87(4):225-32. Review.

[21] De Boer, I.P., Zeestraten, E.C., Lopriore, E., van Kamp, I.L., Kanhai, H.H. & Walther, F.J. Paediatric outcome in Rhesus haemolytic disease treated with and without intrauterine transfusion. *American Journal of Obstetrics & Gynaecology*, 2008: 198(1):54.e1-4.

[22] De Vore GR, Mayden K, Tortora M, Berkowitz RL, Hobbins JC. Dilation of the fetal umbilical vein in rhesus hemolytic anemia: a predictor of severe disease. Am J Obstet Gynecol 1981; 141: 464-66.

[23] Deng YH, Yin AH, He Q, Chen JC, He YS, Wang HQ, Li M, Chen HY. Non-invasive prenatal diagnosis of trisomy 21 by reverse transcriptase multiplex ligation-dependent probe amplification. Clin Chem Lab Med. 2011 Apr;49(4):641-6.

[24] Ehrich M, Deciu C, Zwiefelhofer T, Tynan JA, Cagasan L, Tim R, Lu V, McCullough R, McCarthy E, Nygren AO, Dean J, Tang L, Hutchison D, Lu T, Wang H, Angkachatchai V, Oeth P, Cantor CR, Bombard A, van den Boom D. Noninvasive detection of fetal trisomy 21 by sequencing of DNA in maternal blood: a study in a clinical setting. Am J Obstet Gynecol. 2011 Mar;204(3):205.e1-11. Epub 2011 Feb 18.

[25] Finning K, Martin P, Daniels G. A clinical service in the UK to predict fetal Rh (Rhesus) D blood group using free fetal DNA in maternal plasma. Ann N Y Acad Sci. 2004.Jun;1022:119-23.

[26] Finning KM, Martin PG, Soothill PW and Avent ND, Prediction of fetal D status from maternal plasma: introduction of a new noninvasive fetal RHD genotyping service. Transfusion 42 (2002), pp. 1079–1085.

[27] Finning K, Martin P, Summers J, Daniels G. 2007. Fetal genotyping for the K (Kell) and Rh C, c, and E blood groups on cell-free fetal DNA in maternal plasma. Transfusion. 11: 2126-33.

[28] Formigli L, Papucci L, Tani A, et al. 2000. Aponecrosis: morphological and biochemical exploration of a syncretic process of cell death sharing apoptosis and necrosis. J Cell Physiol. 182:41-9.

[29] Geifman-Holtzman O, Grotegut CA, Gaughan JP. 2006. Diagnostic accuracy of non-invasive fetal Rh genotyping from maternal blood—a meta-analysis. Am J Obstet Gynecol. 2006 4:1163-73.

[30] Geifman-Holtzman O, Grotegut CA, Gaughan JP, Holtzman EJ, Floro C, Hernandez E. 2009. Non-invasive fetal RhCE genotyping from maternal blood. BJOG. 116(2):144-51.

[31] Hahn S, Lapaire O, Tercanli S, Kolla V, Hösli I. Determination of fetal chromosome aberrations from fetal DNA in maternal blood: has the challenge finally been met? Expert Rev Mol Med. 2011 May 4;13:e16.

[32] Hahn S, Rusterholz C, Hösli I, Lapaire O. Cell-free nucleic acids as potential markers for preeclampsia. Placenta. 2011 Feb;32 Suppl:S17-20.

[33] Hughes RG, Craig JIO, Murphy WG, Greer IA. Causes and clinical consequences of Rhesus (D) haemolytic disease of the newborn: a study of Scottish population, 1985–1990. Br J Obstet Gynaecol 1994;101:297–300.

[34] Huppertz B, Kadyrov M, Kingdom JC. 2006. Apoptosis and its role in the trophoblast. Am J Obstet Gynecol. 195:29-39.

[35] Illanes S, Parra M, Serra R, Pino K, Figueroa-Diesel H, Romero C, Arraztoa JA, Michea L, Soothill PW. 2009. Increased free fetal DNA levels in early pregnancy plasma of women who subsequently develop preeclampsia and intrauterine growth restriction. Prenat Diagn. 29(12):1118-2.

[36] Illanes S, Soothill PW. 2006. Fetal therapy. In Progress in Obstetrics and Gynaecology. John Studd (Ed). Elselvier; United Kingdom: 65-78.

[37] Illanes S, Soothill P. 2009. The non-invasive approach for the management of haemolytic disease of the fetus and newborn. Current aspects of the clinical management of haemolytic disease of the newborn and foetus. Expert Review of Hematology 5, 577-582.

[38] Legler TJ, Liu Z, Mavrou A, Finning KM, Hromadnikova I, Galbiati S, Meaney C, Hul; én MA, Crea F, Olsson ML, Maddocks DG, Huang D, Armstrong Fisher S, Sprenger-Haussels M, Soussan AA, van der Schoot CE. 2007. Workshop report on the extraction of foetal DNA from maternal plasma. Prenat Diagn. 27: 824-29.

[39] Legler, T.J., Lynen, R., Maas, J.H., Pindur, G., Kulenkampff, D., Suren, A., Osmers, R. & Kohler, M. Prediction of fetal Rh D and Rh Cc Ee phenotype from maternal plasma with real-time polymerase chain reaction. Transfus Apher Sci, 2002. 27, 217-223.

[40] Li Y, Di Naro E, Vitucci A, Grill S, Zhong XY, Holzgreve W, Hahn S. Size fractionation of cell-free DNA in maternal plasma improves the detection of a paternally inherited beta-thalassemia point mutation by MALDI-TOF mass spectrometry. Fetal Diagn Ther. 2009;25(2):246-9. Epub 2009 Jun 5.

[41] Li Y, Finning K, Daniels G, Hahn S, Zhong X, Holzgreve W. 2008. Noninvasive genotyping fetal Kell blood group (KEL1) using cell-free fetal DNA in maternal plasma by MALDI-TOF mass spectrometry. Prenat Diagn. 28(3): 203-8.

[42] Liley AW Intrauterine transfusion of fetus in haemolytic disease. BMJ II 1963: 1107–1109.

[43] Lindenburg IT, Wolterbeek R, Oepkes D, Klumper FJ, Vandenbussche FP, van Kamp IL. Quality Control for Intravascular Intrauterine Transfusion Using Cumulative Sum (CUSUM) Analysis for the Monitoring of Individual Performance. Fetal Diagn Ther. 2011;29(4):307-14. Epub 2011 Feb 8.

[44] Lo YMD. Fetal RhD genotyping from maternal plasma: Ann Med 1999; 31:308-312

[45] Lo YM, Chan KC, Sun H, Chen EZ, Jiang P, Lun FM, Zheng YW, Leung TY, Lau TK, Cantor CR, Chiu RW. Maternal plasma DNA sequencing reveals the genome-wide genetic and mutational profile of the fetus. Sci Transl Med. 2010 Dec 8;2(61):61ra91.

[46] Lo YM, Corbetta N, Chamberlain PF, Rai V, Sargent IL, Redman CW, Wainscoat JS. 1997. Presence of fetal DNA in maternal plasma and serum. Lancet 350: 485–487.

[47] Lo YM, Tein MSC, Lau TK,Haines CJ, Leung TN, Poon PMK, Wainscoat JS, Johnson PJ, Chang AMZ, Hjelm NM. 1998. Quantitative analysis of fetal DNA in maternal plasma and serum: implications for noninvasive prenatal diagnosis. Am J Hum Genet. 62: 768–775.

[48] Mari G, Deter RL, Carpenter RL, et al. Noninvasive diagnosis by Doppler ultrasonography of fetal anemia due to maternal red-cell alloimmunization. N Engl J Med 2000;342:9-14.

[49] McGlone L, Simpson JH, Scott-Lang C, Cameron AD, Brennand J. 2009. Short term outcomes following intrauterine transfusion in Scotland. Arch Dis Child Fetal Neonatal. 23.

[50] Miura K, Higashijima A, Shimada T, Miura S, Yamasaki K, Abe S, Jo O, Kinoshita A, Yoshida A, Yoshimura S, Niikawa N, Yoshiura K, Masuzaki H. Clinical application of fetal sex determination using cell-free fetal DNA in pregnant carriers of X-linked genetic disorders. J Hum Genet. 2011 Apr;56(4):296-9. Epub 2011 Feb 10.

[51] Müller SP, Bartels I, Stein W, Emons G, Gutensohn K, Köhler M, Legler TJ. 2008. The determination of the fetal D status from maternal plasma for decision making on Rh prophylaxis is feasible. Transfusion, 11: 2292-301.

[52] Murray JC, Karp LE, Williamson RA, Cheng EY, Luthy DA. Rh isoimmunization related to amniocentesis. Am J Med Genet 1983;16:527-34.

[53] Nanal R, Kyle P, Soothill PW. A classification of pregnancy losses after invasive prenatal diagnostic procedures: an approach to allow comparison of units with a different case mix. Prenat Diagn. 2003 Jun;23(6):488-92

[54] National Institute for Clinical Excellence: Technology Appraisal Guidance 156. 2008, review date: may 2011. Routine antenatal anti-D prophylaxis for women who are rhesus D negative. London, NICE.

[55] Nicolaides KH, Fontanarosa M, Gabbe SG, Rodeck CH. Failure of ultrasonographic parameters to predict the severity of fetal anemia in rhesus isoimmunization. Am J Obstet Gynecol 1988; 158: 920-6.

[56] Nicolaides KH, Soothill PW, Clewell WH, Rodeck CH, Mibashan RS, Campbell S. Fetal haemoglobin measurement in the assessment of red cell isoimmunisation. Lancet 1988; 1: 1073-75

[57] Nicolaides KH, Soothill PW, Rodeck CH, Clewell W Rh disease: intravascular fetal blood transfusion by cordocentesis. Fetal Ther. 1986; 1(4): 185-92.

[58] Nicolaides KH, Warenski JC, Rodeck CH. The relationship of fetal plasma protein concentration and Hemoglobin level to the development of hydrops in rhesus isoimmunization. Am J Obstet Gynecol 1985; 152: 341-4

[59] Oepkes D, Seaward PG, Vandenbussche FP, Windrim R, Kingdom J, Beyene J, Kanhai HH, Ohlsson A, Ryan G; DIAMOND Study Group.Doppler ultrasonography versus amniocentesis to predict fetal anemia.N Engl J Med. 2006 Jul 13;355(2):156-64.

[60] Queenan JT. Current management of the Rh-sensitized patient. Clin Obstet Gynecol 1982; 25: 293-301

[61] Rodeck CH, Kemp JR, Holman CA, Whitmore CA, Karnicki J,Austin MA. Direct intravascular fetal blood transfusion by fetoscopy in severe Rhesus isoimmunisation. Lancet I 1981:625– 627.

[62] Rouillac-Le Sciellour, C., Puillandre, P., Gillot, R., Baulard, C., Metral, S., Le Van Kim, C., Cartron, J.P., Colin, Y. & Brossard, Y. Large-scale pre-diagnosis study of fetal RHD genotyping by PCR on plasma DNA from RhD-negative pregnant women. Mol Diagn, 2004. 8, 23-31.

[63] Scheffer P, van der Schoot C, Page-Christiaens G, de Haas M. Noninvasive fetal blood group genotyping of rhesus D, c, E and of K in alloimmunised pregnant women: evaluation of a 7-year clinical experience. BJOG. 2011 Jun 14.

[64] Sehnert AJ, Rhees B, Comstock D, de Feo E, Heilek G, Burke J, Rava RP. Optimal detection of fetal chromosomal abnormalities by massively parallel DNA sequencing of cell-free fetal DNA from maternal blood. Clin Chem. 2011 Jul;57(7):1042-9. Epub 2011 Apr 25.

[65] Socol ML, MacGregor SN, Pielet BW, Tamura RK, Sabbagha RE. Percutaneous umbilical transfusion in severe rhesus isoimmunization: Resolution of fetal hydrops. Am J Obstet Gynecol 1987; 157: 1369-75

[66] Soothill PW, Nicolaides KH, Rodeck CH, Clewell WH, Lindridge J. Relationship of fetal hemoglobin and oxygen content to lactate concentration in Rh isoimmunized pregnancies. Obstet Gynecol 1987; 69: 268-71

[67] Szczepura A, Osipenko L, Freeman K. A new fetal RHD genotyping test: costs and benefits of mass testing to target antenatal anti-D prophylaxis in England and Wales. BMC Pregnancy Childbirth. 2011 Jan 18;11:5.

[68] Tabor A, Bang J, Nørgaard-Pedersen B: Feto-maternal haemorrhage associated with genetic amniocentesis: results of a randomized trial. Br J Obstet Gynecol 1987; 94:528-34

[69] Thein AT, Soothill P. Antenatal invasive therapy. Eur J Pediatr. 1998 Jan; 157 Suppl 1: S2-6

[70] Tounta G, Vrettou C, Kolialexi A, Papantoniou N, Destouni A, Tsangaris GT, Antsaklis A, Kanavakis E, Mavrou A. A multiplex PCR for non-invasive fetal RHD genotyping using cell-free fetal DNA. In Vivo. 2011 May-Jun;25(3):411-7.

[71] Tsui NB, Kadir RA, Chan KC, Chi C, Mellars G, Tuddenham EG, Leung TY, Lau TK, Chiu RW, Lo YM. Noninvasive prenatal diagnosis of hemophilia by microfluidics digital PCR analysis of maternal plasma DNA. Blood. 2011 Mar 31;117(13):3684-91. Epub 2011 Jan 24.

[72] Tynan JA, Mahboubi P, Cagasan LL, van den Boom D, Ehrich M, Oeth P. Restriction enzyme-mediated enhanced detection of circulating cell-free fetal DNA in maternal plasma. J Mol Diagn. 2011 Jul;13(4):382-9. Epub 2011 May 6.

[73] Ubarniak S, 2002. The clinical application of anti-D prophilaxis. In: Alloimmune Disorders of Pregnancy: Anaemia,Thrombocytopenia and Neutropenia in the Fetus and Newborn. Andrew Hadley, Peter Soothill (Ed). Cambridge University Press; Cambridge: 97-121.

[74] Van der Schoot, C.E., Soussan, A.A., Koelewijn, J., Bonsel, G., Paget-Christiaens, L.G. & de Haas, M. Non-invasive antenatal RHD typing. Transfus Clin Biol. 2006.13, 53-57.

[75] Van der Schoot, C.E., Tax, G.H., Rijnders, R.J., de Haas, M. & Christiaens, G.C. 2003. Prenatal typing of Rh and Kell blood group system antigens: the edge of a watershed. Transfus Med Rev. 17: 31-44.

[76] Van Kamp IL, Klumper FJCM, Bakkum RSLA, et al. The severity of immune fetal hydrops is predictive for fetal outcome after intrauterine treatment. Am J Obstet Gynecol 2001;185:668-673.

[77] Vyas S, Nicolaides KH, Campbell S. Doppler examination of the middle cerebral artery in anemic fetuses. Am J Obstet Gynecol 1990; 162: 1066-8

[78] Wataganara T, Bianchi DW. 2004. Fetal cell-free nucleic acids in the maternal circulation: new clinical applications. Ann N Y Acad Sci . 1022: 90–99.

[79] Weiner CP, Wenstrom KD, Sipes SL, Williamson RA. Risk factors for cordocentesis and fetal intravascular transfusion. Am J Obstet Gynecol. 1991 Oct; 165 (4 Pt 1): 1020-5.

[80] Zipursky A, Paul VK The global burden of Rh disease, Arch Dis Child Fetal Neonatal Ed. 2011 Mar;96(2):F84-5. Epub 2010 Oct 30.

Permissions

The contributors of this book come from diverse backgrounds, making this book a truly international effort. This book will bring forth new frontiers with its revolutionizing research information and detailed analysis of the nascent developments around the world.

We would like to thank Dr. Donald S. Silverberg, for lending his expertise to make the book truly unique. He has played a crucial role in the development of this book. Without his invaluable contribution this book wouldn't have been possible. He has made vital efforts to compile up to date information on the varied aspects of this subject to make this book a valuable addition to the collection of many professionals and students.

This book was conceptualized with the vision of imparting up-to-date information and advanced data in this field. To ensure the same, a matchless editorial board was set up. Every individual on the board went through rigorous rounds of assessment to prove their worth. After which they invested a large part of their time researching and compiling the most relevant data for our readers. Conferences and sessions were held from time to time between the editorial board and the contributing authors to present the data in the most comprehensible form. The editorial team has worked tirelessly to provide valuable and valid information to help people across the globe.

Every chapter published in this book has been scrutinized by our experts. Their significance has been extensively debated. The topics covered herein carry significant findings which will fuel the growth of the discipline. They may even be implemented as practical applications or may be referred to as a beginning point for another development. Chapters in this book were first published by InTech; hereby published with permission under the Creative Commons Attribution License or equivalent.

The editorial board has been involved in producing this book since its inception. They have spent rigorous hours researching and exploring the diverse topics which have resulted in the successful publishing of this book. They have passed on their knowledge of decades through this book. To expedite this challenging task, the publisher supported the team at every step. A small team of assistant editors was also appointed to further simplify the editing procedure and attain best results for the readers.

Our editorial team has been hand-picked from every corner of the world. Their multi-ethnicity adds dynamic inputs to the discussions which result in innovative outcomes. These outcomes are then further discussed with the researchers and contributors who give their valuable feedback and opinion regarding the same. The feedback is then collaborated with the researches and they are edited in a comprehensive manner to aid the understanding of the subject.

Apart from the editorial board, the designing team has also invested a significant amount of their time in understanding the subject and creating the most relevant covers. They scrutinized every image to scout for the most suitable representation of the subject and create an appropriate cover for the book.

The publishing team has been involved in this book since its early stages. They were actively engaged in every process, be it collecting the data, connecting with the contributors or procuring relevant information. The team has been an ardent support to the editorial, designing and production team. Their endless efforts to recruit the best for this project, has resulted in the accomplishment of this book. They are a veteran in the field of academics and their pool of knowledge is as vast as their experience in printing. Their expertise and guidance has proved useful at every step. Their uncompromising quality standards have made this book an exceptional effort. Their encouragement from time to time has been an inspiration for everyone.

The publisher and the editorial board hope that this book will prove to be a valuable piece of knowledge for researchers, students, practitioners and scholars across the globe.

List of Contributors

Ezechi Oliver
Chief Research Fellow and Consultant Obstetrician and Gynaecologist Coordinator, Sexual, Reproductive and Childhood Diseases Research Programme, Head of Division, Clinical Sciences Division, Nigerian Institute of Medical Research, Yaba Lagos, Nigeria

Kalejaiye Olufunto
Senior Research Fellow and Haematologist Unit Head, Laboratory Services Unit, Clinical Sciences Division, Nigerian Institute of Medical Research, Yaba Lagos, Nigeria

Ayodotun Olutola and Olugbenga Mokuolu
University of Maryland/Institute of Human Virology, Nigeria

Viviana Taylor, Rosa Uscátegui, Adriana Correa, Amanda Maestre and Jaime Carmona
Universidad de Antioquia/Grupo de Investigación en Alimentación and Nutrición Humana and Grupo Salud y comunidad, Colombia

Savino Biryomumaisho and E. Katunguka-Rwakishaya
Department of Veterinary Medicine, Makerere University, Kampala, Uganda

Albert Mbaya
Department of Veterinary Microbiology and Parasitology, University of Maiduguri, Nigeria

Hussein Kumshe
Department of Veterinary Medicine, University of Maiduguri, Nigeria

Chukwunyere Okwudiri Nwosu
Department of Veterinary Parasitology and Entomology, University of Nigeria, Nsukka, Nigeria

Michela Grosso, Raffaele Sessa, Stella Puzone, Maria Rosaria Storino and Paola Izzo
Dipartimento di Biochimica e Biotecnologie Mediche, University of Naples Federico II, Italy

Antonio M. Risitano
Head of Bone Marrow Transplant Clinical Unit, Department of Biochemistry and Medical Biotechnologies, Federico II University of Naples, Naples, Italy

Chidi G. Osuagwu
Department of Biomedical Technology, Federal University of Technology, Owerri, Imo State, Nigeria

Sevgi Gözdaşoğlu
Ankara University, Turkey

Karina Portillo Carroz and Josep Morera
Department of Pneumology Hospital Germans, Trias i Pujol, Universitat Autónoma de Barcelona, Spain

Adam Bignucolo, Joseph Lemire, Christopher Auger, Zachary Castonguay, Varun Appanna and Vasu D. Appanna
Laurentian University, Canada

Gabriella Donà, Giulio Clari and Luciana Bordin
Department of Biological Chemistry, University of Padova, Italy

Eugenio Ragazzi
Department of Pharmacology and Anesthesiology, University of Padova, Italy

Sebastian Illanes and Rafael Jensen
Fetal Medicine Unit, University of Los Andes, Santiago, Chile